Ion Exchange and
Adsorption Agents in Medicine

Ion Exchange
and Adsorption Agents
in Medicine

The Concept of Intestinal Bionomics

by GUSTAV J. MARTIN, Sc.D.

RESEARCH DIRECTOR,
THE NATIONAL DRUG COMPANY,
PHILADELPHIA

*Illustrated with 15 line drawings
and 11 photographs*

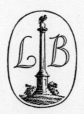

LITTLE, BROWN AND COMPANY
Boston · Toronto

Published simultaneously in Canada
by Little, Brown & Company (Canada) Limited

PRINTED IN THE UNITED STATES OF AMERICA

Foreword

In the early part of 1944, I began the investigation of ion exchange resins for medical use. The first result of that effort was the application of the anion exchangers in the treatment of peptic ulcer; the second was the use of cation exchangers for sodium reduction. Since the launching of these two resin types for general clinical use, a broader and greater sphere of application has arisen, that of conditioning of the gastrointestinal tract. By conditioning, I mean to suggest a state in which toxic chemicals are retained in the intestine and beneficial and nutrient materials permitted entrance into the system. This could well be defined as differential or selective ion exchange and adsorption for medical purposes.

It is my contention, as yet unsubstantiated by clinical observations, that all chronic degenerative disease has as an important component in its etiology the absorption from the intestine of small quantities of toxic chemicals. These agents produce imperceptible but irreversible changes in tissues and in the course of years create gross pathology. I believe that the absorption of these toxic agents can be prevented by proper selection of ion exchange and adsorption materials. As a first effort in substantiation of my major theme, I offer the material of this volume.

Of the many persons who have been of help in the preparation, proofreading and typing of the manuscript, my special thanks are due Henry Hopkins, M.D., who reviewed and corrected the clinical sections of the volume.

GUSTAV J. MARTIN

October, 1954

v

Contents

Ion Exchange and
Adsorption Agents in Medicine

Ions and Solutions

IONIZATION, GENERAL

To UNDERSTAND ion exchange materials is to understand the nature of ions and their behavior in solution. The logical introduction to the field is therefore a brief review of the physical chemistry of ionization. Throughout this summary, it should be held in mind that the behavior of the ion-active groups of insoluble exchangers is identical with that of those same groups attached to soluble molecular units. The simplicity and the complexity of each system are reflected in the other.

The number 6.02×10^{23} is a fundamental constant in physical chemistry, called Avogadro's number. It represents the number of molecules in a gram molecule of any given chemical. A gram molecule is in turn that molecular weight of a given substance expressed in grams; thus, the gram molecular weight of sodium chloride is 58.5, and this weight of sodium chloride would contain 6.02×10^{23} individual molecules of salt.

Avogadro offered the hypothesis that the physical behavior of substances would represent a function of the number of particles involved. Actual measurements of systems such as those of salts in solution showed marked discrepancies from the hypothesis and led van't Hoff to point out the distinctions between solutions of materials like cane sugar, which behaved according to the hypothesis, and solutions of substances like salts, acids and bases, which did not. It remained for Arrhenius (1887) to propose the theory of electrolytic dissociation,

3

which accounted for the abnormal osmotic pressures exerted by solutions of acids, bases and salts. According to this concept, aqueous solutions of acids, bases and salts dissociate into positively and negatively charged particles or ions. The dissociation increases the number of particles in solutions, bringing the behavior of such systems within the scope of Avogadro's hypothesis. Dissociations occur as follows:

$$HCl \rightleftarrows H^+ + Cl^-$$
$$HC_2H_3O_2 \rightleftarrows H^+ + C_2H_3O_2^-$$
$$NH_4OH \rightleftarrows NH_4^+ + OH^-$$
$$NaCl \rightleftarrows Na^+ + Cl^-$$

These equations indicate the dissociation of an acid such as hydrochloric acid into hydrogen and chloride ions; they also indicate the reassociation of these ions into the molecular form of the acid. An equilibrium is established which can be expressed as an equilibrium constant:

$$K = \frac{(H^+)(Cl^-)}{(HCl)}$$

The degree of dissociation of a given electrolyte is a function of its concentration; the more dilute the solution, the greater is the degree of dissociation. At any finite concentration, there are always some undissociated molecules.

Completion of the picture of ionization requires extension of the above concepts, which may tend to confuse, but such extension is essential in the interests of accuracy. With certain strong electrolytes like sodium or potassium chloride, electrical conductance measurements and osmotic phenomena indicate divergence from the electrolytic dissociation concept, and these divergences are clarified by x-ray analysis showing the existence of a completely ionic state even in crystal form. For example, the crystal lattice of potassium chloride exists in the form of ions. For these strong electrolytes, the concept of degree of dissociation loses its significance because complete ionization exists.

However, if complete ionization existed, the properties of salts and strong acids and bases in solutions would be a function of the total number of ions possible, e.g., two for sodium chloride, three for potassium sulfate, four for potassium ferricyanide. This assumption was not in accord with experimental findings and led directly to the formulation of the interionic attraction theory of Debye and Hückel (1923*a, b*). This concept points out that oppositely charged ions attract each other and that this attraction causes deviation from the behavior of ideal solutions. The degree and extent of the interionic attraction varies with concentration and for all practical purposes vanishes in extremely dilute solutions.

The ionization concept came full circle with the introduction of the theory of ionic strength by Lewis and Randall (1923). Ionic strength may be regarded as the effective ionic activity of a given electrolyte. It is a function of valence and is calculated by multiplying the concentration of each ion by the square of its valence, adding all these quantities together and dividing by a factor of two. The introduction of the ionic strength factor into equations dealing with ionic behavior brings into line all deviations from such equations caused by the use of the theoretical ionic concentration factors.

Two types of chemical bonds are generally recognized, the covalent and the ionic. With the covalent type, the over-all structure is established by the sharing of electrons. This is characteristic of the carbon-carbon and the carbon-hydrogen bonds. Ionization is impossible. The ionic type of bond results from actual electron transfer from one atom to another. Such transfer occurs with any electrolyte. For example, the ion formation with potassium bromide results from the transfer of an electron from the potassium to the bromine, and the consequent greater stability of the outer electron shells of each unit. The electron transfer produces the ion, and the interionic attractive forces are due to the respective loss and gain of a single electron. The tendency of all atomic forms is to assume a state corresponding most closely to that of inert and nonreactive rare gases, helium, argon, neon and xenon. They will form anions or cations, respectively, as the gain or loss of an electron tends to confer greater stability in the outer electron shell.

In any consideration of ionization phenomena as applied to biological systems, the formation of various types of complex ions must be considered. The following examples serve to illustrate this point:

$$H_2SO_4 \rightleftarrows H^+ + HSO_4^-$$
$$BaCl_2 \rightleftarrows BaCl^+ + Cl^-$$

Ionization phenomena in a system consisting only of water and phosphoric acid result in the formation of four types of ions, as follows:

$$H_3PO_4 \rightleftarrows H^+ + H_2PO_4^- \rightleftarrows H^+ + HPO_4^{---}$$
$$H^+ + PO_4^{---}$$

From a consideration of this comparatively simple system, the magnitude of the complexities of ionization in a living milieu is enormous.

Another type of complex ion formation follows the interaction of potassium cyanide and silver nitrate:

$$2KCN + AgNO_3 \rightarrow KNO_3 + KAg(CN)_2$$

The complex so formed dissociates as follows:

$$KAg(CN)_2 \rightleftarrows K^+ + Ag(CN)_2{}^-$$

As indicated by Bull (1951), two major factors govern the existence of ions in solution. The first of these is the attraction of ions for each other, which is proportional to the charge on each ion, the distance of the ions from each other, and the dielectric constant of the solvent. In biological systems, the solvent is water with a constant of 78.54 at 25° C., indicating that water decreases the affinity between ions to $\frac{1}{78}$ of that exerted in crystal form. The second factor is ionic hydration, and this will vary in biological systems much as it does in simpler isolated inorganic combinations. Solutes, whether electrolytes or not, form hydrates or solvates in water solution. Whenever a hydrate is formed, the ion plus the water forms a molecular complex acting as a single dissolved unit. The water used up in forming the hydrate is thus withdrawn from the pool of solvent. This factor of ionic hydration is of marked significance in the behavior of ion exchangers.

Some idea of the differences in ionic radii is obtained from the figures of Pauling (1940), given in angstrom units; Li^+, 0.60; Na^+, 0.95; K^+, 1.33; Mg^{++}, 0.65; Ca^{++}, 0.99; Cl^-, 1.81; I^-, 2.16; $SO_4{}^-$, 1.51. Those ions in a given valence series will hydrate to a greater degree as their ionic radii decrease (Bull, 1951); however, the effective number of water molecules associated with anions increases with increasing radii of the anions involved (Stokes and Robinson, 1948).

Ionic hydration is the phenomenon underlying the lyotropic or Hofmeister series, listing relative powers of anion and cation to affect an entire host of biological and physical properties of proteins, colloids, etc. It is perhaps at this point that the extent and degree of ion exchange in biological systems becomes most apparent. Studies of ion exchange resins and similar materials reveal the similarities of their behavior with proteins and other materials in biological systems. This entire scheme of behavior rests in large measure upon ionic hydration. The Hofmeister series for cations is:

$$\text{Th} > \text{Al} > \text{H} > \text{Ba} > \text{Sr} > \overset{0.99}{\text{Ca}} > \overset{1.33}{\text{K}} > \overset{0.95}{\text{Na}} > \overset{0.61}{\text{Li}}$$

and for anions:

$$\text{Citrate} > \text{Tartrate} > \overset{1.51}{\text{SO}_4} > \text{Acetate} > \overset{1.81}{\text{Cl}} > \text{NO}_3 > \text{Br} > \overset{2.16}{\text{I}} > \text{CNS}$$

HYDROGEN IONS, ACIDS AND BASES

In general, the term hydrogen ion concentration refers in fact to the hydrogen ion activity or the apparent hydrogen ion concentration. All physical and chemical methods of measurement give a value corresponding to the hydrogen ion activity.

In recent years, many new concepts have appeared in studies of hydrogen ions. One of these involves the fact of hydration of the hydrogen ion with the formation of hydronium ions. The degree of hydration may progress and an entire series of higher polymers be formed (Huggins, 1936*a*, *b*), thus:

$$H^+ + H_2O \rightleftarrows H_3O^+ + H_2O \rightleftarrows H_5O_2^+ + H_2O \rightleftarrows H_7O_3^+$$

In this and all other systems, the hydrogen ion can be regarded as a proton, infinitely small in size, and capable of penetrating any molecule with which it comes in contact.

Another accepted innovation of the time-honored ionization concept concerns the theory of Brönsted (1923, 1928) and Lowry (1923), who define an acid as any substance capable of yielding protons, and a base as any substance able to accept a proton. The concept is expressed in the following equation:

$$A \rightleftarrows H^+ + B$$

where A is an acid and B is a base. From this it can be stated that the reactions of acids and bases need not necessarily involve the elements of water. Bull (1951) gives as an example of this the reaction of sodium acetate and hydrochloric acid, as follows:

$$CH_3COONa + HCl \rightarrow CH_3COOH + NaCl$$

An acid, HA, will dissociate, forming H^+ and A^-, as expressed by

$$HA \rightleftarrows H^+ + A^-$$

Applying the law of mass action to this system and expressing the concentrations of hydrogen ions and acid anions, we form the equation

$$K_a = \frac{(H^+)(A^-)}{(HA)}$$

which involves the acid dissociation constant, K_a. The above equation states that the product of the concentration of hydrogen ions and the anions from the acid, divided by the concentration of the undissociated acid, is in fact a constant. The magnitude of the constant determines the strength of the acid. If the acid is strong the constant is large, as more dissociation has occurred; if the acid is weak the constant is small, indicating a greater concentration of the acid in the undissociated form. In general, interest is centered in the so-called weak acids and bases, which are not completely dissociated. Consideration of the weak base leads to formulations corresponding to those for the acids:

$$BOH \rightleftarrows B^+ + OH^-$$

Applying the law of mass action to this system, we arrive at the formulation of an equation for the determination of the base dissociation constant:

$$K_b = \frac{(B^+)(OH^-)}{(BOH)}$$

As with the acids, there are weak bases and strong bases: those which dissociate very little and those which dissociate almost 100 per cent or are, in fact, in ionic form prior to solution.

In any consideration of the behavior of weak acids and bases in solution, the factor of the ionization of water must be known. Water dissociates into hydrogen and hydroxyl ions:

$$H_2O \rightleftarrows H^+ + OH^-$$

and this dissociation can be expressed as follows:

$$K_{H_2O} = \frac{(H^+)(OH^-)}{(H_2O)}$$

The value of the water dissociation constant is for a temperature of $25°$ C., 1.008×10^{-14}. The factor for water in the above equation is constant, and therefore the dissociation constant for water represents, in fact, the product of the concentration or activities of hydroxyl and hydrogen ions expressed in gram equivalent weights. The dissociation constant of water is an extremely important factor in biological systems, as it automatically implies that regardless of other components of a given system, the product of hydrogen and hydroxyl ion concentrations must be 10^{-14}. If the system is alkaline, there will be a correspondingly low concentration of hydrogen ions, and vice versa.

The equation given above representing the acid dissociation constant can be written as follows:

$$\frac{1}{(H^+)} = \frac{(A^-)}{K_a(HA)}$$

Further modification of this equation may be made by taking the logarithm of both sides of the equation and expressing it as follows:

$$\log \frac{1}{(H^+)} = \log \frac{1}{K_a} + \log \frac{(A^-)}{(HA)}$$

The logarithm of the reciprocal of the hydrogen ion concentration as expressed above is called pH.

Acetic acid can be used as an example of a weak acid with biological significance. It has a dissociation constant K_a at 25° C. of roughly 10^{-5}. Such constants are frequently expressed in terms similar to that of pH and designated as pK_a. The latter expression is the logarithm of the reciprocal of the dissociation constant, K_a. The pK_a of acetic acid would be roughly 5. Lactic acid has a dissociation constant K_a of approximately 10^{-4} at the above temperature, giving it a pK_a of 4. This means that lactic acid is a stronger acid than is acetic. The smaller the pK_a value, the stronger the acid; the smaller the dissociation constant, the weaker the acid.

Hydrogen ion concentrations can be determined by the indicator method or by the electrometric method. The indicator method depends upon the variation in color assumed by various organic substances with shift in pH. The electrometric method depends upon the electromotive force of a cell whose potential is a direct function of the hydrogen ion concentration.

In dealing with pH values it is good to remember that the scale is not arithmetic, i.e., when a solution is brought from pH 7 to pH 6, the arithmetical increase in hydrogen ion activity is only one-tenth of the increase in going from pH 6 to pH 5 (Bull, 1951).

Biological systems are generally buffered. The term buffer is applied to a substance which tends to resist changes in pH and to increase the amount of acid or alkali needed to cause a unit change in pH. The best buffers are mixtures of weak acids or bases with their corresponding salts. For example, if one adds hydrochloric acid of pH 1.0 to a solution of 0.3 N trisodium phosphate, the following reactions will occur:

$$Na_3PO_4 + HCl \rightarrow NaCl + Na_2HPO_4 \qquad (1)$$
$$Na_2HPO_4 + HCl \rightarrow NaCl + NaH_2PO_4 \qquad (2)$$
$$NaH_2PO_4 + HCl \rightarrow NaCl + H_3PO_4 \qquad (3)$$

The pH of a system in reaction 1 is about 9.0; in reaction 2 about 4.5; and in reaction 3 about 2.5. This means that three equivalents of hydrochloric acid of pH 1.0 have been needed to shift the pH of the sodium phosphate from 10.5 to 2.5.

In a similar manner, the salt of a weak acid can react with a strong acid and prevent the pH from shifting to the degree normally expected:

$$Na_2CO_3 + HCl \rightarrow NaCl + NaHCO_3$$
$$NaHCO_3 + HCl \rightarrow NaCl + H_2CO_3$$

As strong acids are buffered by the salts of weak acids, so strong bases are buffered by the salts of weak bases:

$$NH_4C_2H_3O_2 + NaOH \rightarrow NaC_2H_3O_2 + NH_4OH$$
$$NaH_2PO_4 + NaOH \rightarrow Na_2HPO_4 + H_2O$$

The importance of an understanding of the behavior of weak acids and bases lies in the fact that the cation and anion exchangers currently in use in medical practice are respectively a weak-acid cation exchanger and a weak-base anion exchanger. The effect of pH change on weak-acid and weak-base exchangers is much greater than it is on strong-acid or strong-base exchangers.

BIOLOGICAL ION CONCENTRATIONS

Paleochemistry establishes the probable marine origin of the vertebrate by demonstrating the similarity in ionic composition of sea water and blood. The element magnesium is the only one which is dispro-

TABLE

Ionic Composition of

Ion	Blood		Gastric juice		Bile	
	Mg. %	*MEq./l.*	*Mg. %*	*MEq./l.*	*Mg. %*	*MEq./l.*
Potassium	16–22	4.1–5.6	40	10	10–47	2.6–12
Sodium	330	143	115	50	326–354	142–154
Calcium	9.0–11.5	4.5–5.8	4.1–8.6	2.0–4.3	4–9	2–4.5
Magnesium	1–3	0.83–2.5	2.2–9.4	1.8–7.8	1.82	1.5
Chloride	370	100	500	141	320–355	90–100
Sulfate	19	4.0	Trace	—	0.3	0.06
Phosphate	10	3.1	1.1–4.2	0.34–1.3	12.5	7.3
Bicarbonate	164	27	0–130	0–21	244	40
pH	7.3–7.4		1.2–1.8		7.4–8.5	
Titratable acidity or alkalinity	—	146.6	—	123.3	—	151–181

portionately high in sea water (Macallum, 1926). For general orientation on ionic composition, the blood serum of mammals can be regarded as slightly diluted sea water. A further extension of this generalization is that of regarding the other body fluids as modified blood serum. This concept permits an immediate basis for consideration of the effect of ion exchange resins on blood fluids. As this monograph deals with the gastrointestinal tract primarily, Table 1 is offered, giving ionic composition of sea water, blood, gastric juice, bile, pancreatic juice, small intestinal content, and large intestinal content.

In general, ion exchange resins functioning in an *in vitro* system of comparable ionic composition will behave as they do *in vivo;* however, the complexity of biological fluids is tremendous, and each organic moiety present may modify the ionic behavior of the fluid as well as the exchange function of the resin. *In vitro* studies of ion exchange must therefore be conducted with the milieu comparable in all respects to that found *in vivo*. In the final analysis, the biological fluid itself must form the milieu for study. Frequently, introductory examinations of exchangers can be conducted with artificially prepared ionic compositions.

Obviously, dietary composition and habits will modify the ionic composition of the gastrointestinal tract, and this in turn must be correlated with exchanger function.

1
Biological Fluids

Pancreatic juice		Small intestine		Large intestine		Sea water	
Mg. %	*MEq./l.*	*Mg. %*	*MEq./l.*	*Mg. %*	*MEq./l.*	*Mg. %*	*MEq./l.*
11.7–15.6	3–4	15.6–19.5	4–5	33.6	8.6	37.5–39.1	9.6–10
317	138	322	140	347	151	1012–1044	440–454
4.4–6.4	2.2–3.2	5.0–12.8	2.5–6.4	10.0	5.0	36–40.8	18–20.4
0.34	0.28	1.2–2.4	1–2	1.95	1.6	123–127	101–104.5
213–284	60–80	262–365	74–103	310	87.5	1810–1899	510–535
39.4	8.2	Trace	—	Trace	—	240–255	50–53.2
0.125	0.039	8.3–24.5	2.61–7.66	54.4	17	6.4	2.0
610	100	12–195	2–32	559	91.8	13.4	2.2
7.5–8.8		6.16–7.31		8.03		8.0	
—	50–160	—	158.2	—	164.6	—	550

BIOLOGICAL SIGNIFICANCE OF IONS

The blaze of glory surrounding miracle hormones, vitamins and drugs has dimmed in the minds of many the greater importance of the inorganic ion. The proposal has been made that any protein in the proper environment may assume the characteristics of an enzyme (Sevag, 1945, 1951) and that "the proper environment is doubtless ionic in character." The effect of ions on protein structures and the immediate antagonisms associated therewith form "the dynamic functional systems around which the complex concatenation of living matter is built" (Martin, 1951).

The balance mechanisms forming the antagonisms among ions are of far greater importance than the function of absolute concentrations. Before reviewing briefly this interionic antagonism concept, a summary of the biological significance of individual ions is in order. There can be no doubt that the animal organism is extremely sensitive to ionic content, a fact reflected in the narrow limits for concentration of any given ion in the blood. The factors of absorption, excretion and in some instances storage are functional in the maintenance of blood serum levels. Generally, blood concentrations of ions reflect the tissue concentrations, but in abnormal states this generalization does not apply.

As stated by Martin (1951), anions and cations and their combinations constitute about 1 per cent of the mass of the body. These ions exert a multiplicity of functional characteristics; they are components of enzyme structures and cofactors for enzymes; they control protoplasmic colloidal states, form structural components of the body, and so on.

The function of inorganic ions as components or cofactors of enzymes could hardly be materially modified by ion removal via exchange resins; however, the ratio of ionic concentrations could be materially modified, and it is known that this ratio is determinant in many enzymatic systems. For example, magnesium and calcium ions activate acetylcholinesterase, while potassium inhibits this enzyme (Mendel *et al.*, 1939). Direct antagonism occurs between calcium or magnesium on the one hand and potassium on the other. There are many other examples of ionic antagonism in enzyme systems, but for this brief summary one more will suffice. Northrop (1942), using eserinized brain slices, noted that the formation of acetylcholine was enhanced by potassium ions and inhibited by either calcium or magnesium ions. It seems entirely probable that enzymatic activity would be modified by the restriction of ion intake through the use of exchange resins, assuming that the removal of ions was not such as to leave blood and tissue ratios of these ions unchanged. In other words, the exchangers would have to remove ions selectively and not in proportion to their concentrations in natural biological fluids.

Of considerable interest to the clinician using exchangers is the problem of possible modification of patient reaction to drugs. Whether or not this actually happens in practice is not yet known, but the probability is there. Certainly ionic ratios markedly modify the reaction of the body and of specific tissues to different drugs. Lowering the ratio of calcium to sodium lowers the sympathetic response (Gley, 1928). As an example of the alteration of tissue sensitivity by ions, von Pinter-Kovats (1928) reported that the vasoconstrictor response of the rabbit ear to epinephrine requires the presence of calcium but not potassium. Conversely, drugs may sensitize to ions, as in the case of the veratrum alkaloids, which sensitize tissues to the potassium ion (Goutier, 1950).

One of the earliest clinical states to be recognized as a deviation from the normal in electrolyte balance was tetany. This condition is a reflection of the marked sensitivity of the nervous system to a calcium deficiency. The neuromuscular transmission systems manifest a state of irritability resulting in twitchings and convulsions. In the element calcium and its physiological role we find a unique example of the complexity of the mechanism controlling ionic balance. The physiologically functional calcium of the blood stream is ionic. This is in contrast to the calcium found in this biological fluid in combination in colloidal salts of phosphate and citrate, and to that larger portion of the calcium bound in the form of nonionized and nondiffusible calcium-protein complex. The ionized calcium is controlled in large measure by the parathyroids. In addition to the role of the hormone in the modification of available calcium, vitamin D is involved via the absorption of calcium from the gastrointestinal tract. Limitation of hormonal and vitamin control of ionic calcium to the parathyroid hormone and to vitamin D would be the equivalent of examining but a small central portion of an extremely complex canvas. Almost all hormones and vitamins play some role in the control of electrolyte balance and specifically in the metabolism of calcium. Further, calcium function is correlated with that of phosphate and with virtually all other cations. One final point should be made relative to the role of the kidney; this organ controls in some measure both calcium and phosphorus metabolism, and its failure leads to phosphate retention with resultant lowered ionic calcium and the precipitation of a uremic tetanic state.

To indicate further the concatenation of factors involved in ionic function in biological systems, the problem of magnesium tetany must be mentioned. In this condition, tetany occurs in the presence of a normal or at least noncritical modification of ionic calcium concentration but is associated with modification of ionic magnesium (Orent *et al.*, 1934). The conclusion was reached that disturbed ratios of ionic magnesium and calcium underlay the development of tetany, and this assumption was supported by the findings of Day *et al.* (1936), who observed that animals deprived of both magnesium and calcium survived longer than did those deprived of either element alone.

The control of permeability of cellular structures by ions is of paramount importance. Calcium plays a vital role in this relation. The subject is mentioned here to underline the host of factors surrounding any ionic modification. Briefly, the concept of Danielli (1943), which seems to account best for the role of monovalent and divalent cations in cellular permeability, is that the divalent cation reduces permeability by increasing lateral adhesion in the cellular membrane. The divalent cation produces a cross-binding through union with two anionic groups occurring as part of the cellular membrane. A monovalent cation will not do this, as its sole valence is utilized in combining with a single cellular anionic grouping.

Another problem of great biological importance concerns the penetration of living cells by ions. While no unified picture has been offered in explanation of this phenomenon, it can be stated that ionic concentration occurs in opposition to the concentration gradient; that is, ions pass into the interior of cells even if the concentration of the ion within the cell exceeds that in the external milieu. This active ionic transport is accomplished by the expenditure of work. Bull (1951) gives several examples of this type of transfer. For example, 1500 calories are required for the secretion of 1 l. of gastic juice by the parietal cells of the stomach. The degree of concentration of a given ion within a cell can be enormous, as in the case of a marine alga which concentrates potassium ions to the extent of 500 mEq. per liter from sea water with a potassium ion concentration of 12 mEq. per liter.

The section on fluid and electrolyte balance in Harrison *et al.*, *Principles of Internal Medicine,* is recommended for details concerning potassium and sodium in diseased states. In summary, potassium is the controlling factor for osmolar concentrations of intra-cellular fluids, just as sodium is for extracellular fluids. Cellular mem-branes are relatively impermeable to these ions. Potassium is important for neuromuscular transmission, particularly for that of the heart. With regard to the use of ion exchangers, both excess and deficit of potassium are important.

Potassium deficiency occurs in cases of familial periodic paralysis; in renal disease characterized by retention of chlorides; following the treatment of diabetic coma; during severe diarrhea; following the administration of potassium-free fluids or desoxycorticosterone; as a possible complication of the administration of cation exchange resins. In practice, a portion of the cation exchange resins given for sodium removal are present in the potassium cycle, a precaution rendering im-probable the precipitation of potassium deficit. Symptomatically, stupor and weakness characterize the syndrome. Further, the electro-cardiographic findings show marked abnormality in the T wave.

Potassium excess, a specific indication for cation exchange therapy, occurs in association with renal insufficiency and, in Addison's disease, adrenal cortical hypofunction. Manifestations of potassium excess in-clude cardiac arrhythmias, electrocardiographic changes, probably the twitchings and convulsions seen in the uremic state, and possibly peripheral circulatory failure. In the last instance, the potassium excess may be the result rather than the cause.

As the plasma proteins predominate in the maintenance of osmotic relationships within the blood, so the element sodium is key to the osmotic effects within the tissues. In other words, it is the controlling factor in the extravascular extracellular fluid balance. This fraction of the total body water comprises some 15 to 20 per cent thereof.

Maintenance of serum sodium levels (normally 134 to 141 mEq. per liter) is achieved largely through the kidney's ability to adjust renal excretion. As indicated by Danowski (1951), renal excretion of sodium can be virtually eliminated by reduction of sodium intake.

The steroid hormones elaborated by the adrenal cortex control in large measure the urinary excretion of this ion; those of the desoxy series related to desoxycorticosterone reduce excretion of sodium by increasing tubular reabsorption. The picture is complicated by the natural antagonisms existing among the 11-desoxy and the 11-oxygen-ated steroid hormones, and in addition by the role played by the poste-rior pituitary, the thyroid, and other hormones in ionic equilibrium.

As with all aspects of biochemistry, there is no unidimensional approach to the problem of electrolyte balance. In fact, as stated by Danowski (1951), the concept must be multidimensional. In considering extracellular sodium, the problem is not solely that of sodium balance but also of water balance. One potential danger immediately comes to mind in the consideration of the application of cation exchange resins for sodium removal, and that is the danger of excessive depletion of this ion with resultant hyponatremia. While in fact hyponatremia will not generally ensue following cation exchange therapy, it is obvious that vigilance must be exercised against its appearance under unusual circumstances. One such criterion is the excretion by the patient of urine ample in volume but devoid of chloride and sodium. This is a manifestation of the attempt made by the kidney to maintain normal extracellular concentration of sodium at the expense of loss of body water.

Danowski (1951) emphasizes the fact that "normal or even high sodium concentrations may be present with decreases in the total amount of extracellular sodium, depending on the balance of water during periods of sodium loss." As he points out, knowledge of extracellular sodium stores requires facts on concentration of sodium, volume of extracellular fluid, and the total amount of the ion present.

The circulatory collapse and shock developing coincident with hyponatremia is comparable with that associated with trauma or blood loss and can only be corrected by the reconstitution of the body fluids in respect to ionic sodium. The induction of diuresis, tending to restore blood levels of sodium, or the restoration of fluid volume by sodium-free liquids will not eliminate the defective circulatory factors. The therapy of choice in hyponatremia (Danowski, 1951) is the use of a combination of colloidal solution and saline, providing replacement of electrolyte deficit and colloidal osmotic structure simultaneously.

Edema is etiologically almost invariably associated with sodium retention. It is the direct result of increases in extracellular sodium and the consequent increase in extracellular fluid. Pitting and unusual increase in body weight are most frequently used as diagnostic criteria. Congestive failure and hepatic cirrhosis most commonly manifest this symptom of abnormal electrolyte balance. Virtually without exception, the correction of edema can be brought about by sodium restriction.

In general, low salt diets have been employed as therapeutic procedures. Such diets range in sodium content from around 34 down to 2 mEq., and their efficacy can be attributed to factors other than sodium content. Diuretics such as urea and the mercurials have also

been in general use for the correction of edema through sodium elimination. The danger of hyponatremia with either low salt diets or diuretics far exceeds that in association with the employment of cation exchange resins. Details of such comparison will be given in Chapter 7.
One additional indication for the removal of sodium ions is hypertension. To be sure, the relationship of sodium to vascular disease is not
yet completely established, but the advocates of this relationship have
presented much evidence supporting their views. The material is too
extensive for consideration in this monograph, however.

SUMMATION

The paramount significance of ionic factors in the life process cannot
be overestimated. The origin of life in the aqueous ionic systems comprising the seas of the earth attests to this fact. It has been proposed
that in the proper environment any protein can become an enzyme.
Further, living things are no more than concatenations of intimately
interrelated enzyme systems. From these assertions, the scope and import of ionic milieu in any biological system are apparent.

While absolute values for ionic concentration are of importance, it
is the relative concentrations which are basically determinant. Logical
consideration of the problem of ion balance can never be directed
toward a single ion; it can only be directed toward a single ion in relationship to its naturally synergistic and antagonistic relatives. Two
general concepts must be held in mind at all times. The first is the
theory of biological relativity, which states simply that no single ionic
form possesses in itself a function not shared in some measure by a
closely related ion. The second is the theory of biological antagonism,
which states that the biological effect of a given ion will be modified at
all times by the presence and activity of ions antagonistic to the function
of the ion under consideration.

From these basic premises, one may proceed to the specific problems
of ionic interplay as reflected in electrolyte balance. It is unfortunate
that preoccupation with hormones and vitamins led science to neglect
the even more basic structure of the inorganic ionic world. The hypothesis can be put forward that the vitamins and hormones are no
more than modifiers or regulators of the activities of inorganic ions as
they alter and direct the enzymatic function of macromolecular protein structures.

REFERENCES

ARRHENIUS, S. *Ztschr. physik. Chem.,* 1: 631, 1887.

BRÖNSTED, J. N. *Rec. trav. chim. Pays-Bas,* 42: 718, 1923.

BRÖNSTED, J. N. *Chem. Rev.,* 5: 231, 1928.

BULL, H. B. *Physical Biochemistry.* New York: Wiley, 1951.

DANIELLI, J. F. In Davson, H., and J. F. Danielli, *The Permeability of Natural Membranes.* London: Cambridge University Press, 1943.

DANOWSKI, T. S. *Am. J. Med.,* 10: 468, 1951.

DAY, H. G., H. D. KRUSE, and E. V. McCOLLUM. *J. Biol. Chem.,* 112: 337, 1936.

DEBYE, P., and E. HÜCKEL. *Physik. Ztschr.,* 24: 185, 1923a.

DEBYE, P., and E. HÜCKEL. *Physik. Ztschr.,* 24: 305, 1923b.

GLEY, E. *Arch. sc. biol.,* 12: 39, 1928.

GOUTIER, R. *Brit. J. Pharmacol.,* 5: 33, 1950.

HARRISON, T. R., *et al.* (eds.). *Principles of Internal Medicine.* Philadelphia: Blakiston, 1950.

HUGGINS, M. L. *J. Phys. Chem.,* 40: 723, 1936a.

HUGGINS, M. L. *J. Org. Chem.,* 1: 407, 1936b.

LEWIS, G. N., and M. RANDALL. *Thermodynamics and the Free Energy of Chemical Substances.* New York: McGraw-Hill, 1923.

LOWRY, T. M. *J. Soc. Chem. Indust.,* 42: 43, 1923.

MENDEL, B., D. MUNDELL, and F. STRELITZ. *Nature,* 144: 479, 1939.

MACALLUM, A. B. *Physiol. Rev.,* 6: 316, 1926.

MARTIN, G. J. *Biological Antagonism.* Philadelphia: Blakiston, 1951.

NORTHROP, J. H. *J. Gen. Physiol.,* 25: 465, 1942.

ORENT, E. R., H. D. KRUSE, and E. V. McCOLLUM. *J. Biol. Chem.,* 106: 573, 1934.

PAULING, L. *The Nature of the Chemical Bond.* Ithaca, N. Y.: Cornell University Press, 1940.

SEVAG, M. G. *Immuno-Catalysis.* Springfield, Ill.: Charles C Thomas, 1945, 1951.

STOKES, R. H., and R. A. ROBINSON. *J. Am. Chem. Soc.,* 70: 1870, 1948.

VON PINTER-KOVATS. Z. *Ztschr. ges. exper. Med.,* 62: 634, 1928.

CHAPTER 2

The Chemistry of Anion Exchange Resins

GENERAL CHARACTERISTICS OF ANION EXCHANGE
RESINS

MECHANISM OF ACTION
Ionization
Particle Size
Porosity
Ionic Strength
Kinetics

CONSIDERATION of anion exchange resins resolves itself into two major problems. First, what are anion exchange resins? Second, how do these resins act?

GENERAL CHARACTERISTICS OF ANION EXCHANGE RESINS

The answer to the first question is best approached by a brief review of the manner in which resins of the anion exchange type are formed. In general a modified phenol is condensed with formaldehyde and an amine. This reaction forms a gel which is then heated to produce the fully polymerized resin. Following this the resin is ground, washed, exhaustively leached, dried, and is then ready for use. The specific resin of the anion exchange type used in medicinal products is designated as a polyethylene polyamine methylene—substituted resin of diphenylol dimethylmethane. A resin of this type is made by reacting diphenylol dimethylmethane, phenol and formaldehyde at a temperature of 50° C. The solution formed in sodium hydroxide and water is then mixed with triethylene tetramine. Additional formaldehyde is added and the entire mixture is gradually heated to around 100° C. The gel which forms is dried down in trays and is then crushed, screened, washed, and dried. In the symbols of organic chemistry, this reaction could be represented as seen in Figure 1.

The complexity of anion exchangers used in medicine indicates presentation of the polymer formation by a simpler type. For this purpose a system could be offered wherein a phenol containing an amine radical is reacted with formaldehyde to form first a dimer and subsequently a polymer.

MECHANISM OF ACTION

Until the advent of the high-capacity anion exchange resins, little study had been directed to anion-exchanging materials because the natural exchangers such as clays and alumina had only slight activity. Anion exchange resins used in medicine are weak bases and as such are far more sensitive to pH changes than are the cation exchangers. Anion exchange is not necessarily based on equivalents; thus a resin

FIGURE 1
Anion Exchange Resin Formation

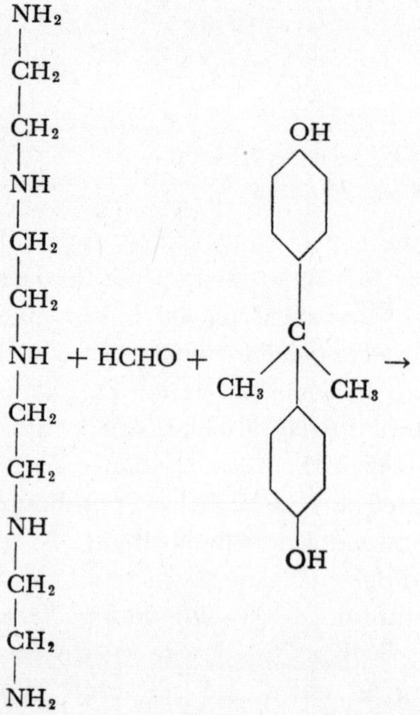

Tetraethylene pentamine + formaldehyde + diphenylol dimethylmethane

FIGURE 1 (*Continued*)

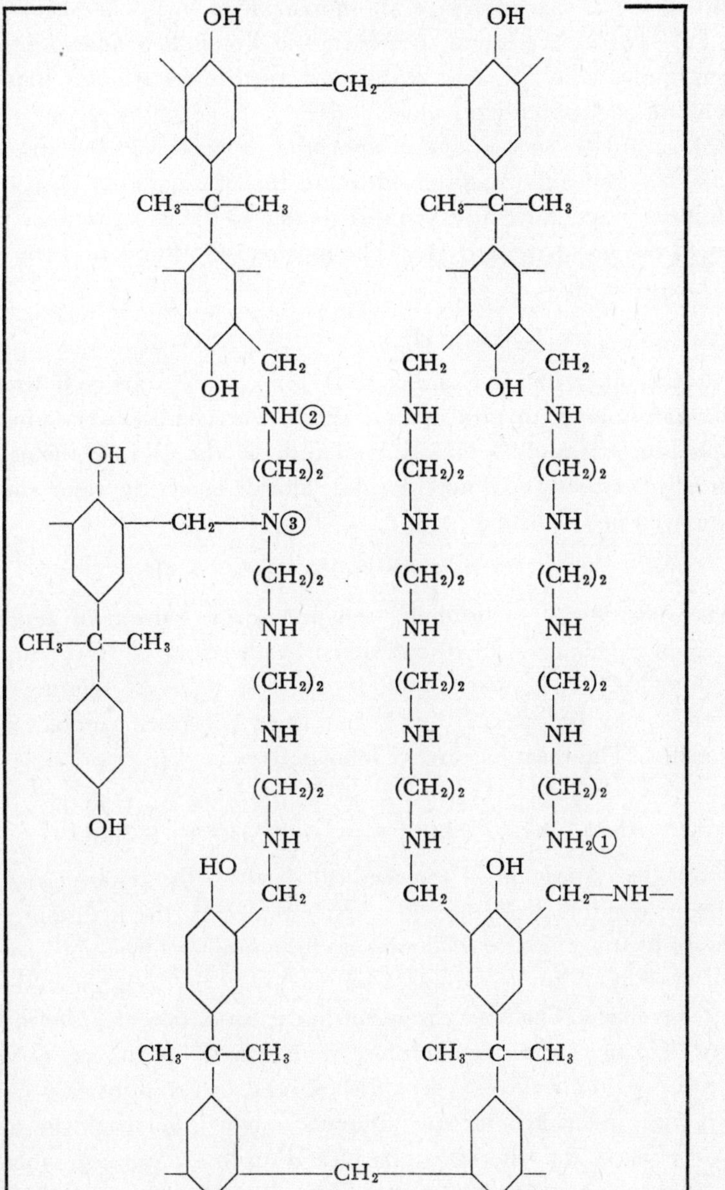

Unit repeat x — 1 times; primary amine group at 1; secondary amine group at 2; tertiary amine group at 3. Unfilled valence lines indicate repeat point of molecular structure.

with hydrochloric acid absorbed thereon when exposed to sulfuric acid will not always exchange an equivalent of hydrochloric acid for one of sulfuric. In general, however, the Freundlich adsorption isotherm applies. Sulfuric acid is absorbed much more strongly than hydrochloric acid on an equivalent basis.

Bishop (1946) measured the absorption of several monobasic acids on alkylene polyamine resins and found that the quantity of acid absorbed per gram of resin was simply related to the ionic product (H^+) (A^-) of the dissolved acid HA. The mechanism of action of the resin was expressed as

$$RNH_2 + H^+ + A^- \rightarrow RNH_3^+A^-$$

On the other hand, Kunin and Myers (1947) observed that an anion exchange resin in a neutral or alkaline condition contains appreciable amounts of the ionized hydroxide, $RNH_3^+OH^-$. If the neutral resin is treated with sodium chloride, chloride enters the resin and the solution becomes alkaline:

$$RNH_3^+OH^- + Cl^- \rightarrow RNH_3^+Cl^- + OH^-$$

The difficulty of determining the precise mechanism of action of the anion exchange resin is underlined by the work of Heymann and O'Donnell (1948), who conclude that in aqueous solutions two processes may be operative and that these processes cannot be distinguished. The reactions are as follows:

$$RNH_2 + H_3O^+ + A^- \rightarrow RNH_3^+A^- + H_2O \tag{1}$$
$$RNH_3^+OH^- + H_3O^+ + A^- \rightarrow RNH_3^+A^- + 2H_2O \tag{2}$$

From the standpoint of the medical scientist, the resolution of this problem is purely academic. If reaction 1 occurs, the hydronium ion gives up hydrogen ion to the amine and the result is formation of water and the resinous amine complex; by reaction 2 precisely the same end point is reached. The reactions result in the formation of water in both cases. Acid neutralization therefore results in the formation of water just as it would if sodium hydroxide had been added to the acid system.

The only point at which a difference might arise would be at the release point of the chloride anion picked up in the stomach when the pH reached 7.5 in the lower gut. Here, if exchange alone occurred, the chloride would simply exchange for the hydroxide ion; however, if this exchange occurred and the complex reverted to a trivalent state, hydrogen ion would be returned to the intestinal juices and it in turn would necessarily be neutralized. Theoretically, the significant point

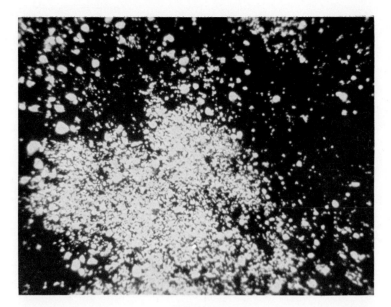

Resin A

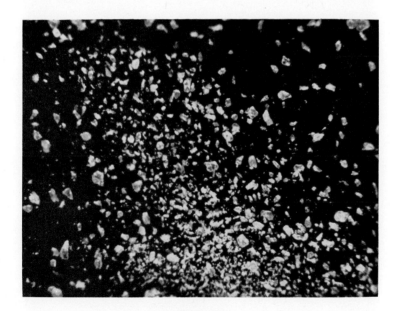

Resin B

FIGURE 2
Photomicrographs of Typical Anion Exchange Resins

would be that in the instances of straight exchange, the resin in the quaternary ammonium chloride cycle passing from the stomach to the gut would cause no shift in the intestinal hydrogen ion concentration. On the other hand, if the valence shift reaction occurred, the pH of the gut would be reduced and there would be a tendency for a reduction in the alkalinity. The probabilities are excellent that the valence shift does not occur, as there is no variation in pH of the intestine as reflected in fecal pH. This, to be sure, is not conclusive in any sense, but it is certainly indicative. In neither type would the chloride be carried out of the body unless the reaction were almost 100 per cent irreversible.

Nachod (1949) took the position that the weak-base anion exchangers react in accordance with equation 1 and that the strong-base anion exchangers react in accordance with equation 2. His concept was based upon the swelling of the weak-base anion exchanger when it takes up hydrochloric acid and the fact that the strong-base anion exchangers swell very little during acid absorption. If the weak-base anion exchangers were in the form $RNH_3^+OH^-$ prior to taking up acid, the degree of swelling would not be marked to the form $RNH_3^+A^-$.

With these basic resins, anion exchange proceeded by equivalents. Kunin and Myers (1947) gave the following order of strength of binding of different anions:

$$SO_4^{--} > CrO_4^{--} > Citrate^{---} > NO_3^- > AsO_4^{---} > PO_4^{---}$$
$$> MoO_4^{---} > C_2H_3O_2^- = I^- = Br^- > Cl^- > F^-$$

As with other exchange materials, anion exchangers can be regarded in terms of the reactions of the corresponding types of simple, organic molecules. The prototype here could be considered to be methyl amine, a soluble organic amine. In aqueous solutions this chemical forms an equilibrium mixture in accordance with the following formulas:

$$CH_3NH_2 + H_2O \rightleftarrows CH_3NH_3^+ + OH^-$$

If one considers the above equation applicable to resinous exchangers, it becomes apparent that when acid is added to the system the hydroxyl ions are replaced by the anion of the acid and the formation of water occurs. As the hydroxyl ion is continuously removed by more acid, the equilibrium shifts to the right and more of the resin amine reacts with water to form the quaternary unit plus hydroxyl.

Anion exchange resins react in any given system in accordance with a multiplicity of factors—particle size, pore size, ionic strength, anionic species, basic strength of the resinous amine, and so on. Each such factor must be considered briefly in order to clarify the behavior characteristics of resins in biological systems. While in some measure these properties are known, it is probable that more remains to be discovered than is now known. In the biological system, the ionic milieu is complex, not only in its inorganic composition, but even more in its organic composition. The interplay of forces will be terrific; the antagonistic phenomena displayed will be legion. The best that can be done in the study of these materials is an attempted extrapolation of present knowledge into the unknown biological sphere.

Ionization

One prime feature of anion exchange action lies in the degree of basic strength shown by the resin itself. There are all types, varying from weak to strong. The significance of this lies in the fact that the weak-base anion exchange resin will be more susceptible to pH shift in the biological system as contrasted to a strong-base anion exchange resin. In the case of the weak-base anion exchanger most commonly employed in medicine, it is possible to derive an equation for reaction in the stomach at pH of 1.0 to 1.5 and the degree of reversal at the pH of the large intestine, which will be around 7.5 to 8.0:

$$RNH_3^+OH^- + Cl^- + H^+ \underset{7.5}{\overset{1.5}{\rightleftarrows}} RNH_3Cl + H_2O \uparrow$$

In the case of the strong-base anion exchanger, the reaction will go to the right at pH 1.5 but its reversal at pH 7.5 will not occur. With the strong-base anion exchanger, it is possible to exchange the chloride of sodium chloride for the hydroxyl of the resin at a pH of 10.0. Theoretically, therefore, the strong-base anion exchanger should retain chloride removed in the stomach throughout the entire pH range of the gastrointestinal tract.

Another feature for consideration in biological systems is the greater affinity of anion exchangers for ions such as phosphate and sulfate as contrasted to chloride. Kunin and Myers (1947) give the capacity at saturation of Amberlite IR-4B (weak-base anion exchanger) as 27.7 mEq. per gram for phosphate contrasted to 9.2 mEq. per gram for hydrochloric acid. Retention of anions on exchangers would therefore favor the phosphate ion. It would theoretically be difficult to remove chloride ions, assuming the presence of phosphate in intestinal fluids.

In general, any typical anion exchange resin will contain primary, secondary and tertiary amine groups; it will therefore automatically possess amine groups of varying basic strength. The basic strength is correlated with the reactivity in the sense that those most weakly basic

FIGURE 3

Correlation between pH and Per Cent Amine Groups Neutralized

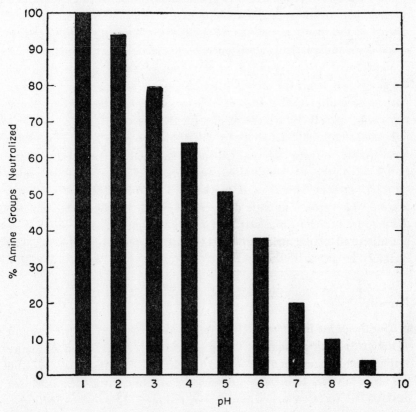

amine groups will be the first to revert to the hydroxide form as the pH shifts to the alkaline side; the stronger base will tend to retain some anion other than the hydroxyl until the pH reaches 8 to 10. Figure 3 illustrates the correlation between pH and the percentage of amine groups neutralized.

Particle Size

From the standpoint of practical application, pore and particle size of resins are interrelated. If the pores are too small to permit free passage of ions into the interstices of the resin particle, only the surface ion-reactive groups can function, and the capacity of the resin will be a direct function of its particle size. Most resins used today, however, are characterized by a pore size of such magnitude as to permit easy passage of ions into the interior of the resin particle. Under these conditions, particle size will not affect the total capacity of the resin but will markedly affect the speed of reaction. In other words, the particle size determines the speed of velocity of the reaction and not the total degree of the reaction, not the total capacity. This might seem to preclude the attachment of significance to the particle size, but clearly time is an element in the practical applications of resins, as the resin will begin to pass from the stomach within 10 to 20 minutes. Further, a patient suffering from pain due to a peptic ulcer will want relief immediately, and therefore the resin with the greatest speed of action is indicated. The fine-particle resin will achieve within a given period a greater percentage of its total capacity than will a grosser-mesh material. Under practical conditions, the capacity of the fine-mesh resin is therefore greater. However, if one were to examine both types *in vitro* it would be found that little difference existed, this being based upon the assumption that time was no factor and that 24 to 48 hours were permitted to elapse prior to the titrations determining the capacity factor.

Porosity

Modifications in porosity are brought about by varying the amount of the cross-linking chemical in the reaction. In the reaction in Figure 1 the cross-linking chemical is the diphenylol dimethylmethane, and therefore in order to increase porosity the amount of the chemical used in the basic reaction would have to be reduced. The number of cross-linkages also determines the capacity of a resinous material to dissolve in water with the formation of a colloidal solution. Water-soluble or water-miscible anion exchange resins are known. Insoluble liquid amines such as methyldinonylamine, methyldioctylamine and trioctylamine are quite active anion exchangers (Smith and Page, 1948). Particle size of the anion exchangers is modified largely by milling, an operation of definite practical limits. Chopping mills must be employed, and the cutting blades of such mills tend to heat, with the result that temperatures are reached which are deleterious to the resin form unless the blades are cooled. It is therefore improbable at present that particle sizes can be achieved which will average less than 200- to 400-mesh. Experimental lots can be made which will average closer to 400-mesh. The particle size at 200-mesh is 74 microns and at 400-mesh about 30 microns.

There is another rather obvious reason for small-particle resins when these materials are applied in medical practice, and that is in relation to patient acceptability. The larger the particle, the more gritty and unpleasant the medication will be and the more difficult patient cooperation will become.

Ionic Strength

The ionic strength effect varies with the basicity of the resin. In general, the ionic strength effect increases as the basicity of the resin decreases. It has already been stated that anion exchange resins applied in medical practice are weak-base resins and therefore the factor of ionic strength becomes dominant. The term ionic strength is one created by Lewis and Randall (1921) and is defined as half the sum of the terms obtained by multiplying the molality (concentration) of each ionic species present in the solution by the square of its valence. In terms applicable to the subject of this monograph, the concept indicates that ionic strength (which means ionic activity for any single ion) varies in accordance with the other ions present in the system. In biological systems, this is a tremendous factor, as the ionic milieu is of great complexity. As a specific example, pH is to be correlated with certain physiological responses, and if care is not taken a secondary salt effect may be responsible for a biological manifestation attributed to pH alone. Presenting this thought in another way, one might state that secondary ions must be considered in any system primarily attributed to pH.

In general, the greater the acid strength and the higher the valence of the anion, the more the system favors replacement of the hydroxyl of the anion exchange resin. This generalization is directly correlated with the strength of the anion exchange base. A weak-base anion exchanger would not react with the anion of a weak acid such as silicic, boric or carbonic. Strong-base anion exchangers will react with these acid anions.

The prime problem from the biological viewpoint is the reactivity of the hydroxyl with ions in solution. This will depend upon many factors, such as base strength of the resin, valence of anions, ion size, and strength of acid in solution. With very basic resins, the hydroxyl ions exhibit a very low tendency to exchange; with weak-base resins, the tendency is very high. For both weak- and strong-base resins, the exchange potential series is the same except for the position of the hydroxyl ion in the series. For the stronger-base resin, the hydroxyl ion is the weakest replacing ion. For the weaker-base resin the hydroxyl ion is the strongest replacing ion. This would account for the complete reversal of ion exchange, resulting in chloride liberation in the intestine by the weak-base anion exchanger. It may also be the factor preventing the strong-base anion exchanger in the hydroxyl cycle from ever taking up other anions in the tract. The strong-base anion exchanger would have to be given in a cycle the anion of which occurred lower in the exchange potential series, and that is difficult to do because chloride is nearly at the bottom of the list. Chloride removal by strong-base anion exchangers would therefore be theoretically almost impossible.

Kinetics

The kinetics of ion exchange in these systems is dependent primarily upon contact. Once the ion which will exchange reaches the ion-reactive grouping of the resin, the exchange itself is almost instantaneous. The time taken to reach the point of reaction is a function of diffusion into the pores of the resin and will therefore be related to particle size, concentration, temperature, degree of saturation of the exchange capacity, and resin hydration. The "parabolic" diffusion law (Barrer, 1941) mathematically expresses the relationship between particle size and reaction rate:

$$\frac{Yt}{Y\infty} = k \sqrt{t}$$

Yt = milliequivalents exchanged or absorbed in time t
$Y\infty$ = milliequivalents exchanged or absorbed at equilibrium

Here k is a constant which varies linearly with the reciprocal of the particle diameter. The smaller the particle, the larger will be the value of the constant and the larger will be the amount of material exchanged in time t. The importance of this equation to medical application of ion exchangers is that it gives an immediate gauge of the speed of action and therefore of the efficacy of resins used in clinical practice.

Under a given set of conditions, a resin with an average particle size of 30 to 40 mesh would take nearly 5 hours to react so that 85 per cent of its amine groups would be involved; the corresponding value of a resin with an average particle size of 200 mesh would be 20 minutes. It will be recalled that in general the resin will remain in the stomach for a period not exceeding 4 hours.

FIGURE 4

Rates of Adsorption of Hydrochloric Acid by Amberlite IR-4B

(From Kunin, R., and R. J. Myers, *J. Phys. Colloid Chem.*, **51:** 1111, 1947)

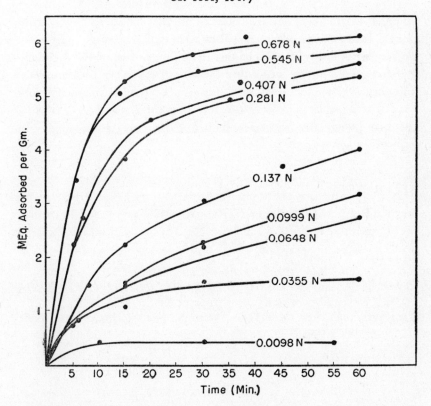

The initial rate of reaction for a system involving an anion exchange resin exchanging its hydroxyl groups for chloride in solution is given by the expression:

$$\left(\frac{dy}{dt}\right)_0 = kC$$

As the reaction progresses, the rate will be a function of the extent of change already completed and will be expressed by the equation:

$$\left(\frac{dy}{dt}\right) = kC(Y\infty - Yt)$$

Figure 4 illustrates the effect of concentration on the rate of reaction. The hydrochloric acid concentration of the stomach is approximately 0.1 N, and, as can be seen from the chart, the reaction rate of this resin would vary from approximately 0.2 mEq. per gram per minute at the outset and would decrease with great speed.

Temperature has a marked effect in determining reaction kinetics, as the energy of activation is approximately 6,000 to 7,000 calories; however, this factor is not important in the well-regulated temperatures of biological systems, where it will be essentially constant.

With weak-base anion exchangers, the dissociation of the exchangeable hydroxyl is of low order and the rate of exchange is of low order unless the exchangers are finely ground or in some manner exhibit large surface area. This will not hold for the strong-base anion exchangers, where dissociation is high and the rate of exchange consequently marked.

REFERENCES

BARRER, R. M. *Diffusion In and Through Solids.* New York: Macmillan, 1941.

BISHOP, J. A. *J. Phys. Chem.,* **50**: 6, 1946.

HEYMANN, E., and I. J. O'DONNELL. *J. Colloid Sc.,* **3**: 479, 1948.

KUNIN, R., and R. J. MYERS. *J. Phys. Colloid Chem.,* **51**: 1111, 1947.

LEWIS, G. N., and M. RANDALL. *Thermodynamics and the Free Energy of Chemical Substances.* New York: McGraw-Hill, 1921.

NACHOD, F. C. *Ion Exchange, Theory and Application.* New York: Academic Press, 1949.

SMITH, E. L., and J. E. PAGE. *J. Soc. Chem. Ind.,* **67**: 48, 1948.

CHAPTER 3

The Chemistry of Cation Exchange Resins

GENERAL CHARACTERISTICS OF CATION EXCHANGE
RESINS

METHODS OF SYNTHESIS

ION EXCHANGE MECHANISMS
In Vitro
In the Body

GENERAL CHARACTERISTICS OF CATION EXCHANGE RESINS

A CATION exchanger is a high molecular weight polymer containing an ion grouping such as phenolic, sulfonic, carboxylic, or phosphonic. In general, the polymeric portion of the molecule is so highly cross-linked as to confer insolubility. While this is of great significance in the application of exchangers to engineering problems, insolubility is unimportant from the standpoint of medical usage. Here the requirement would be for molecular units of such magnitude as to preclude absorption from the gastrointestinal tract while allowing some measure of solubility to improve the acceptability of the medication. Clearly, the patient will accept a liquid resin much more readily than the comparatively gritty, unpleasant solid forms which must be suspended in order to be consumed. The number of cross-linkages therefore becomes of paramount importance, and as this can be modified within the broadest range, it is apparent that an entire series of insoluble and soluble cation exchangers will be available for experimental investigation and ultimate medical application.

The significance of the ionic groupings present will depend entirely upon the strength of the acid concerned. This will be considered in the section devoted to the kinetics of these molecules. Inasmuch as the resin form, whether soluble or not, will be nonabsorbable, it is clear that factors of toxicity cannot enter except in the sense of removal of es-

31

sential food elements. Any acid grouping such as arsenic could be used
with impunity. It is interesting to speculate upon the possible use of a
resin containing ion-active arsenical groupings. One might reasonably
anticipate the use of such material as an intestinal antiseptic.

Stability of the resin, a major consideration in the design of such
materials for engineering purposes, is of little significance relative to
possible medical applications. The resins for medical use need remain
stable under physiological conditions for periods of only 24 to 48 hours.
Fundamentally, the stability of these polymers is such that no problems
of storage are encountered.

The cross-linkages are determinant in the degree of swelling which
will occur when the resin is wet; thus if there is one cross-linkage for
every 100 atoms in the chain the resin will swell tenfold (Nachod,
1949). From the physiological standpoint, the laxative or bulking
effect of a given resin would in some measure be a function of the
number of cross-linkages. The implication apparent in the statement
on swelling characteristics is that certain members of the resin group
with comparatively few cross-linkages would make excellent laxatives.
Certainly no currently used laxative possesses the power to increase
its bulk by a factor of ten. It is to be expected therefore that resins
will appear in the category of laxatives in the near future.

In general, resins used in medicine are of two types; those with
carbon-to-carbon linkages and those with carbon-to-nitrogen linkages:

$$\left[\begin{array}{ll} -C-C-C-C- & \text{(straight hydrocarbon type)} \\ -C-N-C-N- & \text{(amine linkages)} \end{array} \right]$$

Restriction of development in the field of engineering application of
resins led to these types, as stability was a major feature, but in physiological systems it is extremely probable that other linkage types may be
employed. This indicates the magnitude of the problem still confront-
ing investigators in the field. There are doubtless hundreds of resin
forms which should be investigated in this connection.

The most fundamental generalization which can be made in regard
to ion exchange resins is that the ionic character of the reactive grouping is the same in the resin as it is in the simple organic compound.
Two general classes of cation-reactive groupings have been applied in
medicine, the carboxylic and the sulfonic. The carboxylic type cor-
responds to a weak acid and the sulfonic type to a much stronger
acid. As this is true of the resin forms, so it is true of simple organic

compounds. Benzene sulfonic acid is much stronger than benzoic; phenol sulfonic acid is stronger than salicylic.

In constructing an exchanger, it appears that the best idea is to put in as many ion-active groups as possible. For engineering purposes, there must be a balance between the cross-linkages and the number of ion-active groups. The balance is a factor in the swelling characteristic. Again, the physiological application of such materials may well indicate more ion-reactive groups and fewer cross-linkages. In favor of this is the fact that pore size will be reduced if there are more cross-linkages. This tightening up of the entire structure would decrease the diffusion rate of ions through the resin particle, slowing up ion exchange. Reduction of particle size would compensate in some measure for decreased pore size, but the ideal situation would be small particles and large pores, providing optimum exchange potential.

METHODS OF SYNTHESIS

With the foregoing factors under consideration, the synthesis of the cation exchange resin follows general principles. One procedure involves the incorporation of the ionic groups into the resin structure as the resin polymerizes. The ionic groups are part and parcel of the monomeric unit. The second general procedure involves the formation of the polymer with subsequent introduction of ionic groups. A resin for application in the medical world is made by the first procedure, as the result is a truly homogeneous product.

As an example of the formation of a carboxylic type of cation exchanger, Figure 5 shows the reaction of an alkylacrylic acid monomer with formaldehyde and divinyl benzene to form a resin the structure of which is actually three-dimensional. Divinyl benzene is the cross-linking agent, forming the resin by coupling linear polymers into the macromolecular complex. With more formaldehyde the condensation continues to form a chain, and finally cross-linkage occurs and the ion exchange resin is created.

The details of a specific resin formation as given by Kunin and Myers (1950) refer to a German sulfonic cation exchanger, Wofatit K. In the formation of this resin, benzaldehyde-2,4-disulfonic acid is added to a mixture of water and resorcinol. The solution is heated, cooled and rendered alkaline, and formaldehyde is added. The mixture is stirred and heated until the gel stage is reached. Finally, the resin as formed is crushed, washed, dried and regenerated.

In the case of the carboxylic types, the details are essentially the same except that the initial material is 1,3,5-resorcylic acid and this is reacted with formaldehyde.

Selectivity in ion exchange is the ultimate goal. The probabilities of achievement are excellent. As an example of this, Skogseid (1946)

FIGURE 5

Formation of Carboxylic Cation Exchange Resin

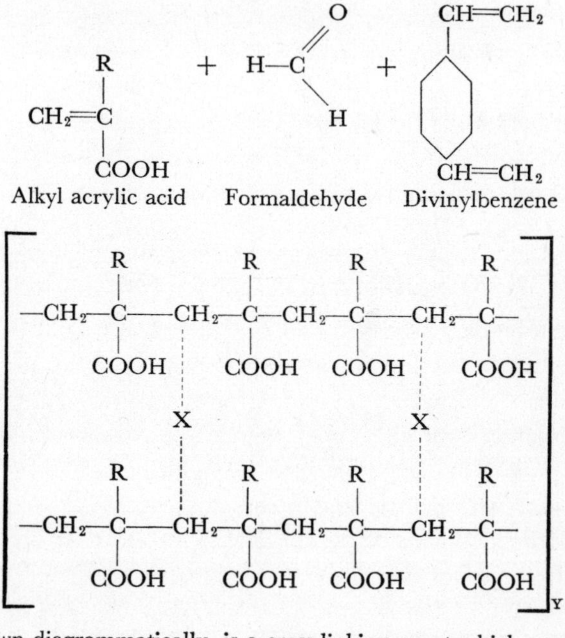

Alkyl acrylic acid   Formaldehyde   Divinylbenzene

X, as shown diagrammatically, is a cross-linking agent which may be divinylbenzene, trivinylbenzene, etc. By cross-linking, or tying the linear polymers together, a three-dimensional polymer is obtained. This increases chemical stability, and, more important, decreases markedly the water sensitivity of the resin.

prepared a resin based upon nitrated and reduced polystyrene. The structure given by Kunin and Myers (1950) for this resin is:

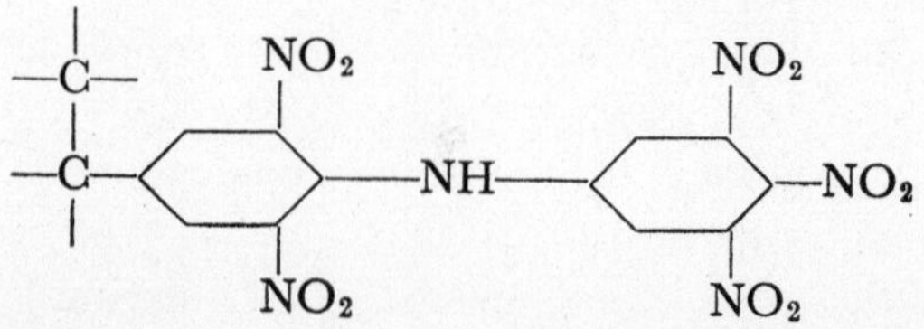

The remarkable attribute of the resin is its specificity for potassium. As indicated by Kunin and Myers, this selectivity is related to the separation of potassium from sodium by the precipitation of the insoluble hexanitrodiphenylaminate:

$$O_2N-\underset{NO_2}{\overset{NO_2}{\bigcirc}}-\underset{N}{\overset{K}{N}}-\underset{NO_2}{\overset{NO_2}{\bigcirc}}-NO_2$$

The demand for a resin specific for potassium is great in the field of lower nephron nephritis, a condition in which potassium is specifically contraindicated. The foregoing example illustrates the future potential for developments in this field.

ION EXCHANGE MECHANISMS

Work on ion distribution between exchangers and solution is usually carried out by adding an exchanger saturated with cation A to a solution containing cation B, shaking, filtering out the resin, and then determining by analysis the distribution of cation. The time required for the system to reach a state of equilibrium varies greatly, in fact from minutes to months. Exchange occurs within the pores of the gel-like structure of the exchanger, which fact introduces the possibility of an error, inasmuch as a certain amount of the cation in solution will remain within the pore system and give values indicating greater exchange than actually occurred. This situation holds for the synthetic aluminum silicates, the synthetic resins and the sulfuric-treated coals. The naturally occurring exchangers such as clays have a large external surface, and exchange is mainly a surface phenomenon.

The phenomenon of hysteresis also occurs. Here the exchanger saturated with cation A will not form a true equilibrium with the cation B in solution. The exchanger will retain more of the cation A than it would if a true equilibrium were reached. The generalization may be made that the characteristics of a cation exchange material will in some measure be determined by the cation fixed on the exchanger (Renold, 1935; Walton, 1943). For one thing, the gel structure will be modified in accordance with the fixed cation (Walton, 1943). The significance of this in biological systems is that one cannot assume that an exchanger in the sodium cycle will obey physical laws precisely as it will in the calcium cycle.

In general, ion exchange with cation exchangers proceeds by equivalents; i.e., one gram equivalent weight of a cation replaces or is exchanged for one gram equivalent weight of another cation. The term gram equivalent weight is defined as that weight expressed in grams determined by dividing the atomic weight by the valence of the unit under consideration. As an example, calcium has a valence of two and an atomic weight of 40.08, giving an equivalent weight of 20.04.

In Vitro

There are many mathematical formulations covering ion exchange, and in general these equations are of value in any consideration of the biological applications of exchangers. The exchange mechanism roughly follows the Freundlich adsorption isotherm. Walton (1949) proposes as most useful the equation of Rothmund and Kornfeld (1918, 1919):

$$\frac{m_{AX}}{m_{BX}} = K \left[\frac{(A^+)}{(B^+)} \right]^p$$

In this equation, m_{AX} and m_{BX} represent moles of cations A and B fixed on a gram of the resin, and (A^+) and (B^+) molar concentrations of these cations in the solution. K and p are constants which vary with the ions under consideration. As this equation would hold only for cations of the same valence, it is modified to cover ions of different valence, as follows:

$$\frac{m_{CaX}}{m^2_{NaX}} = K \left[\frac{Ca^{++}}{(Na^+)^2} \right]^p$$

Here the symbols have the same significance, and the equation is applied specifically to an exchange system involving sodium and calcium ions. As Walton (1949) indicates, the value of these equations lies in the fact that almost all exchange distribution data can be expressed as straight-line graphs by plotting $\log (m_{AX}/m_{BX})$ against $\log ([A^+]/[B^+])$.

With the resinous exchangers, practically all of the exchange occurs within the pores of the gel-like structure. It is consequently possible to consider the exchange as a partition of ions between the two phases, solid and liquid; between the gel and the solution. Under these conditions, the law of mass action can be applied and the exchange reaction written as:

$$A^+ + BX \rightleftarrows AX + B^+$$

In terms of ionic activities, the mathematical expression of the exchange becomes:

$$\frac{a_{AX} \cdot a_{B^+}}{a_{BX} \cdot a_{A^+}} = K$$

The term ionic activity refers to the apparent fraction of the material ionized. Ordinarily, it is less than actual concentration. The activity or capacity of an ion to function in exchange is not strictly a function of its concentration but rather of that fraction of its concentration which is "active." If one assumes that activities are directly proportional to equivalent concentrations, the above equation becomes:

$$\frac{m_{AX}}{m_{BX}} = K \frac{[A^+]}{[B^+]}$$

Because of the complexity of biological systems, applications of mathematical equations are extremely difficult. With the cation ex-

TABLE 2
Ionic Composition of Gastric Juice

Ions	Mg. %	MEq./l.
Potassium	40	10
Sodium	115	50
Calcium	4.1–8.6	2.0–4.3
Magnesium	2.2–9.4	1.8–7.8
Chloride	500	141
Sulfate	Trace	—
Phosphate	1.1–4.2	0.34–1.3
Bicarbonate	0–130	0–21
Titratable acidity or alkalinity	—	123.3

changers, exchange would occur in the stomach, in the small intestine and in the large intestine. For review purposes, the ionic composition of gastric juice is given in Table 2.

In the Body

Exchange in the stomach will occur only with the strong-base sulfonic types of cation exchangers, but both strong- and weak-base exchangers will undergo exchange reactions in the small intestine. Table 3 gives the ionic composition of intestinal juices.

From these tables it is apparent that exchange phenomena in biological systems are extremely complex. Therefore the value of consideration of mathematical equations governing ion exchange lies in orientation rather than in the immediate prospect of application to the system under study. The ionic activity of a given ion species will be modified by the other cations and anions present, whether organic or inorganic. Furthermore, pH factors will often whirl the entire structure into a cloud of confusion; nevertheless, a beginning must be made, an avenue of attack must be opened. No study can be regarded as complete until it has been subjected to detailed mathematical analysis.

TABLE 3
Ionic Composition of Content of Small Intestine

Ion	*MEq./l.*
Potassium	4–5
Sodium	140
Calcium	2.5–6.4
Magnesium	1–2
Chloride	74–103
Sulfate	Trace
Phosphate	2.61–7.66
Bicarbonate	2–32
Titratable acidity or alkalinity	158.2

From a consideration of gastric and intestinal juice composition, it is apparent that the exchanging powers of different cations, particularly when those cations are simple metallic ions, are of paramount importance in predicting the effect of an exchanger. The exchanging power of various cations, when those cations are simple metallic cations, is constant for different exchangers. The higher the valence of the cation, the more strongly it is bound; thus divalent cations are bound more strongly than the univalent. In each valence series, the strength of binding increases as the atomic weight increases. For the alkali and the alkaline earth cations, the replacing powers are in the following order:

$$Li^+ < Na^+ < K^+ < Rb^+ < Cs^+$$
$$Mg^{++} < Ca^{++} < Sr^{++} < Ba^{++}$$

The fundamental aspect of ion affinities lies in degree of hydration;

the more hydrated the ion, the less strongly it is bound. Expressed in another manner, as the radius of the hydrated ion decreases, the more strongly it will be absorbed. The implication contained in these experimental findings is that the affinity of the exchanger for members of a given valence series remains the same but is in effect modified by the hydrated state of the ion in solution. As the concentration of alcohol is increased in an essentially aqueous system, the variation in ionic hydrations decreases and so do the differences in affinity of an exchanger for the ions under study (Wiegner, 1931).

Considering the potential application of soluble cation exchangers, polymeric units with few cross-linkages, it is of great interest to note the work of Samuelson (1944), who found that a resin which swells greatly in solution permits entrance into its pores of cations of all hydration degrees, and that with such resins cation affinities in a given valence series vanish. Walton (1949) concludes that differences in exchanging power will be greater with exchangers which are rigid and dense, such as the aluminosilicates, and of lesser degree in the more elastic, less dense type of exchanger such as the synthetic resin. This might well be interpreted to indicate that resins with a lower degree of cross-linkage will in fact possess a generally uniform affinity for cations in a given valence series. If this is true, the known greater affinity of cation exchangers *in vivo* for potassium in contrast to sodium would be eliminated, and another reason supporting the value of soluble cation exchangers in medical work would be forthcoming.

There are three special types of cations the involvement of which in biological systems is certain: the complex cation, the organic cation and the hydrogen ion. The first of these, the complex cation, is of importance because many elements such as copper, cobalt and nickel form such complexes and as a result are trapped in units the radii of which prevent their entrance into the pores of other than loose-mesh exchangers. The organic cations fit into this same picture, the correlation of pore size of the exchanger and radius of the cation determining whether or not exchange will take place. The point of prime consideration in the biological system would be in the intestine, where (assuming cation formation) many nutrient materials might be removed if exchange occurred.

The hydrogen ion presents a special case, as many cation exchangers which hold ions by electrostatic force combine with hydrogen ions to form a covalent molecule. The two types of cation exchangers of the resin group currently employed in medical practice represent respectively a weak acid, the carboxylic type, and a strong acid, the sulfonic type. The position of hydrogen in an exchange series will determine whether or not a resin given in a cycle other than the hydrogen will exchange in the stomach. Further, it will determine whether or not the hydrogen cycle form of the resin will exchange. In the case of the strong-acid sulfonic type of resin, the hydrogen ion falls between lithium and sodium (Boyd *et al.*, 1947*a, b*). The interpretation of this fact in terms of the biological system is that the sulfonic type of resin will exchange hydrogen ions for either univalent or multivalent metallic cations in the stomach at a pH of 1.5. As some cation absorption occurs in the stomach, the probability of excessive depletion with the sulfonic type of cation exchanger is greater than with a weak-acid exchanger of the carboxylic type. In this case, the affinity of hydrogen ion for the carboxylic radical is of such magnitude as to preclude its displacement. Further, if the carboxylic type of resin is fed in the potassium or other metallic cation cycle, the metallic cation will be replaced by the hydrogen of the gastric juice and the resin will be converted almost 100 per cent into the hydrogen cycle form. The weak-base carboxylic type of cation exchange resin more nearly parallels the behavior of the synthetic aluminum silicate, where the hydrogen ion is held with a strength approximately equal to that of barium (Jenny, 1927).

Expressed in another manner, the effect of pH on exchange involving the strong-acid sulfonic types will be slight; the effect of pH on exchange systems involving a weak-acid carboxylic type of cation exchanger will be great.

Generally, temperature has little effect on ion exchange reactions. In biological systems, this factor would be constant in any event. A similar situation holds for the anionic composition of the medium under study, in that little or no effect is exerted.

Walton (1949) points out that the process of cation exchange represents a change in the environment of the ion but does not cause any modification in its electric charge. One ion passes into and another out of the negatively charged matrix of the exchanger.

Another approach to understanding of the action of exchangers is offered by Bauman (1949) through the application of the Donnan equilibrium concept, which applies to any system in which one of the ions is constrained in its movements. In biological systems, the restriction of movement usually involves a particle which will not pass through a semipermeable membrane. In the case of the resin, the ion unit attached to the resin, the anionic fraction, cannot pass from the resin phase to the solution phase, and the Donnan theory becomes applicable. The close parallel of the membrane system and the resin system is shown in Figure 6. In both systems, the chloride ion concentration will be greater in the phase not containing the fixed anion. In the resin system, the chloride ion concentration will be greater in the solution phase and less in the resin phase. In the membrane system, the chloride ion concentration will be less on the side containing the protein. In both systems, the cation concentration represented by $Na^+ + H^+$ is higher on the side containing the fixed anion. In the case

FIGURE 6
Donnan Concept Involving Membrane and Resin

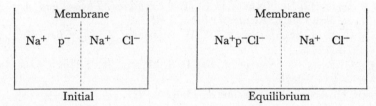

System initially sodium proteinate on one side of membrane with sodium chloride on the other. The protein anion will not diffuse.

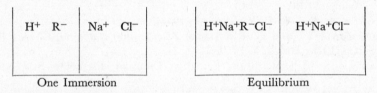

System on immersion is hydrogen cycle resin put into a sodium chloride solution. Essentially parallels situation in intestinal tract.

of the resin, the cationic concentration in the resin phase will be higher than in the solution.

The exchange rate of cationic materials is controlled by two factors: the surface exchange speed and the ionic diffusion rate. The determinant in biological systems is dual. The degree of significance of the surface exchange speed is a function of the particle size; the smaller the particle size, the greater the surface area exposed and the more significant the factor of surface exchange rate. With fine-mesh resins, this is the dominant factor until the critical limiting concentration of external phase is reached (0.1 N) (Boyd *et al.*, 1947*b*). At this point ionic diffusion is the rate-controlling factor.

Diffusional driving force will also come into consideration. The stronger the acid, the higher will be the diffusional driving force; thus a resin containing sulfonic acid radicals when treated with sodium hydroxide will be neutralized almost instantaneously. With a carboxylic type of resin, there will be a lag phase of some 2 to 4 hours. The rate is determined by hydrogen ion concentrations within the particle, and in the case of a weak acid this is very small. With the stronger acid, the hydrogen ion concentration is very high and the diffusion driving force is high.

REFERENCES

BAUMAN, W. C. In Nachod, F. C., *Ion Exchange, Theory and Application*. New York: Academic Press, 1949.

BOYD, G. E., J. SCHUBERT, and A. W. ADAMSON. *J. Am. Chem. Soc.*, 69: 2818, 1947a.

BOYD, G. E., A. W. ADAMSON, and L. S. MYERS, JR. *J. Am. Chem. Soc.*, 69: 2836, 1947b.

JENNY, H. *Kolloidchem. Beihefte*, 23: 428, 1927.

KUNIN, R., and R. J. MYERS. *Ion Exchange Resins*. New York: Wiley, 1950.

NACHOD, F. C. *Ion Exchange, Theory and Application*. New York: Academic Press, 1949.

RENOLD, A. *Kolloid-Beihefte*, 43: 1, 1935.

ROTHMUND, V., and G. KORNFELD. *Ztschr. anorg. allgem. Chem.*, 103: 129, 1918; 108: 215, 1919.

SAMUELSON, O. Dissertation, Kungliga Tekniska Högskolan, Stockholm, 1944.

SKOGSEID, A. Dissertation, Norges Tekniske Högskole, Trondheim, 1946.

WALTON, H. F. *J. Phys. Chem.*, 47: 371, 1943.

WALTON, H. F. In Nachod, F. C., *Ion Exchange, Theory and Application*. New York: Academic Press, 1949.

WIEGNER, G. *J. Soc. Chem. Ind.*, 50: 65 T, 1931.

CHAPTER 4

Biochemical Applications
of Ion Exchange Materials
Restricted to Those Underlying
the Medical Applications

VITAMINS

AMINO ACIDS

INORGANIC IONS

NUCLEIC ACIDS AND RELATED COMPOUNDS

CARBOHYDRATES

BLOOD COAGULATION

MACROMOLECULES

VIRUSES AND BACTERIA

ANTIBIOTICS

PHARMACEUTICALS

GENERAL COMMENT

REMARKABLE advances in resin chemistry are to be anticipated, and with these advances the selectivity of resins will be increased. It is therefore important to consider the biochemical applications of ion exchange materials, since these will be related to medical usage in the future. As the removal of cationic impurities by resinous exchangers was correlated with relevance to sodium removal in the patient with cardiac edema, so a now current biochemical application will form the basis for tomorrow's medical usage.

The obvious correlative of this line of thinking is that, in the light of our present knowledge of biochemical usage, certain undesirable effects of exchange resins may be related to metabolite removal. The application of cation exchangers for sodium removal automatically carried with it the well-known capacity of these agents to remove potassium. The procedure for the correction of this situation by the replacement of potassium will be applied in the future, with necessary resin cycles administered to prevent the precipitation of deficiency states.

Approaching present and future medical use of resins from the standpoint of present biochemical knowledge, we are led immediately to the necessity of considering soluble and insoluble exchange materials, as well as the ion exchange characteristics of chelators whether soluble or insoluble. Oral administration of resinous exchangers for modification of gastrointestinal tract biochemistry will doubtless have its corollary in the parenteral use of soluble ion exchange chemicals.

VITAMINS

In the early periods of research on the vitamin B complex, isolation procedures by precipitation, filtration, washing, and similar methods were soon replaced by adsorption on fuller's earth (Windaus *et al.*, 1932). With the development of knowledge in this field, it became known that the adsorption of B complex factors on the naturally occurring silicates was at least partially due to base exchange phenomena. These earlier observations led naturally to the application of cation exchange resins for this purpose. Herr (1945), utilizing the principles of chromatographic adsorption and base exchange, separated thiamin from riboflavin. The latter molecule cannot act as a cation and therefore is separable from the thiamin. For practical purposes the technic was found wanting, as high concentrations of mineral acids (30 to 37 per cent) were required for removal of the vitamin (thiamin) from the resin.

Any vitamin forming a cationic unit will be removed from a solution of proper pH by a cation exchanger, and similarly any vitamin forming an anion will under proper conditions be removed by an anion exchanger. Pyridoxine would be removed by a cation exchanger, and ascorbic acid would be removed by an anion exchanger. Further, a vitamin such as B_{12} is removed by virtue of its molecular magnitude rather than through its ionic form (Pfiffner *et al.*, 1946).

The probability of removal of vitamin nutrients by adsorption and ion exchange materials is very real, as demonstrated by Messerli (1922), who found that rats and pigeons fed a diet of decorticated rice developed an avitaminosis more rapidly and more severely if either charcoal or kakolin was added to the diet. Melnick *et al.* (1945) extended such studies to the human being and found that while fuller's earth did reduce markedly the availability of thiamin, kaolin did not interfere with the utilization of this factor. These investigators emphasized the fact that continuous use of large doses of adsorbing agents should not be assumed to be free of the danger associated with insufficient vitamin intake, unless tests have been conducted.

Resinous ion exchangers possess characteristics which would lead one to suspect that they might interfere with the absorption of vitamins from the gastrointestinal tract. In laboratory tests with animals and in extensive clinical trials over periods of years, there has been no evidence of any alteration of vitamin nutrition by the exchangers (see Chapters 5, 6, and 7). In the case of the anion exchangers, the sequence of acid-pH gastric content followed by alkaline or neutral intestinal juices completely reverses any exchange which occurs with liberation of any adsorbed vitamins. Explanation of the failure of cation exchangers to remove nutrients is not immediately apparent; factors of concentration and the complexity of intestinal content probably are involved. In any event, the potential interference with vitamin nutrition by the resinous exchangers has been proved to be, in fact, nonexistent. This situation obtains for other materials such as kaolin and natural and synthetic sodium aluminum silicates. While the currently employed exchange and adsorption agents do not modify vitamin nutrition, the warning of Melnick *et al.* (1945) should be held in mind and actual proof obtained before any new materials are applied clinically over prolonged periods.

AMINO ACIDS

Possible interference with amino acid nutrition by adsorption and exchange materials could take two lines. The first of these would involve inhibition of the action of proteolytic enzymes and the second would involve prevention of absorption of certain amino acids. There are, in general, three types of amino acids; basic amino acids, including arginine, histidine, lysine and possibly tryptophane; dicarboxylic amino acids, such as glutamic and aspartic acids; and finally the neutral amino acids, such as glycine, alanine, and valine. The characteristics of acidity or basicity would determine possible reaction with anionic and cationic resinous material, but other features might be involved in straight adsorption reactions. The aromatic amino acids, tyrosine, tryptophane and phenylalanine, are to be regarded as a class in the consideration of adsorption phenomena relative to the amino acids.

The basic amino acids can be removed from protein hydrolysates and similar preparations by a variety of materials. Whitehorn (1923) found that arginine, lysine and some histidine could be brought out on Permutit, a sodium cycle synthetic zeolite (sodium aluminum silicate). Decalso (Nelson *et al.*, 1946) and silica gel (Schramm and Primosigh, 1944) possess similar power. In addition to the inorganic zeolites, Lloyd's reagent, classified as a bleaching earth, functions effectively in basic amino acid adsorption (Ackermann and Fuchs, 1936). Still another general class of materials for basic amino acid isolation is the metallic oxides. For example, Wieland (1942) used aluminum oxide for the removal of basic amino acids from neutral solutions.

Cation exchange resins were first applied in the isolation of the basic amino acids by Block (1942, 1945) and Freudenberg *et al.* (1942). From their observations, these investigators developed a technic for fractionation of amino acids into three groups: the acidic amino acids, held by the anion exchange resins; the basic amino acids, held by the cation exchange resins; and the neutral amino acids, which should not be held by either type of exchanger. Not only anion exchange resins but also aluminum oxide and similar materials will remove the acid amino acids.

Thus it is clear that exchangers and adsorption agents will remove both basic and acidic amino acids from solutions. In addition, as a complicating factor for consideration in the application of such materials in the medical world, it is known that the aromatic amino acids can be removed by activated charcoal and that certain cation exchange resins may have a specificity for a single amino acid such as tryptophane (Turba *et al.*, 1943).

Despite the fact that exchangers and adsorption agents can remove single amino acids or groups of amino acids from solutions, there is no existing evidence that any of these materials interfere in any manner with the absorption of amino acids from the gastrointestinal tract. The evidence both laboratory and clinical has established that no deficiencies occur following the use of either anion, cation, or combinations of such resins for prolonged periods. Again, as is the case with the vitamins, it follows that any dicarboxylic acid removed by anion exchangers in the acid medium of the stomach will be released again in the neutral or alkaline pH of the intestine. Perhaps the complexity of intestinal content prevents removal of other amino acids by cation exchangers. In any event, testing both clinical and laboratory was essential before these or any other such materials could be safely used.

INORGANIC IONS

The removal of cations by cation exchange resins is considered in detail in Chapter 6. In summary, such resins will remove cations in a largely nonselective manner. Relative specificities of currently available cation exchange resins are not of sufficient degree to consider any resin as specific. For practical purposes, the aspects of selectivity are achieved by restoring those cations not designated for removal. In each instance of application, laboratory and clinical studies must be performed to determine the spectrum of ions or the single ion which must be added to the diet to correct for losses via the resin. Generally, in the adult, potassium is the only cation which must be restored. In the infant or growing child, both potassium and calcium represent essential supplements to the regimen. Calcium requirements of the growing organism render delicate the balance of this element.

The removal of anions by anion exchange resins is considered in Chapter 5. In summary, pH factors cause a reversal of the absorption of anions by the resins. The acid pH of the stomach permits the absorption and the neutral or basic pH of the intestine reverses the process. It is firmly established that monovalent anions such as chloride are not removed from the body by the resins. Whether or not polyvalent anions such as phosphate are removed remains a debated issue. McChesney (1952) has reported the removal of 0.3 to 0.6 mEq. of phosphate per gram of resin administered. While this is a comparatively minor amount of phosphate in terms of total intake, the point has academic interest. The phosphate content of the diet would determine the concentration of this anion in the intestinal juices. Degree of removal by a resin would in turn be directly proportional to concentration in the tract. In other words, a high phosphate content diet would lead in animal experiments to a situation in which the resin might remove many times more phosphate than it would under clinical conditions. Clearly, the diet of the patient would determine the comparative adsorptive characteristics of the resin as applied. More work will have to be carried out using diets of varying phosphate content before positive statements can be made relative to phosphate removal by anion exchange resins. To mention but one other complicating factor in such experiments, the anionic spectrum—the concentrations of other polyvalent and monovalent anions—would be a major determinant in the experimental findings.

NUCLEIC ACIDS AND RELATED COMPOUNDS

Adenosine triphosphate (ATP), one of the highest phosphate potential compounds known, is prepared by a simplified procedure involving ion exchange (Polis and Meyerhof, 1947). The ATP is obtained as the sodium salt, free of contaminating heavy-metal traces, by exchange between a sodium cycle cation exchange resin and the ATP solution containing heavy-metal cations. Beiler and Martin (1952) have used resin exchangers in the direct isolation of adenosine triphosphate from complex and relatively crude extracts.

Smith and Wender (1948) have described a method for the separation of small amounts of xanthine and guanine involving the absorption of xanthine and guanine at acid pH and the subsequent removal of the xanthine by elution. Their work does not demonstrate the effect of the cation exchanger used on purines and pyrimidines in complex mixtures, but it does indicate that absorption can occur.

Cohn and his associates (1950a, b, 1951) have published extensively on the application of ion exchange materials to the separation and preparation of yeast nucleic acid derivatives. The technic consists of hydrolysis of ribonucleic acid, removal of sulfuric acid and the major portion of the guanine plus inorganic phosphate by neutralization with barium hydroxide, separation of the adenine, guanine, and the two pyrimidine nucleotides by acid elution from a strong-base anion exchanger, and finally crystallization or precipitation of each pyrimidine nucleotide from the portion of the column effluent in which it occurs. This ion exchange procedure for the preparation of uridylic and cytidylic acids does not result in a more highly purified product but is much more practical.

In general, the technic of Cohn may be applied to the separation of desoxyribonucleotides as well as to the ribonucleotides (Hurst *et al.*, 1951; Sinsheimer and Koerner, 1951; Volkin *et al.*, 1951).

The intestinal juices contain nucleases, nucleotides and nucleosidases. From their activity, nucleic acids are broken down into nucleotides, nucleosides and finally into purines, pyrimidines and sugars. The potentiality exists that certain strong-base anion exchange resins and some strong-acid cation exchange resins may alter the absorption of nucleic acid derivatives from the gastrointestinal tract. If this should occur, it is improbable that detrimental effects would ensue, as the body has the potential for the synthesis of purines and pyrimidines and is therefore not dependent upon exogenous sources. This point is, however, not entirely settled, and clinical situations may exist in which intestinal adsorbents would interfere with nucleic acid anabolism.

CARBOHYDRATES

The application of resinous exchangers for the purification of sugars is primarily for demineralization. The generalization can be made that sugar molecules are not absorbed by exchangers, as they are nonionic. Molecular units of the type of glucose-1-phosphate do not follow this rule. The molecule is a strong acid with a high exchange capacity, and it can be removed by acid-binding resins (McCready and Hassid, 1944). The glucose-1-phosphate is subsequently eluted with a weak alkali and isolated as the crystalline dipotassium salt. This is a most important biochemical; its relative ease of preparation, using exchange resins, has made possible much research otherwise necessarily deferred because of scarcity of the chemical.

This example of exchange involving a carbohydrate derivative is given to indicate the potentialities of modification of the milieu of the intestinal tract by ion exchange resins which could alter bacterial metabolism, change phosphorylation reactions, or prevent absorption of such phosphorylated molecules. With the resins at present employed in medical practice, there is no evidence of any modification of carbohydrate metabolism or of carbohydrate absorption, but with the development of new resin types the potentialities for selective interference in any specific metabolic pattern will increase.

BLOOD COAGULATION

Steinberg (1944) first proposed the use of a cation exchanger in the sodium cycle for the removal of calcium from the blood to prevent its coagulation. The calcium removal was accomplished either by passing the blood over a column of the resin or by simply mixing the resin with the blood sample. Detailed analysis indicated that the resin-treated blood did not differ significantly from oxalated blood.

TABLE 4
Influence of Oxalate or Resin Treatment upon Properties of Blood

(From Steinberg, A., *Proc. Soc. Exper. Biol. Med.*, **56**: 124, 1944)

Determination	Specimen	Resin-treated	Direct* or oxalate
RBC (million/cu. mm.)	1	4.85	4.78
	2	4.76	4.60
	3	3.73	3.52
	4	4.09	4.05
	5	5.21	5.00
Hemoglobin (Gm./100 cc.)	1	14.8	14.5
	2	13.5	13.2
	3	12.5	11.6
	4	14.5	14.2
	5	14.0	13.5
Sediment rate (mm./hr.)	1	3.5	9.2
	2	8.0	13.5
	3	15.0	22.0
Hematocrit (%)	1	37.0	32.0
	2	33.0	28.5
WBC (per cu. mm.)	1	6,250	5,200
	2	7,400	6,700
	3	10,500	8,800
Platelet count (per cu. mm.)	1	310,000	260,000
	2	240,000	220,000
	3	375,000	320,000
	4	270,000	250,000
Prothrombin time (sec.)	1	16.8	21.2
	2	24.2	25.6
	3	13.6	15.4
	4	15.4	17.2

* Direct refers to finger puncture.

Using a purified form of the resin, Amberlite IR-100, Stefanini (1948) treated blood samples and found that such treatment decreased the sedimentation rate but otherwise did not seem to modify the morphological, chemical or physical properties of blood. Spe-

TABLE 5
Serological and Biochemical Studies of Resin- and Oxalate-treated Blood

(From Steinberg, A., *Proc. Soc. Exper. Biol. Med.*, **56**: 124, 1944)

Determination	Resin-treated	Oxalated*†
Sugar (mg. %)	111.2	114.0
Urea nitrogen (%)	14.3	13.8
Uric acid (%)	4.1	4.4
Total protein (Gm.)	7.31	7.25
A/G ratio	2.03	2.16
Albumin (Gm.)	4.90	4.75
Globulin (Gm.)	2.41	2.20
Fibrinogen	0.268	0.324
Nonprotein nitrogen (mg. %)	29.1	26.4
Inorganic phosphorus (mg. %)	2.6	2.2
Sugar (24 hrs.) (mg. %)	22.5	45.0
Specific gravity, whole blood	1.0623	1.0608
Specific gravity, plasma	1.0285	1.0278
Oxygen capacity (cc.)	22.73	21.99
Cephalin-cholesterol flocculation test	Negative	Negative
Creatinine (mg. %)	1.2	1.2
Cholesterol (mg. %)	182.0	194.0
Serology†		
Wassermann	Negative	Negative
Wassermann	++++	++++
Kahn	Negative	Negative
Kahn	++++	++++
Mazzini	Negative	Negative

* Average of five samples.
† Serum for serology.

cifically, there was no change in prothrombin, fibrinogen, or in the labile factor of Quick (1947). Recalcified samples of treated blood were found to clot in a shorter time than did native blood, but as indicated by Stefanini this is a characteristic of oxalated and citrated blood also.

It remained for Applezweig and Rice (1949) to determine the amount of calcium removed from blood by the resin treatment. They report some 80 per cent of the blood calcium as being removed; this would leave a residual calcium content adequate to promote coagulation, and as the sample did not coagulate it was assumed that the calcium remaining must be in a bound or nonionized form. Prior to the date of the work of Applezweig and Rice, Quick (1947) had employed resins to study the quantitative relationship between calcium and prothrombin. He reached the conclusion that the optimum or critical concentration of calcium for maximum prothrombin activity was less than the amount of free or ionized calcium. Recently this same group (Hussey *et al.,* 1950) made a study of the influence of heparin and sodium citrate on the absorption of calcium by Amberlite IR-100, sodium cycle. Heparin did not modify the decalcifying action of the ion exchanger. Citrate produced an effect which bore an inverse linear relationship from the standpoint of molarity of the sodium citrate to the amount of calcium removed from the preparations tested.

Anion exchange resins have no effect on the coagulability of blood; cation exchange resins under certain conditions prevent, via calcium withdrawal, the coagulation of blood. The inference might be contained in these facts that anion exchange resins could be freely used in any condition involving gastrointestinal pathology associated with hemorrhage. The literature proves this to be correct. But what of the use of the cation exchangers under such conditions? The chances are remote that any hemorrhagic situation would occur contraindicating the use of cation exchange resins; the amounts of resin present would have to be very great, and the degree of removal of calcium essential to the prevention of coagulation could hardly be achieved under the conditions of practical applications of these agents. In summary, therefore, the anion exchangers would not modify coagulation in any manner and could be used in the treatment of any state of gastrointestinal pathology where indicated, even in the presence of hemorrhage. In Chapter 5 we have reviewed a large number of cases of patients with hemorrhaging gastric ulcer who were treated with anion exchange resins with highly satisfactory results. There is no recorded instance of interference by a cation exchange resin with clotting of blood in intestinal areas. One case (see Chapter 6) has been reported in which the physician felt that the use of a sulfonic type of cation exchange resin was contraindicated due to ulcer recurrence. Even in this case, hemorrhage was not a factor.

MACROMOLECULES

The gonadotropic hormone of the anterior pituitary can be isolated from urine by shaking the urine with Permutit for several hours and then eluting with dilute ammonium hydroxide (Lejwa, 1932). A similar application of adsorption* and elution technics has been made by Katzman *et al.* (1943) for the preparation of gonadotropic hormone concentrates with potencies of 85,000 I.U. per milligram. Another interesting procedure involving exchangers is applied to the purification of the oxytocic hormone, separation from the pressor principles of posterior pituitary extract (Potts and Gallagher, 1944). Still another example of the application of the technic of ion exchange in the separation of macromolecules is that involving the separation of pectin methylesterase and pectin polygalacturonase from commercial pectinase (McColloch and Kertesz, 1945).

In the preceding instances macromolecular units are separated by direct exchange of absorption and elution. There is another basic application of exchangers which involves modification of ionic strength through the use of resinous exchangers. One of the most ingenious of such applications is that for the production of therapeutic fractions of human blood serum (Reid and Jones, 1949). The separation of blood serum protein fractions in significant quantities depends on the relative solubility of the proteins in different media. One mechanism of separation involves decreasing ionic strength of the solution by removal of salts or by dilution. Until Reid and Jones used exchangers, salt removal was carried out exclusively by means of dialysis. The exchangers were ideally suited to mechanisms of lowering ionic strength. Alpha, beta and gamma globulin fractions can be produced by progressive reduction of ionic strength. For example, alpha globulin predominates in solutions of ionic strength 0.001. The laboratory operation is simple and involves no special equipment; the blood sample is mixed with the cation exchanger and then with the anion exchanger until ionic strength has been reduced to the point at which a fraction separates. In general, this will occur in the sample after the resins have been removed; it is then only a problem of centri-

---

* Throughout the book, the attempt has been made to use the term adsorption only in reference to the physical surface phenomenon. On the other hand, the exchange occurring in resins is referred to as absorption. The ions cannot be said to be adsorbed; rather they are absorbed into the interstices, into the pores of the resin where the exchange reaction occurs.

fuging, obtaining the fraction, and subsequently proceeding to a more drastic reduction in ionic strength for removal of further fractions.

From these examples of the separation technics for macromolecular units, it is seen that exchange materials can directly absorb or so change the ionic milieu as to cause precipitation of the least soluble macromolecule involved. Exchangers might therefore be expected to alter the macromolecular composition of the fluids contained in the gastrointestinal tract by either one or both of these basic mechanisms. The fact that resinous ionic exchangers and similar material do in fact so modify gastrointestinal biochemistry was to have been anticipated. The manner in which these agents function against enzymes is considered in detail in Chapters 5 and 6. Generally, anion exchangers as well as cation exchangers, through absorption, inactivate proteolytic and perhaps other enzymes.

VIRUSES AND BACTERIA

The use of ion exchange resins in the purification of viruses has taken two lines. The first was employed by Muller (1950) and involved the removal of nitrogenous impurities from the neurotropic viruses. The impurities were taken out on a cation exchanger while the virus was contained in the effluent. Far more interesting from the standpoint of medical use of resins is the second approach, which involved the absorption of a virus directly onto an anion exchanger. LoGrippo (1950) used a strong-base anion exchange resin and with it was able to extract poliomyelitis virus from human feces and the Theiler virus from mouse feces. The removal of virus was almost quantitative. Approximately 20 per cent of resin (Amberlite XE-67) was required to remove the virus from human feces.

This work is of tremendous importance in the application of resinous exchangers and adsorbents to medical practice. Virus adsorption onto resin particles would render them noninfective and strongly suggests the use of such material as a prophylactic measure against any virus disease known to gain entrance into the human body through the gastrointestinal tract. The poliomyelitis virus is known to follow this path into the body. While it is true that the quantitative aspects of this approach would for the present seem difficult of practical attainment, the future will doubtless see the development of resins with ever increasing capacity and specificity. One might even speculate on the probability that reduction of the infecting virus dose through removal on resins might bring into balance the invasive forces and the defensive mechanisms of the body, permitting immediate victory for the host.

Gunnison and Marshall (1937) found an apparent adsorption *in vitro* of *Escherichia coli, Clostridium welchii* and *Lactobacillus acidophilus* by particulate kaolin, Lloyd's reagent, calcium carbonate, aluminum hydroxide and barium sulfate. Charcoal effectively removed *L. acidophilus* but did not significantly affect *Esch. coli* or *Cl. welchii.* The general impression given by these authors is that alterations in intestinal flora produced by the administration of inert particulate agents are not due to adsorption of bacterial cells.

Recently Martin *et al.* (1952) attempted to obtain quantitative results on bacterial adsorption by resins. The bacteria most commonly associated with gastrointestinal disturbances were used in an experimental design in which aliquot portions of 16- to 24-hour broth cultures of the organisms were shaken with the adsorbent for two hours at 37° C., filtered, measured turbidimetrically and compared with suitable controls. The results are presented in Table 6. The table indicates that sodium aluminum silicate was the most effective agent of those tested for the removal of bacteria. The anion exchange resin was only slightly effective at the highest concentrations employed.

While the therapeutic significance of the adsorption of bacteria by particulate therapeutic agents is debatable in view of the enormous numbers of bacteria in the gastrointestinal tract, the removal of bacterial toxins and the alteration of the flora of the gut by these agents is beyond question. Braafladt (1923) demonstrated the neutralizing effect that kaolin had on toxins and toxic products of pathogenic bacteria. His technic involved treating the cultures, centrifuging and then injecting the supernatant fluid into animals. Adsorption was offered as the explanation of the successful use of kaolin in Asiatic cholera, bacillary dysentery, acute enteritis, typhoid, meat poisoning and botulism. Kaolin combined with toxins and toxic products of *Vibrio cholerae, Bacillus dysenteriae* (Shiga), *B. enteritidis, B. diphtheriae, B. botulinus, B. typhosus,* and *B. paratyphosus B,* and seemed to combine with toxic products of putrefactive and proteolytic bacteria. Kaolin changed the composition of the bacterial flora of the gut from one predominantly proteolytic to one predominantly aciduric. Braafladt even used kaolin in gastrointestinal disturbance in tuberculous patients, with marked success. In 1950, Moss and Martin studied the adsorption of bacterial toxins by inert particulate materials. The results

TABLE 6
Adsorption of Bacterial Cells by Exchange Materials

Agent and conc. (mg./cc.)	Turbidity readings*				
	S. typhosa	S. schottmuelleri	S. dysenteriae	Esch. coli	Staph. aureus
Weak-base anion exchange resin					
1	144	234	124	290	107
5	141	220	144	290	106
10	141	172	171	278	89
25	112	179	137	266	55
Sodium aluminum silicate					
1	52	106	27	192	46
5	10	44	X	—	X
10	X	X	X	X	X
25	X	X	X	X	X
Anion exchange resin + sodium aluminum silicate					
1 (each)	68	93	81	188	13
5 (each)	30	47	34	90	X
10 (each)	X	—	—	44	X
25 (each)	X	X	X	X	X
Aluminum hydroxide					
1	—	118	108	252	78
5	—	86	82	108	56
10	—	X	41	110	61
25	—	X	X	89	26
Organism control reading	144	224	124	294	108

* X designates that the agent was probably effective in almost complete removal of organisms.

are given in detail in Chapter 7. The conclusions of this work indicated the necessity for the use of multiple adsorption agents, as no single material possessed optimal capacity in the various systems studied.

The effect produced by any given adsorption or exchange agent or by any combination thereof will be multiple but will follow three general mechanisms. First, there will be removal of bacterial cells. Second, the toxic chemicals elaborated by the bacteria will be adsorbed or absorbed. Third, the composition of the intestinal content will be modified, with resultant alteration in the nutrients available for bacterial growth. This will tend to alter the bacterial flora. It seems probable that the continued use of exchangers and adsorption agents will modify the intestinal flora, and that in general the shift will be from a proteolytic to an aciduric type.

ANTIBIOTICS

The major import of knowledge concerning the absorption or adsorption of antibiotics by resins and similar materials lies in the poten-

TABLE 7

The Adsorption of Commercial Penicillin on a Weak-Base
Anion Exchange Resin

Time in contact with the resin (min.)	pH of filtrate after exper.	Units of penicillin per ml. of filtrate	Units of penicillin adsorbed per Gm. of resin
1	3.48	850	230,000
5	3.27	340	332,000
10	2.98	250	350,000
20	2.84	300	340,000

tial dangers of concomitant use of these agents with antibiotics if adsorption actually occurs. In such eventuality the physician would be administering an antibiotic which would be adsorbed onto the resin and thus remain in the gastrointestinal tract, producing no systemic effect whatever. In some measure, such dangers do exist.

The exchange resins have become a part of the standard procedures involved in the isolation of various antibiotics. Cruz-Coke *et al.* (1945) applied both cation and anion exchange resins in the isolation of streptomycin. The Carter technic involved the use of alkaline alumina. Another antibiotic, streptothricin, is concentrated and purified through the use of cation exchangers both of the resinous and of the silicate types (Kocholaty and Junowicz-Kocholaty, 1947).

The results of experiments conducted by Martin and Sullivan (1949) are here presented in some detail, as they indicate the quantitative aspects of penicillin removal by anion exchange resins *in vitro*. The results shown in Table 7 were obtained from experiments in which 0.1 gm. of acid-washed anion exchange resin was stirred with 20 ml. of sodium penicillin (commercial mixture) solution containing 2,000 units per milliliter. The resin was removed by filtration and the

TABLE 8

The Adsorption of Penicillin-G on a Weak-Base Anion Exchange Resin

Time in contact with the resin (min.)	*pH of filtrate after exper.*	*Units of penicillin per ml. of filtrate*	*Units of penicillin absorbed per Gm. of resin*
1	3.35	522	296,000
5	3.16	400	320,000
10	3.16	310	338,000
20	3.02	320	336,000

filtrate analyzed. The results of a similar set of experiments with penicillin-G are given in Table 8.

From these results it seems that adsorption occurs to an appreciable extent and that apparent equilibrium is quickly and easily obtained. It is of particular interest to note that the anion exchanger did not adsorb penicillin at pH 7 to 8. Experiments of this type were carried out by washing the acid-treated resin with 0.5 M sodium bicarbonate solution in the usual way before proceeding.

It was of interest to determine the conditions under which the penicillin could be removed from the penicillin-resin combination. Table 9 gives the results, which indicate quite clearly that acid would not remove as much of the penicillin from the resin as would base. This is not surprising, in view of the previously noted fact that the resin will not adsorb penicillin at a pH of 7 to 8, whereas adsorption readily takes place from acid solution.

It is apparent from this and similar experiments that antibiotics may well be adsorbed, and that their absorption into the systemic circulation may be modified by resinous exchangers and related materials. The use of antacids with antibiotics has been common practice, as the broad-spectrum antibiotics are known to produce a high incidence of gastrointestinal upsets, including loss of appetite, nausea, vomiting and epigastric pain. In 1949, Schoenbach *et al.* reported the effectiveness of aluminum hydroxide gels in relieving aureomycin-induced nausea, and Di Gangi and Rogers found that the antibiotic was strongly adsorbed onto the antacid. Subsequently, the adsorption

TABLE 9

The Removal of Penicillin from 0.1 Gm. of a Resin Containing 397,000 Units of Penicillin per Gram after Stirring with 20 Ml. of the Indicated Solution

Solution used for penicillin removal	*Time of stirring (min.)*	*pH of filtrate after exper.*	*% of penicillin removed from resin*
0.01 M HCl	20	2.1	12.0
0.1 M NaHCO$_3$	60	8.7	41.0
0.1 M NaHCO$_3$	120	8.8	41.0
0.05 M Na$_2$CO$_3$	20	10.3	23.9
0.5 M Na$_2$CO$_3$	20	10.9	20.2

of aureomycin onto aluminum hydroxide gels has been amply confirmed (Bartholomew and Nichols, 1950; Rogers *et al.*, 1952; Seed and Wilson, 1950; Waisbren and Hueckel, 1950; Greenspan *et al.*, 1951; Williams and Weekes, 1951; Paul and Harrington, 1952).

Williams and Weekes (1951) determined blood levels of aureomycin in a series of patients given a combination of aluminum hydroxide, magnesium trisilicate and gastric mucin (Mucoitin) or an aluminum hydroxide preparation. With the mucin combination, there was no interference with the absorption of aureomycin, as contrasted with the marked reductions noted in the aluminum hydroxide gel series. This was a unique finding and suggested that the mucin must in some manner coat the aluminum hydroxide particles and modify their adsorptive characteristics. One would wonder if some modification in antacid capacity might not follow. If the administration of aureomycin was delayed for 30 minutes following the administration of alumina gel, there was no marked interference with absorption of the antibiotic. This marked difference between concomitant administration and 30-minute-interval dosage may be due to adsorption by the gel of the aureomycin in the acid content of the stomach when the two are given simultaneously. The reversal of such adsorption would not proceed

TABLE 10

Serum Aureomycin Levels 5 to 6 Hours after a Single Dose of Aureomycin in Gammas per Milliliter

(From Greenspan, R., *et al., Am. J. Dig. Dis.,* **18:** 35, 1951)

Subject No.	Control No. 1 (750 mg. aureomycin)	Control No. 2 (750 mg. aureomycin)	Amphojel (30 ml.) (750 mg. aureomycin)	Carmethose (30 ml.) (750 mg. aureomycin)
1	2.5	2.5	0.3125	2.5
2	4.0	4.0	0.01625	5.0
3	2.0	2.0	0.625	2.0
4	2.3	2.0	1.0	2.0
5	5.0	4.0	0.625	4.0
6	2.0	2.0	0.25	2.0
7	4.28	1.25	1.25	4.0

Subject No.	Control No. 1 (1000 mg. aureomycin)	Control No. 2 (1000 mg. aureomycin)	Amphojel (30 ml.) (1000 mg. aureomycin)	Carmethose (30 ml.) (1000 mg. aureomycin)
8	5.0	4.0	0.625	4.0
9	8.0	8.0	1.25	4.0*
10	4.0	2.5	0.0625	4.0

* Gastritis.

with any degree of speed and would result in a net loss of aureomycin. When the antacid is given before the antibiotic, the pH of the gastric content will be elevated (less acid), a condition apparently less favorable to adsorption.

Another antacid which does not interfere with the absorption of aureomycin is sodium carboxymethylcellulose (Carmethose) (Greenspan *et al.,* 1951). Actually Carmethose is a combination of sodium carboxymethylcellulose and magnesium oxide, and here once again the speed of action of one ingredient, namely the magnesium oxide, on the acid of the stomach may so modify pH conditions as to create a situation unfavorable to adsorption. The sodium carboxymethylcellulose antacid effectively controlled the side effects precipitated by the aureomycin. The authors concluded that "Carmethose is an ion exchange buffer, combining with hydrochloric acid in the stomach and then releasing it in the intestine." From this they imply that ion exchangers would not adsorb antibiotics. Table 10 and Figure 7 summarize the results reported in substantiation of these conclusions.

Terramycin hydrochloric acid as well as aureomycin hydrochloric acid strongly adsorbed on aluminum hydroxide gel, even to the extent

FIGURE 7
Effect of Antacids on Serum Aureomycin Levels
(From Greenspan, R., *et al.*, *Am. J. Dig. Dis.*, **18**: 35, 1951)

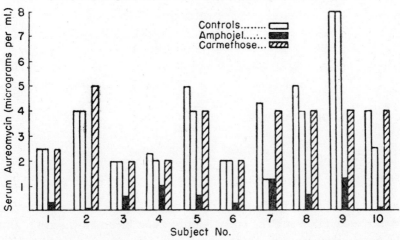

of 25 to 90 per cent (Paul and Harrington, 1952). Another antacid, dihydroxyaluminum aminoacetate, was also found to adsorb the antibiotics. Bismuth subsalicylate, however, did not inactivate either terramycin hydrochloric acid or aureomycin hydrochloric acid. While the studies were conducted *in vitro,* the probability is that similar findings would be noted *in vivo.*

Martin *et al.* (1952) studied antibiotic adsorption by cation exchangers *in vitro.* Aqueous solutions of penicillin-G were treated with various amounts of the carboxylic cation exchange resin by stirring at room temperature for varying time intervals. The filtrates from these mixtures were assayed for residual penicillin. At a maximum mixing time of 1 hour, 1 Gm. of the resin removed a little over 110,000 units of penicillin from a solution containing 500,000. Under similar conditions, the resin removed only traces of streptomycin, aureomycin or Chloromycetin. When a sulfonic type of cation exchange resin was used similar results were obtained. In the case of penicillin-G, however, some 90 per cent of the penicillin was removed, indicating a much more marked tendency for penicillin adsorption or absorption.

In vivo studies gave the results presented in Table 11. It is apparent that the penicillin was strongly bound to the resin and that the fluids of the gastrointestinal tract failed to elute the penicillin to any significant extent. Subsequently, attempts to remove the penicillin from the resin by chemical means (acids and bases) failed.

There can be little question but that each antibiotic must be studied in relation to every possible adsorption for exchange material with

TABLE 11
Absorption of Penicillin from a Penicillin–Sulfonic Cation Exchanger Combination

Sample	Units of penicillin per ml. of blood			
	1 hr.	2 hrs.	4 hrs.	6 hrs.
Penicillin–sulfonic type of resin combination	0–trace	0	0	0
Penicillin (plain)	1.2–1.83	0.8	0.3	0.3

which it is likely to be used. The high incidence of gastrointestinal disturbance following the oral administration of broad-spectrum antibiotics renders essential the application of procedures to control these unpleasant side effects. The adsorption and exchange agents offer the logical approach and will be used extensively for this purpose. It will be most unfortunate if through improper use with particulate exchange materials the antibiotics are retained in the gut when the physician believes he is getting a general systemic effect. Further study will clearly indicate the safe combinations and their use will improve antibiotic therapy, as patient acceptance and side effects are one and the same.

PHARMACEUTICALS

Whitehorn (1923) first reported that Permutit (a natural cation exchange material) removed adrenalin from solution. Subsequently he studied the adsorption of some 52 different organic compounds by this agent. All strong nitrogenous bases could be separated with relative ease from weaker bases and from nonbasic substances. The bases were removed more effectively from neutral solutions than from acid or alkali. Organic bases dissolved in organic solvents were also adsorbed. Whitehorn recommended a saturated aqueous solution of potassium chloride for the elution of the bases. Recoveries of 85 to 92 per cent were possible.

The original application of adsorption for the manufacture of alkaloids was made by Fink (1937), who employed a mixture of kaolin and asbestos for the isolation of the alkaloids of cinchona. In recent years the resinous exchangers have been employed for this purpose. Applezweig (1944) and Applezweig and Ronzone (1946) employed a sulfonic type of cation exchanger for the recovery of atropine, scopolamine, morphine, totaquine, quinine and similar compounds. Studies by Sussman *et al.* (1945) resulted in the use of exchangers for the recovery of totaquine from cinchona bark and scopolamine from the *Datura* plant. As indicated by Applezweig and Nachod (1949), the basis of this interaction lies in the formation by the alkaloids of large cations, which, once attached to the exchanger, must be removed by special technics involving solvent extraction. Certain curare alkaloids, such as d-tubocurarine chloride, have been obtained by exchange using anionic materials (Bashour, 1946).

In order to ascertain the possible *in vivo* application of the adsorption of atropine by cationic and anionic exchangers, Sullivan and Martin (1950) gave toxic doses of atropine to mice, alone and in combination with an anion exchange resin or tragacanth. The results are presented in Table 12.

The L.D.-50 reduction resulting from the concomitant administration of an anion exchange resin doubtless indicates adsorption and retention of the atropine in the gastrointestinal tract, where it is slowly released and thus does not build up a comparable blood level. This technic of adsorption and slow release has found clinical application in a combination product, anion exchanger plus homatropine methylbromide, which provides continuous release of an antispasmodic, thus reducing the incidence of side effects inherent in the use of antiacetylcholine drugs (Sullivan and Martin, 1951).

Digitoxin in all probability will be administered on occasion with resins. With this thought in mind, Beiler *et al.* (1952) investigated the possibilities of adsorption of this drug onto the resin. Four types of resins were employed: a strong-base and a weak-base anion exchanger, a sulfonic type of cation exchanger, and a carboxylic type of cation exchanger. Because of the insolubility of digitoxin in water, methanol was used as the solvent least likely to alter ionic reactions. In this menstruum, there was no detectable adsorption of the digitoxin by any of the resins. Parallel findings have been reported by Chambers *et al.* (1952). Work of this type does not guarantee that resin therapy would not interfere with the use of digitoxin, but it does make the potentiality a remote one.

TABLE 12

Acute Toxicity of Atropine Sulfate as Affected by an Anion Exchange Resin*

(Oral Administration in Mice)

Group No.	No. mice in group	No. dead in group	Mg./Kg.	L.D.	Time (hrs.)
		Atropine alone			
1	10	10	1000	100	24
2	10	9	1200	90	24
		Atropine + anion exchange resin			
3	10	7	1000	70	24
4	10	6	1200	60	24
		Atropine + tragacanth—no resin			
5	10	10	1000	100	24
6	10	10	1200	100	24

* Resin = 250 mg. per cubic centimeter in 0.5 per cent tragacanth for suspension. Each mouse in groups 3 and 4 received 250 mg. of resin.

Khellin is a coronary vasodilator likely to be used in conjunction with resin therapy. As with the broad-spectrum antibiotics, this drug tends to produce gastrointestinal upsets, which in turn indicate therapy with exchangers and adsorption agents. Martin *et al.* (1952) have investigated the absorption of khellin from the gastrointestinal tracts of dogs when the drug was given alone and when in combination with resins. The dogs were given 200 mg. of khellin dissolved in 50 ml. of 30 per cent alcohol. The controls received khellin alone; the experimentals received khellin plus one or more exchange or adsorption agents. The results are given in Table 13. The method for the determination of khellin was not completely satisfactory, but the results permit the conclusion that the adsorption and ion exchange materials employed did not prevent the absorption of khellin. Ancillary to this conclusion is the assumption that resins and similar materials may be used with khellin in any indicated condition.

From the material reviewed in this section dealing with pharmaceuticals, it is apparent that studies should be conducted with each and every drug to be used in conjunction with an exchange or adsorption agent. In general materials such as khellin and digitoxin might be assumed to be satisfactory for concomitant administration with resins,

TABLE 13

The Effect of Exchangers and Adsorption Agents on the
Absorption of Khellin from the Gastrointestinal Tract in Dogs

	Khellin concentration (mg. %)		
*Agent**	½ *hr.*	*1 hr.*	*1½ hrs.*
Control	0	4	7.5
Anion exchange resin	7.5	15	15
Sodium aluminum silicate	0	11	11
Magnesium aluminum silicate	0	0	5
Combinations of all three agents (Resion)	13	7	5

* The amounts of exchange and adsorption agents given were as follows: anion exchange resin, 5 Gm.; sodium aluminum silicate, 5 Gm.; magnesium aluminum silicate, 1 Gm.; combination (Resion) contained 1.5 Gm. each of anion exchange resin and sodium aluminum silicate, plus 0.2 Gm. of magnesium aluminum silicate.

as they are essentially nonionic, but in every instance it should be remembered that exchangers are also adsorption agents and as such might remove drugs which are completely nonionic. Study of each combined system should be made.

One point of great importance for the future of exchangers and adsorption agents used in combination with drugs lies in the possibility that initial adsorption or absorption might result in subsequent slow release of the drug, thus giving a more constant blood level and extending the period during which effective blood levels are maintained following a single administration of the drug. Atropine absorbed on an anion exchange resin is slowly released, permitting much better control of its beneficial antispasmodic characteristics. There will doubtless be an entire series of agents falling into this category.

GENERAL COMMENT

The discussion of the biochemical applications of resinous exchangers and related materials gives in some measure the background for the application of these agents in the world of medicine. It is interesting to speculate briefly on the future in this field, since it will be related to the creation of new forms of resins.

Of great importance to the general economy is the development of plastic semipermeable membranes by Ionics, Inc., of Cambridge, Massachusetts. These ion exchange resins in membrane form permit, through combination with electric power, the deionization of salt waters at prices which lend themselves to practical application. The operation of these systems is less expensive than the usual compression stills and should permit vast areas of the world now virtually uninhabitable to be converted into synthetic oases.

The obvious parallel between these membranes and those of such importance to the biological structure suggests a vast future field for study in fundamental biological and medical research. One rather probable application will be in the design of more efficient artificial kidneys. One is inclined to speculate on the potentiality for the creation of an entirely synthetic gastrointestinal tract. In any event, the future holds great promise for the application of membranes composed of ion exchange resins.

Another new and exciting development lies in the family of polymers based on hydroquinone, which will exchange electrons with their environment. Enzymatic mechanisms, in general, can be designated as conducting systems for the transfer of electrons. Now we have available resins which can be used to conduct oxidation-reduction reactions. The pioneering efforts of Harold Cassidy of Yale University in this field should yield industrial and medical applications. He points out that proton transfer (hydrogen ion transfer) has been in use for some time. The medical application of proton transfer lies in the field of ulcer therapy and the use of anion exchangers. Similarly, sodium removal via cation exchangers represents another application of proton transfer involving resins. Biochemists are already studying the use of films of this electron transfer polymer as models for the effect of redox potentials on fluid transfer through membranes and for the study of the driving forces involved in fluid transport.

The potentialities for design of new resins are virtually unlimited. Recently, Broser and Lautsch (1951) have copolymerized styrene and methylpheophorbide, the latter chemical being a degradation product of chlorophyll. Similarly, protoporphyrin dibenzyl ester (a derivative of a hemoglobin degradation product) will be copolymerized with styrene. The resins formed from these reactants contain the pigments distributed over the chains. It is not possible at present to predict applications of such unique polymeric units, comprising as they do natural and synthetic monomers in polymeric form. In any event, they serve to illustrate the future of this unique world of resins.

REFERENCES

ACKERMANN, D., and H. G. FUCHS. *Ztschr. physiol. Chem.*, **240**: 198, 1936.

APPLEZWEIG, N. *J. Am. Chem. Soc.*, **66**: 1990, 1944.

APPLEZWEIG, N., and F. C. NACHOD. In Nachod, F. C., *Ion Exchange, Theory and Application*. New York: Academic Press, 1949.

APPLEZWEIG, N., and M. RICE. In Nachod, F. C., *Ion Exchange, Theory and Application*. New York: Academic Press, 1949.

APPLEZWEIG, N., and S. E. RONZONE. *Ind. Eng. Chem.*, **38**: 576, 1946.

BARTHOLOMEW, L. G., and D. R. NICHOLS. *Proc. Staff Meet., Mayo Clin.*, **25**: 370, 1950.

BASHOUR, J. T. U.S. Patent 2,409,241, October 15, 1946.

BEILER, J. M., M. GRAFF, and G. J. MARTIN. Unpublished data, 1952.

BLOCK, R. J. *Proc. Soc. Exper. Biol. Med.*, **51**: 252, 1942.

BLOCK, R. J. U.S. Patent 2,386,926, October 16, 1945.

BRAAFLADT, L. H. *J. Infect. Dis.*, **33**: 434, 1923.

BROSER, W., and W. Lautsch. *Naturwissenschaften*, **38**: 208, 1951.

CARTER, H. E., R. K. CLARK, JR., S. R. DICKMAN, Y. H. LOO, P. S. SKELL, and W. A. STRONG. *J. Biol. Chem.*, **160**: 337, 1945.

CHAMBERS, M. A., L. P. ZILL, and G. R. NOGGLE. *J. Am. Pharm. A. (Scient. Ed.)*, **41**: 461, 1952.

COHN, W. E. *J. Am. Chem. Soc.*, **73**: 1539, 1951.

COHN, W. E., and C. E. CARTER. *J. Am. Chem. Soc.*, **72**: 2606, 1950a.

COHN, W. E., and C. E. CARTER. *J. Am. Chem. Soc.*, **72**: 4273, 1950b.

COHN, W. E., and E. VOLKIN. *Nature*, **167**: 483, 1951.

CRUZ-COKE, E., F. GONZALES, and W. HULSEN. *Science*, **101**: 340, 1945.

DI GANGI, F. E., and C. H. ROGERS. *J. Am. Pharm. A. (Scient. Ed.)*, **38**: 646, 1949.

FINK, H. U.S. Patent 2,072,089, March 2, 1937.

FREUDENBERG, K., H. WALCH, and H. MOLTER. *Naturwissenschaften*, **30**: 87, 1942.

GREENSPAN, R., H. MacLEAN, A. MILZER, and H. NECHELES. *Am. J. Dig. Dis.*, **18**: 35, 1951.

GUNNISON, J. B., and M. S. MARSHALL. *J. Bacteriol.*, **33**: 401, 1937.

HERR, D. S. *Ind. Eng. Chem.*, **37**: 631, 1945.

HURST, R. O., J. A. LITTLE, and G. C. BUTLER. *J. Biol. Chem.*, **188**: 705, 1951.

HUSSEY, C. V., A. J. QUICK, M. STEFANINI, C. F. CONSOLAZIO, and F. SARGENT. *J. Biol. Chem.*, **184**: 105, 1950.

KATZMAN, P. A., M. GODFRID, C. K. CAIN, and E. A. DOISY. *J. Biol. Chem.*, **148**: 501, 1943.

KOCHOLATY, W., and R. JUNOWICZ-KOCHOLATY. *Arch. Biochem.*, **15**: 55, 1947.

LEJWA, A. *Biochem. Ztschr.*, **256**: 236, 1932.

LoGRIPPO, G. A. *Proc. Soc. Exper. Biol. Med.*, **74**: 208, 1950.

McCHESNEY, E. W. *J. Lab. Clin. Med.*, **39**: 629, 1952.

McCOLLOCH, R. J., and Z. I. KERTESZ. *J. Biol. Chem.*, **160**: 149, 1945.

McCREADY, R. M., and W. Z. HASSID. *J. Am. Chem. Soc.*, **66**: 560, 1944.

MARTIN, G. J., M. GRAFF, and J. M. BEILER. Unpublished data, 1952.

MARTIN, G. J., and J. N. MOSS. Unpublished data, 1952.

MARTIN, G. J., J. N. MOSS, and J. M. BEILER. Unpublished data, 1952.

MARTIN, G. J., and M. J. SULLIVAN. Unpublished data, 1949.

MELNICK, D., M. HOCHBERG, and B. L. OSER. *J. Nutrition*, **30**: 233, 1945.

MESSERLI, N. *Arch. internat. physiol.*, **19**: 103, 1922.

MOSS, J., and G. J. MARTIN. *Am. J. Dig. Dis.*, **17**: 18, 1950.

MULLER, R. H. *Proc. Soc. Exper. Biol. Med.*, **73**: 239, 1950.

NELSON, J. A., W. D. McFARLANE, and M. BOULET. *Federation Proc.*, **5**: 148, 1946.

PAUL, H. E., and C. M. HARRINGTON. *J. Am. Pharm. A. (Scient. Ed.)*, **41**: 50, 1952.

PFIFFNER, J. J., S. B. BINKLEY, E. S. BLOOM, and A. D. EMMETT. U.S. Patent 2,407,096, Sept. 3, 1946.

POLIS, B. D., and O. MEYERHOF. *J. Biol. Chem.*, **169**: 389, 1947.

POTTS, A. M., and T. F. GALLAGHER. *J. Biol. Chem.*, **154**: 349, 1944.

QUICK, A. J. *Am. J. Physiol.*, **148**: 211, 1947.

REID, A. F., and F. JONES. *Am. J. Clin. Path.*, **19**: 10, 1949.

ROGERS, C. H., T. O. SOINE, and C. O. WILSON. In Rogers, C. H., Soine, T. O. and Wilson, C. O., *Inorganic Pharmaceutical Chemistry* (5th ed.). Philadelphia: Lea and Febiger, 1952.

SCHOENBACH, E. B., M. S. BRYER, and P. H. LONG. Conference on Aureomycin. *Ann. New York Acad. Sc.*, **51**: 987, 1949.

SCHRAMM, G., and J. PRIMOSIGH. *Ber deut. chem. ges.*, **77B**: 417, 1944.

SEED, J. C., and C. E. WILSON. *Bull. Johns Hopkins Hosp.*, **86**: 415, 1950.

SINSHEIMER, R. L., and J. F. KOERNER. *Science*, **114**: 42, 1951.

SMITH, S. C., and S. H. WENDER. *J. Am. Chem. Soc.*, **70**: 3719, 1948.

STEFANINI, M. *Proc. Soc. Exper. Biol. Med.*, **67**: 22, 1948.

STEINBERG, A. *Proc. Soc. Exper. Biol. Med.*, **56**: 124, 1944.

SULLIVAN, M. J., and G. J. MARTIN. *Am. J. Pharm.*, **122**: 48, 1950.

SULLIVAN, M. J., and G. J. MARTIN. U.S. Patent 2,554,072, May 22, 1951.

SUSSMAN, S., A. B. MINDLER, and W. WOOD. *Chemistry and Industry,* 57: 455, 1945.

TURBA, F., M. RICHTER, and F. KUCHAR. *Naturwissenschaften,* 31: 508, 1943.

VOLKIN, E., J. X. KHYM, and W. E. COHN. *J. Am. Chem. Soc.,* 73: 1533, 1951.

WAISBREN, B. A., and J. S. HUECKEL. *Proc. Soc. Exper. Biol. Med.,* 73: 73, 1950.

WHITEHORN, J. C. *J. Biol. Chem.,* 56: 751, 1923.

WIELAND, T. *Naturwissenschaften,* 30: 374, 1942.

WILLIAMS, M. L., and D. J. WEEKES. *Rev. Gastroenterol.,* 18: 128, 1951.

WINDAUS, A., R. TSCHESCHE, H. RUHKOPF, F. LAQUER, and F. SCHULTZ. *Ztschr. physiol. Chem.,* 204: 123, 1932.

CHAPTER 5

Anion Exchange Resins in the
Treatment of Peptic Ulcers

ETIOLOGY OF PEPTIC ULCER AS IT RELATES TO EXCHANGERS

CURRENTLY, the major application of anion exchange resins lies in the management of peptic ulcer. It is not the purpose of this monograph to review gastric physiology, biochemistry or pharmacology, or to cover etiological factors except as they apply to the direct use of anion exchangers in the resolution of the problem. The logic of the use of resins in peptic ulcer lies in the acceptance of the only points about

70

which experts in the field agree: (1) pepsin and hydrochloric acid are etiological factors; and (2) control of peptic activity and reduction of free hydrochloric acid concentrations permit healing of the ulcerations.

Let us consider first the evidence for the involvement of pepsin and hydrochloric acid in the development of ulcers. This in no sense implies abandonment of other features (i.e., psychogenic and neurogenic), nor does it imply lack of belief in proposals concerning mucosal ischemia. The etiology of peptic ulcer is doubtless multiple in nature, involving several positive features perhaps combined with negative features. It seems probable that all disease is of multiple etiological origin, and peptic ulcer is no exception. Involvement of pepsin and gastric acid has been generally conceded, but emphasis on the relative significance of each has been shifting.

Emphasis on the dominant role of hydrochloric acid came from Dragstedt (1942) and Mann and Bollman (1932). This concept was underlined by the production of ulcers in nearly all species of animals by injection of histamine in beeswax (Hay *et al.*, 1942). Histamine is known to stimulate the secretion of a gastric juice high in acid and low in pepsin.

The tendency toward shift in emphasis from acid to pepsin was initiated by the demonstration of Vanzant *et al.* (1933) that the secretion of the enzyme was increased in ulcer patients and that a direct correlation existed between symptomatic severity and enzyme concentration. In the laboratory, substantiation of this concept came from Schiffrin and Warren (1942), who (using perfused isolated loops of small intestine from cats) produced typical ulcerations with hydrochloric acid and pepsin (not with acid alone), and from Matzner *et al.* (1936), who produced ulcers in rats by feeding the enzyme and the acid. Extension and confirmation of these observations have been recorded (Driver *et al.*, 1945; LeVeen, 1947).

Doubtless much of the confusion clouding any attempt to place prime emphasis is associated with inadequacy in methods for the determination of peptic activity. LeVeen (1946) and LeVeen and Hallinger (1947) have emphasized this from the standpoint of the laboratory as well as the clinic. It seems logical therefore to present at this point the salient features of the action of pepsin. This principal proteolytic enzyme of the gastric juice has an optimum pH for activity of 1.5 to 2.5. This is of great importance, because any agent shifting pH in gastric juice to a higher range will automatically reduce peptic activity regardless of its direct action on the pepsin itself. Further, at neutral and alkaline pH values, the inactivation of pepsin is irreversible.

Gastric mucosa does not contain pepsin but does contain its precursor, pepsinogen, which is autocatalytically converted at pH values higher than 6.0. In the course of the conversion, a pepsin inhibitor is formed (Herriott, 1941). It is clear that the point of conversion or activation of pepsinogen would be of paramount importance in the study of gastric ulcer etiology; moreover, the pepsin inhibitor concentration would be key to the degree of peptic activity. It is not difficult to imagine transformation of inactive to active proteolytic enzyme without inhibitor formation or with varying degrees of inhibitor formation.

LeVeen and Hallinger (1947) studied inhibitor concentrations in normal individuals and peptic ulcer patients, finding that 99 per cent of the pepsin present in both groups was inhibited. This is a manifestation of biological antagonism, and its localization to mucosal strata may well be a basic feature of etiological import. While these investigators observed no differences in degree of inhibitor activity between the groups, this does not mean that localized tissue differences would not be found. In gastric juice, it was concluded that peptic activity in the ulcer patient exceeded that of the normal subject largely by virtue of the effect of pH. Determinations were made with and without dilution of gastric juice; only at high dilutions was the inhibitor effect largely nullified.

Pepsin acts upon a large assortment of proteins, producing proteoses, peptones and polypeptides. These breakdown products in turn act as inhibitors of the enzymatic activity. Thus two types of inhibitors—one formed during conversion of pepsin to pepsinogen and a second formed by action of pepsin on its natural substrate—tend to control activity of the enzyme, and in both cases dilution reduces this inhibitory effect. The logical correlative appears to be that fluid intake should be restricted in the peptic ulcer patient. LeVeen and Hallinger (1947) emphasize that through simple dilution the digestive power of gastric juice can be elevated by a factor of five thousand.

The elaboration and secretion of pepsin and hydrochloric acid into the gastric lumen is controlled by a series of component structures. These are mentioned only to indicate the complexity of the pathological physiology operative in the ulcer patient. There are a central nervous system component, a peripheral parasympathomimetic unit, and finally the parietal and zymogenic cells of the gastric glands. The

TABLE 14
Pepsin Activity of Gastric Juice in 30 Duodenal Ulcer Subjects and 21 Normal Subjects

(From LeVeen, H. H., and L. Hallinger, *J. Clin. Investigation*, **26**: 767, 1947)

Total pepsin activity (pepsin equivalents per ml.)		Active pepsin fraction (pepsin equivalents per ml.)		pH of gastric juice		Resting peptic activity (pepsin equivalents per ml.)	
Normal	Ulcer	Normal	Ulcer	Normal	Ulcer	Normal	Ulcer
2,500	2,500	2.6	1.2	5.12	1.35	0.5	1.5
3,400	3,900	1.7	1.0	3.25	2.55	0.8	0.7
4,300	3,000	0.6	1.1	1.85	2.15	0.6	0.9
4,300	5,200	4.4	1.2	1.50	1.45	5.9	1.5
313	2,700	1.1	1.3	4.90	1.10	0.8	1.9
7,500	3,600	2.2	1.7	1.50	2.20	2.8	1.1
188	2,500	0.6	1.3	7.45	1.40	0	1.6
1,900	6,200	1.7	1.6	4.55	1.50	0.6	2.1
6,100	940	1.0	1.8	1.80	2.10	0.9	1.3
250	4,900	0	1.3	6.45	2.0	0	1.1
6,100	2,500	1.5	1.0	1.50	1.50	1.9	1.1
8,600	6,200	1.3	1.2	1.60	2.30	1.5	0.8
4,300	8,700	1.2	1.4	1.80	1.50	1.1	1.7
3,900	5,400	1.1	1.9	1.55	1.45	1.3	2.5
3,900	4,800	1.1	1.0	2.55	3.10	0.7	0.6
3,600	11,200	1.2	1.8	2.70	1.50	0.8	2.2
2,800	3,600	0.9	1.0	1.55	1.40	1.0	1.1
6,100	2,500	0.8	1.0	2.25	1.50	0.7	1.1
7,500	4,900	2.8	1.3	1.40	1.30	4.2	1.7
1,600	4,100	1.1	1.0	3.55	1.50	0.6	1.1
2,800	1,300	5.6	1.9	3.70	1.80	1.1	1.8
	1,000		1.3		1.30		1.8
	5,200		1.6		1.55		1.9
	3,600		0.9		1.50		1.0
	4,300		1.1		1.65		1.1
	3,400		0.6		1.40		0.7
	3,900		1.3		1.50		1.5
	4,900		1.4		1.25		2.0
	3,000		1.1		1.60		1.1
	2,500		0.9		1.50		1.0

stimulus to the central nervous system may be psychogenic, gastric or intestinal. Clearly, the individual variations possible in a multiple component system are legion. Control of peptic activity and gastric concentration will depend not only upon their removal from but also upon their speed of formation in the stomach. Dosage will logically be highly variable. Further, it seems appropriate to attempt the blockage of the central nervous component, the peripheral parasympathomimetic com-

FIGURE 8

Postulated Stratification of Enzymes in Parietal Cell and Mechanism of Hydrochloric Acid Formation

(From Patterson, W. B., and D Stetton, Jr., *Science,* 109: 256, 1949)

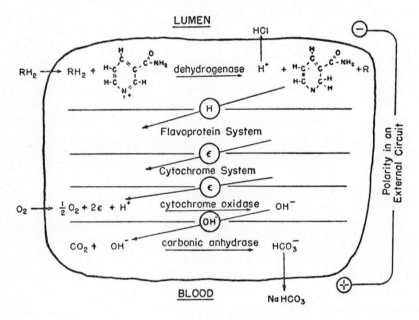

ponent, as well as to control by removal or neutralization the hydrochloric acid and pepsin at the end point, namely the gastric juice.

In considering an approach to resin application, let us briefly outline the mechanism of hydrochloric acid formation. The proposals of Patterson and Stetten (1949) seem most nearly to integrate experimental facts recorded to date. Their hypothesis is based upon two facts: the hydrogen ions of the gastric juice arise from the reduction of pyridine nucleotide, and there is a stratification within the parietal cells of the oxidation-reduction enzyme systems. This concept is most easily presented by Figure 8, from their work.

The purpose of presentation of the complexities of acid and enzyme formation and control thereof lies in the conclusion that no single approach represents a final answer to ulcer therapy. Certainly the multiple approach through the use of barbiturates to control the central nervous system component, of antispasmodics to control the parasympathomimetic component, and finally of antacids and antipepsins to control the peptic activity at the end organ seems the rational one, and in general it is used. With this review as background, the use of resinous exchangers can be more clearly considered.

LABORATORY BACKGROUND FOR THE USE OF ANION EXCHANGE RESINS IN MEDICINE

Acid-neutralizing Power

The acid-neutralizing power of the anion exchange resin used as an antacid is 10 mEq. per dry gram of resin. The term acid neutralizing power is in some ways a misnomer, as the acid is not neutralized in the sense of being converted into water through reaction with a base. Further, the removal of acid by the resin is not truly ion exchange; it is rather a reversible molecular absorption. The equation expressing the reaction is:

$$RNH_2 + HCl \rightleftarrows RNH_3Cl$$

Expressed in other terms, it requires 1 Gm. of resin to bring 50 ml. of 0.1 N hydrochloric acid or 50 ml. of gastric juice to pH 4.0 (Martin and Wilkinson, 1946). In reference to gastric physiology, considering the gastric residuum during the interdigestive period to average 30 to 50 ml. of 18.5-unit* free acidity, 0.4 Gm. of resin would bring the pH to 4.0. The corresponding figures for the peptic ulcer patient are 67 ml. of 28-unit free acid and approximately 0.5 Gm. of resin. It is to be remembered that at pH 4.0 no free acid is present.

Estimates of the total gastric juice secretion in a 24-hour period vary, but 2 to 3 l. seems a reasonable figure. If this were all 50-unit juice and if 50 per cent of it would need to be reduced by the resin, it would require from 10 to 15 Gm. to accomplish the desired result. These figures are presented to permit subsequent comparison of the theoretical values with clinical observation.

* Unit = cubic centimeters of 0.1 N sodium hydroxide to neutralize 100 cc. = milliequivalents of acid per liter of juice.

The speed of buffering or of acid removal is determined by the time needed for contact. The reaction occurs instantaneously once the reactive group of the resin and the acid molecule are within those distances required for the functioning of short-range chemical forces. This is reflected in the fact that rate of acid removal by resin depends on stirring. Martin and Wilkinson (1946) report that an increase in the

FIGURE 9

Neutralization of Gastric Juice by Amberlite IR-4 (200-Mesh)

(From Martin, G. J., and J. Wilkinson, *Gastroenterology,* 6: 316, 1946)

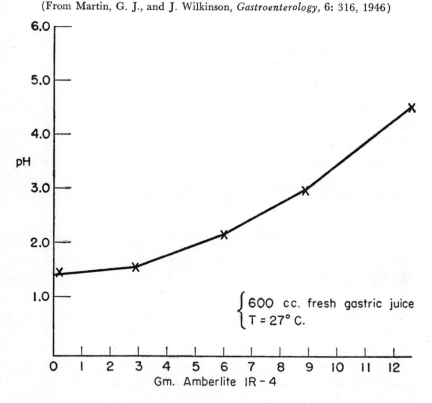

speed of stirring by a factor of eleven resulted in a 218-fold increase in the rate of acid removal. *In vivo,* the parallel phenomenon would be peristaltic waves, the physiological stirring mechanism. Another factor of paramount importance to speed of acid removal is particle size of the resin. As can be seen from Figure 10, 200-mesh resin reacted many thousandfold times more quickly with acid than did 40-mesh material (Martin and Wilkinson, 1946). One might state

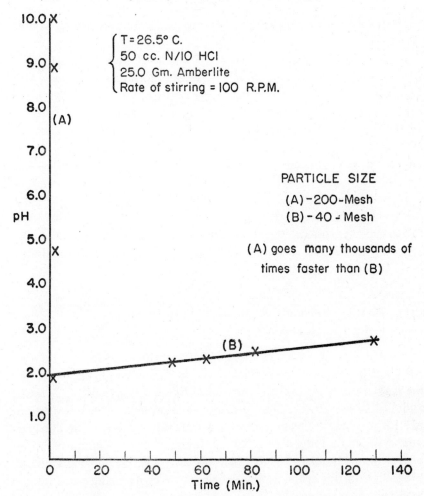

FIGURE 10
Dependence of Rate of Acid Neutralization
on Particle Size of Amberlite

(From Martin, G. J., and J. Wilkinson, *Gastroenterology*, **6**: 316, 1946)

that the greater the mesh and the finer the particle size of the resin, the more efficacious it should be *in vivo*. There is, however, a practical limit to the effectiveness of modern milling equipment, and it is this factor which dictates the speed of reaction possible. Since it is improbable that more efficient milling mechanisms will be devised within the near future, 200- to 400-mesh resins of particle size ranging from 74 to 30 microns and averaging 50 microns are likely to remain the best available. The question arises with particles of this extremely small size whether or not they will pass through the wall of the gastro-intestinal tract. It is estimated that particles of diameters approximately 4 to 5 millimicrons will pass through the mucosa of the tract. This means that the smallest resin particles are still approximately one thousand times larger than the size of the maximum unit which would penetrate.

Explanation of the greater speed of action of finer resin particles lies in the fact that with the smaller particle more reactive groups are exposed on the surface. With the larger particle, the major portion of the reactive groups is within the porous gel-like structure, and the acid must diffuse into the capillaries of the gel before it can come in contact with the reacting moiety. This diffusion requires time, ranging from minutes to hours depending upon the distance it must travel into the capillaries.

A point of interest in a consideration of the merit of resins as ant-acids is that of comparative speed of action. Martin and Wilkinson (1946) demonstrated that the resin brought about a reduction in acidity with a speed roughly paralleling that seen with various alum-inum hydroxide gels.

Effect of Anion Exchange Resins on Certain Important Physiological Substances

Anion exchange resins of the polyamine formaldehyde type do not adsorb either thiamin or riboflavin at pH values paralleling those of the gastrointestinal tract (1.5 for stomach, 8.5 for intestine) (Martin and Wilkinson, 1946). One vitamin, ascorbic acid, was adsorbed at pH 1.5, but desorption was complete with shift of pH to the alkaline side. A similar situation held for the inorganic salts, sodium chloride and sodium phosphate, with quantitative recovery following shift of pH to 8.5. In this instance, adsorption is "molecular" and not a mani-festation of exchange (Wilkinson and Martin, 1946). The adsorption of sodium phosphate occurred from hydrochloric acid solutions, but that of sodium chloride occurred only from a nitric acid solution. Physiologically, it is to be assumed that sodium chloride adsorption would not occur. The adsorption of sodium chloride from nitric acid solution is due to the formation of a double salt of sodium chloride and the quaternary ammonium salt form of the resin. This was estab-lished by studies (Wilkinson and Martin, 1946) demonstrating the

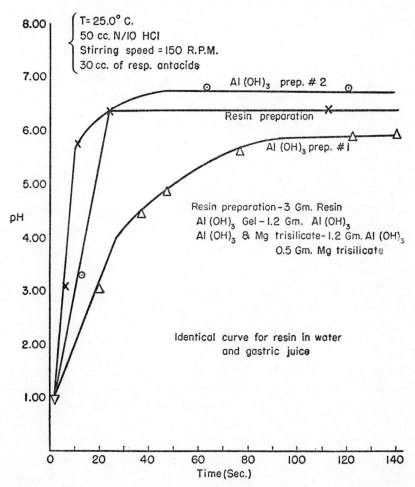

FIGURE 11
Comparative Rate of Acid Neutralization for Antacid Suspensions
(Amberlite IR-4 in Bentonite, etc.)

(From Martin, G. J., and J. Wilkinson, *Gastroenterology*, 6: 316, 1946)

proportionality between adsorbed nitrate (HNO_3) and chloride, an essential feature if the law of mass action applies.

Effect of Anion Exchange Resins on Enzymes

Pepsin. Gastrointestinal enzymes of prime consideration in peptic ulcer therapy are pepsin, trypsin and lysozyme, the pepsin for reasons which have been reviewed here. Segal *et al.* (1945) studied the problem of pepsin inactivation by anion exchange resins and reached the conclusion that the sole effect was due to pH changes, which would in turn modify enzymatic activity. They employed acid-exhausted resins. In other words all of the reactive groups of the resin molecule were rendered inactive by virtue of prior treatment with hydrochloric

FIGURE 12

Proportionality Between Adsorbed Nitrate (HNO₃) and Chloride
as Required by the Law of Mass Action for the Dissociation
of the Postulated Double Salt of Sodium Chloride
and Quaternary Ammonium Salt

(From Wilkinson, J., and G. J. Martin, *Arch. Biochem.,* 10: 205, 1946)

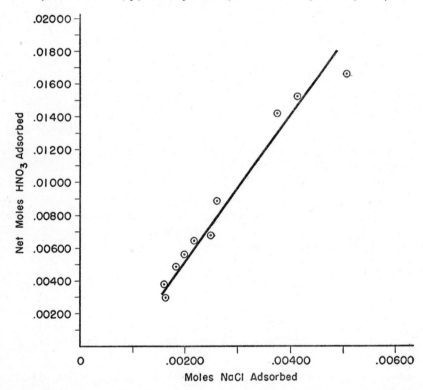

acid. In the experiments of Martin and Wilkinson (1946) and Wilkinson and Martin (1946), reactive resin forms were employed and these led to reduction in peptic activity. The criticism was raised that pH shift could account for the results observed. To attempt a resolution of this divergence of opinion, Alpert and Martin (1949) re-evaluated the entire problem. Shifts of pH were blocked by buffering reaction solutions. Careful readjustments were made of minor changes in pH prior to determination of peptic activity. Generally, 15 mg. of resin or other test material were added to 5 ml. of a solution of pH 1.5 to 1.6 containing 1.5 mg. of N.F. pepsin. In a system of this type, it would require 100 mg. of resin to shift the pH to a value at which enzyme inactivation would occur. Under these conditions, various anion exchange resins gave values indicating 30 to 100 per cent inactivation of the pepsin. Cation exchange resins in the hydrogen cycle under similar testing conditions gave values varying from 0 to 49 per cent. Comparative figures for other substances are given in Table 15.

Controversial aspects of this problem are probably due to the resin used and even to the specific sample of resin used. It cannot and should not be assumed that one anion exchange resin is precisely like another even though they are obtained from the same manufacturer. Resins are only relatively well defined, and while lots made at different times are essentially identical they do differ in some respects. Those released for medical use are qualified as standard by virtue of proper control and rejection of any lots which do not conform.

The inactivation of pepsin is a surface phenomenon, as shown by the power of sodium alkyl sulfate to enhance the effect of the anion exchange resins (Alpert and Martin, 1949). In this case, the tendency of the surface-active agent would be to reverse the pH effect of the resin. There are at least four mechanisms of pepsin inactivation: (1) pH shift to values of 5.0 or higher, (2) surface adsorption, as seen with charcoal, (3) mass action of end products, as seen with protein hydrolysates, and (4) complex formation such as occurs with gentian violet. In the case of the anion exchange resins it is proposed that two factors are operative: surface adsorption and pH. The latter is involved in a restricted sense of the pH shift which occurs at the particle surface, where the pepsin molecule is adsorbed, but not in that which occurs in the surrounding medium. The degree of such inactivation will vary markedly and would not occur with an acid-exhausted resin because no surface pH shift would be operative.

Trypsin. As there is at present no evidence that trypsin is involved in the etiology of duodenal ulcer, and it is certain that this enzyme is essential to protein digestion, any antacid material used in the treatment of ulcers should inhibit pepsin but not trypsin and the other proteolytic enzymes of the intestine. Alpert and Martin (1950) investigated the trypsin-inhibiting qualities of thirty-five different adsorption

TABLE 15

The Inhibitory Action of Chemical Agents on Peptic Activity

(From Alpert, S., and G. J. Martin, *Am. J. Dig. Dis.*, **16:** 10, 1949)

Substance tested	Conc. (mg./5 cc.)	Conc. 1:3000 N.F. Pepsin (mg./5 cc.)	% Inhibition (heterogeneous mixture)	% Inhibition (supernatant liquid)
1. Insoluble polyamine anion exchange resin A, commercial sample, 200-mesh	15	1.5	89	99
2. Insoluble polyamine anion exchange resin A, commercial sample, 200-mesh	13	1.5	61	75
3. Insoluble polyamine anion exchange resin A, commercial sample, 200-mesh	10	1.5	50	79
4. Insoluble polyamine anion exchange resin A, commercial sample, 200-mesh	5	1.5	41	50
5. Insoluble polyamine anion exchange resin A, commercial sample, 200-mesh	2	1.5	30	30
6. Insoluble polyamine anion exchange resin B, commercial sample, 200-mesh	15	1.5	95	100
7. Insoluble polyamine anion exchange resin C, commercial sample, 200-mesh	15	1.5	100	100
8. Insoluble polyamine anion exchange resin D, commercial sample, 200-mesh	15	1.5	65	100
9. Cation exchange resin A, hydrogen-activated commercial sample, 200-mesh	15	1.5	26	None

TABLE 15 (*Continued*)

Substance tested	Conc. (mg./5 cc.)	Conc. 1:3000 N.F. Pepsin (mg./5 cc.)	% Inhibition (heterogeneous mixture)	% Inhibition (supernatant liquid)
10. Cation exchange resin B, hydrogen-activated commercial sample, 200-mesh	15	1.5	40	40
11. Cation exchange resin C, hydrogen-activated commercial sample, 200-mesh	15	1.5	49	49
12. Cation exchange resin D, sodium-activated commercial sample, 60-mesh	15	1.5	75	44
13. Synthetic sodium aluminum silicate, 200-mesh	15	1.5	0	75
14. Activated bauxite (essentially Al_2O_3)	15	1.5	88	94
15. Fuller's earth (essentially SiO_2)	15	1.5	99	99
16. Synthetic magnesium silicate	15	1.5	75	94
17. Activated charcoal	15	1.5	100	100
18. Diatomaceous earth	15	1.5	19	19
19. Bauxite	15	1.5	44	58
20. Magnesium trisilicate	15	1.5	84	84
21. Filtrol adsorbent	15	1.5	88	84
22. Yeast protein hydrolysate	32	3.0	—	86
23. Lactalbumin hydrolysate	40	3.0	—	88
24. Methionine	16	3.0	—	56
25. Glycine	16	3.0	—	78
26. Sulfonated product of fatty acids and aliphatic compounds (anionic detergent)	15	1.5	—	84
27. Decyl benzene sodium (anionic detergent)	15	1.5	—	75

TABLE 15 (*Continued*)

Substance tested	Conc. (mg./5 cc.)	Conc. 1:3000 N.F. Pepsin (mg./5 cc.)	% Inhibition (heterogeneous mixture)	% Inhibition (supernatant liquid)
28. Cetyl dimethyl benzyl ammonium chloride (cationic detergent)	15	1.5	—	19
29. Sodium oleate (anionic detergent)	15	1.5	100	—
30. Bentonite	15	1.5	100	100
31. Bentonite	10	1.5	100	100
32. Bentonite	6	1.5	100	100
33. Bentonite	4	1.5	99	99
34. Bentonite	2	1.5	61	83
35. Sodium alkyl sulfate (principally lauryl)	15	1.5	100	100
36. Sodium alkyl sulfate (principally lauryl)	10	1.5	—	100
37. Sodium alkyl sulfate (principally lauryl)	5	1.5	—	100
38. Sodium alkyl sulfate (principally lauryl)	2	1.5	—	100
39. Sodium alkyl sulfate (principally lauryl)	1	1.5	—	84
40. Sodium alkyl sulfate (principally lauryl)	0.5	1.5	—	53
41. Graphite powder	15	1.5	None	None
42. Al(OH)$_3$ powder	15	1.5	89	92
43. Salicylic acid	15	1.5	63	—
44. Nicotinyl salicylic acid	15	1.5	41	26
45. l (+) histidine HCl	15	1.5	None	—
46. l (+) tyrosine	15	1.5	None	None
47. 9-Aminoacridine HCl	15	1.5	None	—
48. Gentian violet	15	1.5	81	—
49. Oil black (dye)	15	1.5	None	None
50. Bentonite	5	1.5	72	72
Insoluble polyamine resin A	5	—	—	—
51. Bentonite	7.5	1.5	93	93
Insoluble polyamine resin A	7.5	—	—	—
52. Bentonite	5	1.5	88	100
Insoluble polyamine resin A	10	—	—	—

TABLE 15 (*Continued*)

Substance tested	Conc. (mg./5 cc.)	Conc. 1:3000 N.F. Pepsin (mg./5 cc.)	% Inhibition (heterogene-ous mixture)	% Inhibition (supernatant liquid)
53. Bentonite	7.5	1.5	100	100
Sodium alkyl sulfate	7.5			
54. Bentonite	7.5	1.5	97	97
Synthetic sodium aluminum silicate	7.5			
55. Insoluble polyamine resin	14.5	1.5	94	100
Sodium alkyl sulfate	0.5			
56. Insoluble polyamine resin	14	1.5	99	100
Sodium alkyl sulfate	1			
57. Insoluble polyamine resin	13	1.5	100	100
Sodium alkyl sulfate	2			
58. Insoluble polyamine resin	10	1.5	100	100
Sodium alkyl sulfate	5	—	—	—

and antacid materials. With one exception (certain anion exchange resins), all material tested reduced markedly the hydrolytic power of the enzyme. Aluminum compounds and magnesium trisilicate are capable of blocking both enzymes. Of marked interest is the observation that some anion exchange resins inactivate both enzymes. This is further proof of the statement that one cannot consider the resins as a group and that each must be investigated individually.

Lysozyme. Lysozyme is an enzyme capable of depolymerizing the high molecular weight mucopolysaccharides contained in many cell walls and constituting mucin, a normal constituent of gastric and intestinal juices. Meyer *et al.* (1948*a*, *b*) attributed to the enzyme a primary role in peptic ulcers and in ulcerative alimentary disease. The premise was that lysozyme destroyed the protective coating of mucin over the mucosal surfaces and that secondarily pepsin and hydrochloric acid acted. While recent reports (Jerzy Glass *et al.*, 1950; Reifenstein *et al.*, 1950; Moeller *et al.*, 1951) do not substantiate the concept of the etiological significance of lysozyme in peptic ulcer and in

TABLE 16
Inhibition of the Activity of Trypsin by Adsorptive Agents

(From Alpert, S., and G. J. Martin, *Rev. Gastroenterol.*, **17**: 251, 1950)

Adsorbent	% Adsorbed using 0.1 Gm. adsorbent per 100 cc. trypsin sol. (8 mg./100 cc.)	% Adsorbed using 0.4 Gm. adsorbent per 100 cc. of same trypsin sol.
1. Insoluble polyamine anion exchange resin A, commercial sample, 200-mesh	None	None
2. Insoluble polyamine anion exchange resin B, commercial sample, 200-mesh chloride salt	45	73.0
3. Insoluble polyamine anion exchange resin C, commercial sample, 200-mesh	None	None
4. Insoluble polyamine anion exchange resin D, commercial sample, 200-mesh	31.0	39.0
5. Insoluble polyamine anion exchange resin E, commercial sample, 200-mesh	31.0	39.0
6. Insoluble polyamine anion exchange resin F, commercial sample, 200-mesh	45.0	45.0
7. Cation exchange resin A, hydrogen-activated commercial sample, 200-mesh	73.0	82.0
8. Cation exchange resin B, hydrogen-activated commercial sample, 200-mesh	73.0	87.0
9. Cation exchange resin C, hydrogen-activated commercial sample, 200-mesh	45.0	82.0
10. Cation exchange resin D, hydrogen-activated commercial sample, 200-mesh	73.0	82.0
11. Cation exchange resin E, hydrogen-activated commercial sample, 200-mesh	15.0	31.0
12. Cation exchange resin F, carboxylic acid type of commercial sample, 200-mesh	15.0	31.0

TABLE 16 (*Continued*)

Adsorbent	% Adsorbed using 0.1 Gm. adsorbent per 100 cc. trypsin sol. (8 mg./100 cc.)	% Adsorbed using 0.4 Gm. adsorbent per 100 cc. of same trypsin sol.
13. Cation exchange resin G, carboxylic acid type of commercial sample, 200-mesh	31.0	73.0
14. Cation exchange resin H, sodium-activated commercial sample, 200-mesh	39.0	73.0
15. Cation exchange resin C, sodium-activated commercial sample, 200-mesh	None	73.0
16. Cation exchange resin I, sodium-activated commercial sample, 200-mesh	45.0	73.0
17. Colloidal magnesium aluminum silicate gel	62.0 (conc., 1 cc./100 cc.)	82.0 (conc., 4 cc./100 cc.)
18. Synthetic magnesium silicate	82.0	89.0
19. Synthetic sodium aluminum silicate, 200-mesh	82.0	87.0
20. High-capacity synthetic sodium aluminum silicate 200-mesh	31.0	45.0
21. Polyamine anion exchange resin A (10%) Synthetic sodium aluminum silicate (10%) (suspended in colloidal magnesium aluminum silicate gel)	73.0 (conc., 1 cc./100 cc.)	>89.0 (conc., 4 cc./100 cc.)
22. Activated charcoal A	82.0	>89.0
23. Activated charcoal B	86.0	>89.0
24. Activated charcoal C	89.0	89.0
25. Activated bauxite (essentially Al_2O_3)	82.0	87.0
26. Fuller's earth (essentially SiO_2)	82.0	89.0
27. Diatomaceous earth	None	73.0
28. Kaolin (English)	73.0	82.0
29. Talc	45.0	89.0
30. Bentonite	73.0	82.0

TABLE 16 (*Continued*)

Adsorbent	% Adsorbed using 0.1 Gm. adsorbent per 100 cc. trypsin sol. (8 mg./100 cc.)	% Adsorbed using 0.4 Gm. adsorbent per 100 cc. of same trypsin sol.
31. Bauxite	73.0	82.0
32. Filtrol adsorbent	73.0	87.0
33. Aluminum hydroxide gel	73.0	73.0
	(conc., 1 Gm./100 cc.)	(conc. 4 Gm./100 cc.)
34. Magnesium trisilicate	82.0	>89.0
35. Aluminum hydroxide powder	73.0	90.0

ulcerative colitis, there is no disagreement on the tremendous variation in concentrations of this enzyme under various life situations and emotional states (Grace *et al.*, 1949, 1950).

It seems therefore that the final word has not been said on the importance of the enzyme in gastrointestinal pathology and that evidence on the inhibition of the action of this factor should be valuable. In this reference, Moss and Martin (1948) studied lysozyme inhibition by various surface-active agents and by a series of adsorption materials including anion exchange resins. The resins were inactive unless combined with a bentonite and a zeolite which were in themselves active; however, the tripartite combination exerted an antilysozyme activity far in excess of that accountable from a consideration of individual activities.

MEDICAL AND CLINICAL SECTION

Introductory

There is little question that peptic ulcer can best be treated by the multiple approach. Few clinicians today dispute this point and all of the reports dealing with the use of anion exchange resins in peptic ulcer treatment emphasize the necessity of a polyphasic regimen. The purpose of this monograph is not to review the relative merits of antispasmodics, dietary regimens, psychotherapies and similar adjuvants but to underline the discussion of the anion exchangers with the statement that there is no ideal therapy and that no single therapeutic agent is sufficient unto itself for all cases.

The clinical reports which will be considered are without exception based upon radiologically diagnosed peptic ulcer. It is the consensus of clinicians that no other criterion is acceptable.

A fundamental premise acceptable to all clinicians is that the prime and immediate responsibility is to provide symptomatic relief from pain and regression of the ulcer crater by medical means if possible. Another such premise is that one-third of uncomplicated duodenal ulcers will heal spontaneously without any special treatment (Hall and Hornisher, 1950). Certainly, the principles of Sippy—rest, neutralization of free acid, and relief of spasm—are basic (Jordan, 1947).

Therapeutic Effect

Therapeutically, anion exchange resins in the hands of Spears and Pfeiffer (1947) gave 96.6 per cent pain relief and in excess of 70 per cent ulcer crater healing. In this series, aside from restrictions on the use of alcohol, tobacco and coarse or highly seasoned food, no dietary limitations were imposed, and no medications other than the anion exchange resins were used. It is remarkable that the relief of pain following the administration of the resin in capsules occurred in general within 5 to 10 minutes. These authors emphasize that the relief of pain does not necessarily indicate healing. It is the present author's opinion that the evidence they present is not conclusive on this point. Healing of an ulcer crater will involve many factors other than the protection of the area from acid and enzyme; such factors as protein nutrition, amino acid supply, capillary strength and spasticity will play a vital role. Spears and Pfeiffer (1947) felt that failure of the resin to produce relief from the symptoms of pain was virtually diagnostic of disease other than peptic ulcer.

The studies of Kraemer (1948) were conducted over an extended period following his initial report (Kraemer and Lehman, 1947). The findings parallel in the broader sense those of Spears and Pfeiffer. The dosage regimen was modified in that dietary restriction was more rigid and both atropine sulfate and phenobarbital were used. In this group, 100 duodenal ulcer patients were observed for periods of from 1 to 17 months. Eighty-five per cent of all ulcer patients on the regimen were kept symptom-free.

Emphasis is placed by Kraemer (1948) on the advisability of keeping patients on ulcer regimens (continued use of antacids and antispasmodics) for many years in order to prevent recurrences. Recurrence of gastric ulcer is regarded as an invitation to malignancy, and the rationale of continued measures to guard against this probability can hardly be denied. It is here that above all else the patient must be assured of a regimen involving an absolute minimum of side effects; the anion exchange resins offer a resolution of the problem from the standpoint of the antacid to be elected.

Another feature of the Kraemer report lies in his use of resins in ulcer patients who have severe hemorrhages. He lists 6 such patients who responded well to resin therapy. Many physicians are reluctant to use particulate matter in such patients, but certainly Kraemer has proved that this objection does not apply to anion exchange resins.

Confirmation of the symptomatic relief afforded by anion exchange resins to the peptic ulcer patients came with the report of Peters (1948). As was done in the Kraemer series, Peters used dietary restriction and antispasmodics in addition to the resin, and found that some 88 per cent of his series of 25 cases were satisfactorily controlled. With relatively small doses of resin, he found relief of pain occurred in 5 to 15 minutes and continuous relief within 4 days. The period of observation in this series was from 2 to 11 months. The opinion is expressed by Peters that the resins give at least as good clinical results as other antacids, without the undesirable side effects. Although he warns that complications may develop in patients while under treatment with resin, this situation obtains for any therapeutic regimen employed.

Using anion exchangers as medication, Weiss (1948) gave an average figure of 10 to 14 days as ulcer regression time (from initiation of treatment to radiological cure). Symptomatic relief occurred in from 1 to 8 days. Comparison of healing time with that attributable to aluminum preparations and other conventional methods led Weiss to conclude that the resins were superior. Of his series of 44, 3 were gastric ulcer patients and failed to respond to resin therapy. It is not improbable that the use of capsules is not indicated in gastric ulcer treatment where immediate effect is desired. With these patients, resin powder or suspension should be employed, as no element of time will then need to elapse before the resin is free to act.

Recurrence rate following the use of anion exchange resins seems identical with that following any similar drug. For example, Marks (1949) reported 2 recurrences, one in 3 months and one in the first week following discontinuance of therapy. His series comprised some 30 patients. It does not seem reasonable to assume that recurrence rate can be correlated with the drug or antacid used, since recurrence will

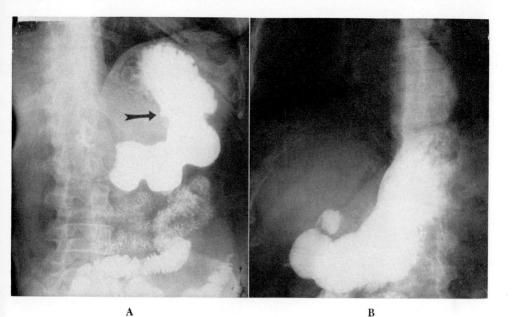

A. Case 1. X-ray upon admission. Note ulcer niche on lesser curvature.
B. Case 1. X-ray taken prior to discharge. Niche has receded.

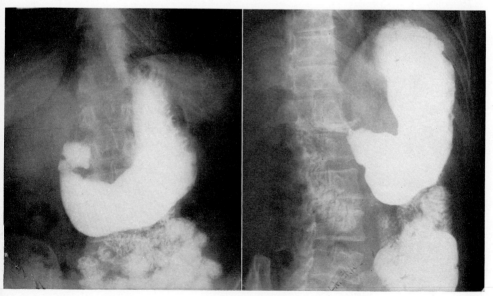

C. Case 1. Readmitted 1 week after being discharged.
D. Case 1. Recent x-ray, negative.

FIGURE 13

(From Weiss, S., *et al.*, *Rev. Gastroenterol.*, **16**:501, 1949*a*)

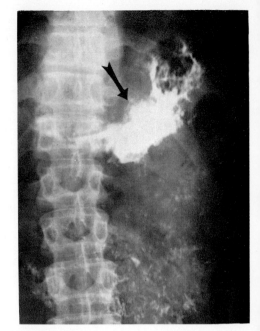

E. Case 2. Mucosal study, 4 days
prior to hospitalization.

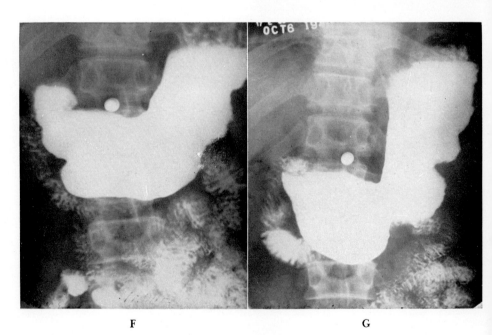

F   G

F. Case 2. Fifteen days after hospital admission. No evidence of niche seen
in E.

G. Case 2. Four and one-half months later.

FIGURE 13 (*Continued*)

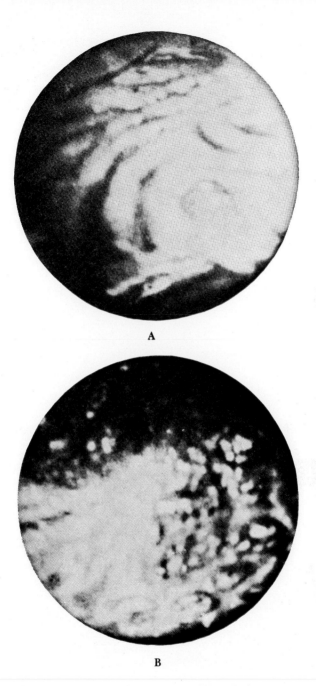

A. Gastrophotograph of mucosa coated by Resinat.
B. Gastrophotograph of mucosa coated by other substance.

FIGURE 14

(From Weiss, S., *et al.*, *Rev. Gastroenterol.*, **16**:501, 1949*a*)

depend in large measure upon the emotional and general health status of the patient in the intervening period.

The premise that the peptic ulcer patient is a psychosomatic problem cannot be denied. The report of Martin (1949) serves to emphasize this aspect. Of 100 peptic ulcer patients in this series, 61 were diagnosed as psychiatrically normal and 39 as abnormal. The results of a multiphasic approach involving resins gave 87 per cent radiological cures in the normal and only 30 per cent in the psychiatrically abnormal group. The entire group consisted of veterans, among whom peptic ulcer exceeds all other gastrointestinal diseases as a cause for discharge from the army (Kantor, 1942). Martin's series consisted of patients who had had x-ray diagnosed ulcers for periods of 2 or more years. All of these patients had been subjected to various other forms of standard therapy. Ninety-one per cent were afflicted by duodenal ulcers. A weight gain averaging 11 lbs. occurred in 77 of the patients under treatment for a period of 6 months. In explanation of the relative ineffectiveness of the therapeutic regimen in the psychiatric patient, Martin offers the observation that such patients will not follow the prescribed regimen.

The work of Demole and Wissmer (1949) and Demole *et al.* (1950) is of such preliminary nature as to add nothing to the scope of the general subject.

The results of Weiss *et al.* (1949a, b), covering 120 patients, establish the period for symptomatic relief following resin use at 48 to 72 hours and the time interval for complete regression of ulcer crater at 2 to 4 weeks. This work emphasizes the coating action of the exchange resins as revealed by gastroscope and the gastrophotor. (Figures 13 and 14.)

As detailed case histories often give valuable information not subject to generalization, two case histories (Cases 1 and 2) from the paper of Weiss *et al.* (1949a) and two (Cases 3 and 4) from the report of Bergen and Greenberg (1950) are here reproduced.

Case 1

F.G., age 66, housewife, white. First developed stomach trouble about nine years ago. At that time, she had positive x-ray evidence of peptic ulcer with all the clinical symptoms. Since then she has had recurrent attacks of pain in midepigastrium, controlled by medication and diet. For the past four months, patient had almost steady pain in midepigastrium and right upper quadrant extending to the back and occurring one hour after eating. The pain was relieved by

TABLE 17
**Case Histories of 100 Peptic Ulcer Patients Treated
with Anion Exchange Resin**

(From Martin, C. L., unpublished data, 1949)

Patient No.	Age at 1st diag.	Status*	Date pos. x-ray diag., start of treatment	Type of ulcer†	Hematemesis or melena‡	Psychiatric diagnosis§	No. days before ulcer symptoms relieved	X-ray evidence of healing‖	Lbs. gained in about 6 mos.	Comments
1	24	NC,US	3/48	D	HM	N	1	N	—	No constipation
2	30	NC,US	3/48	D	—	N	None	—	—	Patient entered T.B. sanitarium 4/48
3	28	NC,US	3/48	D	—	N	3	N	15	Severe constipation cleared in 2 wks.
4	30	NC,O	3/48	D	—	P	None	C	—	Entered Letterman G.H. 11/43, x-ray neg.
5	31	NC,US	3/48	D	—	N	2	S	11	Mental inst. 3 wks.' treatment
6	37	NC,US	3/48	D	—	P	1	DS & C	−6	Divorced month before x-ray
7	22	NC,O	3/48	D	—	N	3	N	9	Constipation on Al(OH)₃ cleared in 2 wks. with Resinat
8	24	C	3/48	D	H	N	6	C	4	None
9	31	C	3/48	D	—	N	1	N	22	Constipation on Al(OH)₃ cleared in 3 wks. with Resinat

* NC,O—noncombat, overseas; NC,US—noncombat, U.S.; C—combat, enemy fire.
† D—duodenal; S—stomach; M—marginal.
‡ H—hematemesis; M—melena.
§ N—normal; P—psychoneurosis; S—schizophrenia.
‖ N—no ulcer visualized; C—crater formation still present; S—scarring of duodenum; CS—crater and spasm; DS—duodenal spasm.

TABLE 17 (*Continued*)

Patient No.	Age at 1st diag.	Status*	Date pos, x-ray diag., start of treatment	Type of ulcer†	Hematemesis or melena‡	Psychiatric diagnosis§	No. days before ulcer symptoms relieved	X-ray evidence of healing‖	Lbs. gained in about 6 mos.	Comments
10	38	NC,US	3/48	D	—	P	None	DS & C	−4	X-ray neg. Ft. Lewis 1/44. Heavy psychic overlay
11	24	NC,US	3/48	D	—	N	4	C	−8	Constipation on $Al(OH)_3$ relieved in 1 wk. with Resinat
12	23	NC,US	3/48	D	—	P	1	N	12	Heavy psychic overlay
13	41	NC,O	3/48	D	—	P	1	DS & C	1	Heavy psychic overlay
14	32	NC,O	3/48	D	HM	N	4	N	16	Nausea intermittent on Resinat
15	36	NC,O	3/48	D	—	N	2	N	8	Constipation cleared in 1 wk. with Resinat
16	23	NC,O	3/48	D	—	N	3	N	15	Relief 1 wk. Resinat. Constipation on $Al(OH)_3$
17	31	NC,US	3/48	D	—	N	3	N	8	No constipation
18	33	NC,US	3/48	D	M	N	1	N	11	No constipation
19	28	NC,US	3/48	D	M	N	1	C	−1	None
20	30	C	3/48	D	—	P	None	C	−6	Patient did not follow treatment
21	40	NC,US	3/48	D	—	P	None	C	1	X-ray neg. Letterman G.H. 7/43. Did not follow treatment

* NC,O—noncombat, overseas; NC,US—noncombat, U.S.; C—combat, enemy fire.
† D—duodenal; S—stomach; M—marginal.
‡ H—hematemesis; M—melena.
§ N—normal; P—psychoneurosis; S—schizophrenia.
‖ N—no ulcer visualized; C—crater formation still present; S—scarring of duodenum; CS—crater and spasm; DS—duodenal spasm.

TABLE 17 (*Continued*)

Patient No.	Age at 1st diag.	Status*	Date pos. x-ray diag., start of treatment	Type of ulcer †	Hematemesis or melena‡	Psychiatric diagnosis§	No. days before ulcer symptoms relieved	X-ray evidence of healing‖	Lbs. gained in about 6 mos.	Comments
22	23	NC,O	3/48	D	—	N	1	N	16	No constipation
23	21	NC,US	3/48	D	—	N	1	N	8	No constipation
24	33	NC,O	3/48	D	HM	N	2	DS	9	No constipation
25	34	NC,US	3/48	D	—	N	2	DS	16	No constipation
26	33	NC,US	2/48	D	—	P	2	S	9	Treatment started 4/48
27	36	NC,US	3/48	D	H	S	None	C	−14	Treatment started Apr. Remission of schizophrenia
28	29	NC,O	4/48	D	—	N	3	N	4	Constipation on Al(OH)₃ cleared in 2 wks. with Resinat
29	41	NC,US	4/48	D	—	N	1	N	9	No constipation
30	37	NC,US	4/48	D	—	P	3	C	0	Constipation
31	34	NC,O	1/48	S	H	N	2	N	18	Treatment started 4/48
32	27	NC,US	4/48	D	—	P	3	C	8	Took Resinat 1 mo. only
33	34	NC,US	4/48	D	—	N	1	N	4	No constipation
34	30	NC,US	4/48	D	—	P	None	C	0	Heavy psychic overlay
35	33	NC,O	4/48	D	—	P	1	C	−8	G.I. study neg. San Diego N.H. 7/43. No constipation
36	21	NC,US	4/48	D	HM	N	6	N	9	Constipation not relieved with Resinat

* NC,O—noncombat, overseas; NC,US—noncombat, U.S.; C—combat, enemy fire.
† D—duodenal; S—stomach; M—marginal.
‡ H—hematemesis; M—melena.
§ N—normal; P—psychoneurosis; S—schizophrenia.
‖ N—no ulcer visualized; C—crater formation still present; S—scarring of duodenum; CS—crater and spasm; DS—duodenal spasm.

TABLE 17 (*Continued*)

Patient No.	Age at 1st diag.	Status*	Date pos. x-ray diag., start of treatment	Type of ulcer†	Hematemesis or melena‡	Psychiatric diagnosis§	No. days before ulcer symptoms relieved	X-ray evidence of healing‖	Lbs. gained in about 6 mos.	Comments
37	29	NC,US	11/47	D	—	N	2	N	16	Regimen started 4/48. No constipation
38	22	NC,O	4/48	D	—	P	3	N	8	Constipation relieved in 2 wks. with Resinat
39	25	NC,O	4/48	D	—	P	1	N	5	Constipation on Al(OH)$_3$ relieved in 1 wk. with Resinat
40	27	NC,US	4/48	D	—	N	7	S	9	Discharged 11/43. Apparent ulcer cure
41	26	NC,US	4/48	D	H	P	None	DS	3	G.I. series neg. 3/42 U.S. Nav. Hosp., Seattle
42	33	NC,O	4/48	D	H	N	2	N	8	No constipation
43	31	NC,US	4/48	D	H	P	14	DS	0	No constipation
44	30	NC,US	4/48	D	—	N	1	N	9	Constipation on Al(OH)$_3$ relieved in 2 wks. with Resinat
45	30	NC,O	4/48	D	—	N	2	N	20	No constipation
46	27	NC,O	4/48	D	—	N	1	DS	14	No constipation
47	22	NC,US	3/48	D	—	P	3	S	30	Treatment started 4/48. No constipation
48	22	NC,US	3/48	D	M	P	1	N	9	Treatment started 4/48. No constipation

* NC,O—noncombat, overseas; NC,US—noncombat, U.S.; C—combat, enemy fire.
† D—duodenal; S—stomach; M—marginal.
‡ H—hematemesis; M—melena.
§ N—normal; P—psychoneurosis; S—schizophrenia.
‖ N—no ulcer visualized; C—crater formation still present; S—scarring of duodenum; CS—crater and spasm; DS—duodenal spasm.

TABLE 17 (*Continued*)

Patient No.	Age at 1st diag.	Status*	Date pos. x-ray diag., start of treatment	Type of ulcer†	Hematemesis or melena‡	Psychiatric diagnosis§	No. days before ulcer symptoms relieved	X-ray evidence of healing‖	Lbs. gained in about 6 mos.	Comments
49	22	NC,US	1/48	D	—	P	1	DS	6	Treatment started 4/48. Constipation stopped 1 wk. Resinat
50	26	NC,O	4/48	D	M	N	2	N	10	Diarrhea relieved
51	24	NC,O	4/48	D	—	N	6	N	11	No constipation, some nausea
52	23	NC,US	4/48	D	H	N	2	S	4	No constipation
53	31	NC,US	4/48	S	—	P	14	DS	7	Heavy psychic overlay. No constipation
54	33	NC,O	4/48	D	—	N	3	N	3	Constipation on Al(OH)₃ relieved in 2 wks. with Resinat
55	38	NC,O	4/48	D	—	P	1	N	3	Constipation on Al(OH)₃ relieved in 2 wks. with Resinat
56	38	NC,O	4/48	D	—	P	3	DS	1	No constipation, no diarrhea
57	37	NC,US	4/48	D	—	N	7	N	0	No constipation, no diarrhea
58	30	NC,US	4/48	D	M	N	2	N	18	No constipation, no diarrhea
59	23	NC,O	4/48	D	M	N	1	N	3	Constipation on Al(OH)₃ relieved in 2 wks. with Resinat

* NC,O—noncombat, overseas; NC,US—noncombat, U.S.; C—combat, enemy fire.
† D—duodenal; S—stomach; M—marginal.
‡ H—hematemesis; M—melena.
§ N—normal; P—psychoneurosis; S—schizophrenia.
‖ N—no ulcer visualized; C—crater formation still present; S—scarring of duodenum; CS—crater and spasm; DS—duodenal spasm.

TABLE 17 (*Continued*)

Patient No.	Age at 1st diag.	Status*	Date pos. x-ray diag., start of treatment	Type of ulcer†	Hematemesis or melena‡	Psychiatric diagnosis§	No. days before ulcer symptoms relieved	X-ray evidence of healing‖	Lbs. gained in about 6 mos.	Comments
60	40	NC,US	4/48	M	M	P	None	C	−3	Gastroenterostomy 10/44, poorly functioning anastomosis. No relief
61	21	NC,US	4/48	D	—	N	2	DS	9	Constipation continued
62	34	NC,O	4/48	D	—	N	1	N	8	No constipation, no diarrhea
63	23	NC,US	4/48	D	—	P	None	Vagotomy	−3	Since operation, excessive gas, excessive burning bowel movements. Blacking-out spells
64	31	NC,O	4/48	S	—	N	1	N	11	No constipation, no diarrhea
65	38	NC,US	4/48	D	—	N	5	N	8	Constipation on Al(OH)₃ relieved in 1 wk. with Resinat
66	40	NC,O	5/48	D	—	N	1	DS	3	Treated overseas with cure. Recurrence 1948
67	28	NC,O	5/48	S	—	P	None	No x-ray	—	X-ray neg. Letterman G. H. 4/44, moved to N.Y. after 1 wk.

* NC,O—noncombat, overseas; NC,US—noncombat, U.S.; C—combat, enemy fire.
† D—duodenal; S—stomach; M—marginal.
‡ H—hematemesis; M—melena.
§ N—normal; P—psychoneurosis; S—schizophrenia.
‖ N—no ulcer visualized; C—crater formation still present; S—scarring of duodenum; CS—crater and spasm; DS—duodenal spasm.

TABLE 17 (*Continued*)

Patient No.	Age at 1st diag.	Status*	Date pos. x-ray diag., start of treatment	Type of ulcer†	Hematemesis or melena‡	Psychiatric diagnosis§	No. days before ulcer symptoms relieved	X-ray evidence of healing‖	Lbs. gained in about 6 mos.	Comments
68	28	NC,US	5/48	D	—	P	None	Vagotomy	0	Diarrhea, excessive gas, bloating, postoperatively
69	29	NC,O	5/48	D	—	N	5	N	5	No constipation, no diarrhea
70	41	NC,US	5/48	M	—	N	7	C	0	Gastroenterostomy 6/47. No constipation
71	24	NC,O	5/48	D	HM	N	1	DS & C	3	No co-operation after 1st wk.
72	32	C	5/48	D	—	N	3	N	8	No constipation, no diarrhea
73	41	NC,US	5/48	D	H	P	None	C	−3	Diarrhea, due to mucous colitis not controlled
74	31	NC,O	5/48	D	—	P	3	C	−4	No constipation, no diarrhea
75	26	NC,O	5/48	D	—	P	None	C	−9	G.I. series neg. Ft. Ord 5/44. Heavy psychic overlay, financial, family troubles
76	33	C	5/48	D	—	N	3	N	8	No constipation
77	30	NC,O	5/48	D	—	N	3	DS	8	Constipation on Al(OH)$_3$ cleared in 1 wk. with Resinat

* NC,O—noncombat, overseas; NC,US—noncombat, U.S.; C—combat, enemy fire.
† D—duodenal; S—stomach; M—marginal.
‡ H—hematemesis; M—melena.
§ N—normal; P—psychoneurosis; S—schizophrenia.
‖ N—no ulcer visualized; C—crater formation still present; S—scarring of duodenum; CS—crater and spasm; DS—duodenal spasm.

TABLE 17 (*Continued*)

Patient No.	Age at 1st diag.	Status*	Date pos. x-ray diag., start of treatment	Type of ulcer†	Hematemesis or melena‡	Psychiatric diagnosis§	No. days before ulcer symptoms relieved	X-ray evidence of healing‖	Lbs. gained in about 6 mos.	Comments
78	33	NC,O	5/48	D	—	P	None	C	1	Did not follow treatment
79	22	NC,US	5/48	D	H	N	7	N	8	No constipation
80	36	NC,US	5/48	D	HM	P	None	DS & C	0	X-ray neg. San Diego N.H. Heavy psychic overlay
81	38	NC,US	5/48	D	—	N	1	N	2	No constipation
82	30	NC,US	5/48	S	—	N	1	N	16	Constipation on Al(OH)$_3$, cleared in 1 wk. with Resinat
83	26	NC,US	5/48	D	—	N	1	N	5	No constipation
84	26	NC,O	5/48	D	H	P	None	C	1	Followed treatment
85	23	NC,US	6/48	D	H	N	2	S	8	No constipation
86	31	NC,US	6/48	D	H	S	None	DS & C	0	X-ray neg. Letterman G.H. 10/44
87	31	NC,O	6/48	D	—	N	2	S	8	Constipation continued with Resinat
88	22	NC,US	6/48	D	—	P	2	S	6	No constipation
89	37	NC,O	6/48	D	—	P	2	C	-5	No constipation
90	30	NC,O	6/48	D	—	N	1	N	1	No constipation
91	23	NC,US	6/48	S	—	N	1	C	3	No constipation
92	25	NC,O	6/48	S	—	N	1	N	8	Constipation relieved with Resinat

* NC,O—noncombat, overseas; NC,US—noncombat, U.S.; C—combat, enemy fire.
† D—duodenal; S—stomach; M—marginal.
‡ H—hematemesis; M—melena.
§ N—normal; P—psychoneurosis; S—schizophrenia.
‖ N—no ulcer visualized; C—crater formation still present; S—scarring of duodenum; CS—crater and spasm; DS—duodenal spasm.

TABLE 17 (*Continued*)

Patient No.	Age at 1st diag.	Status*	Date pos. x-ray diag., start of treatment	Type of ulcer†	Hematemesis or melena‡	Psychiatric diagnosis§	No. days before ulcer symptoms relieved	X-ray evidence of healing‖	Lbs. gained in about 6 mos.	Comments
93	37	NC,US	6/48	D	—	P	None	C	−1	No complaint of stomach until 5/45, when small crater found. Didn't co-operate
94	30	C	6/48	D	HM	N	1	N	4	No constipation
95	27	NC,O	6/48	D	—	P	None	DS	18	No constipation
96	31	NC,O	6/48	D	—	P	None	DS	8	Diarrhea stopped with Resinat
97	24	NC,US	6/48	D	H	N	3	N	7	No constipation
98	32	NC,US	6/48	D	—	N	3	N	18	Constipation on $Al(OH)_3$ relieved in 1 wk. with Resinat
99	33	NC,O	6/48	D	H	N	1	N	31	No constipation, no diarrhea
100	26	C	6/48	D	HM	N	3	N	9	No constipation, no diarrhea

* NC,O—noncombat, overseas; NC,US—noncombat, U.S.; C—combat, enemy fire.
† D—duodenal; S—stomach; M—marginal.
‡ H—hematemesis; M—melena.
§ N—normal; P—psychoneurosis; S—schizophrenia.
‖ N—no ulcer visualized; C—crater formation still present; S—scarring of duodenum; CS—crater and spasm; DS—duodenal spasm.

milk and alkalis. The patient also complained of heartburn, nausea and vomiting, and reported a loss of six pounds within the past four months. No tarry stool or jaundice was present.

Physical examination: Patient was well developed, slightly pale and dehydrated. Her past history contributed nothing remarkable. Blood pressure 190/90; tenderness upon pressure in midepigastrium and right upper quadrant; no masses felt in the abdomen. Blood studies: Hemoglobin: 79 per cent; Red Blood Cells: 3,970,000; White Blood Cells: 7,600—Differential: Polymorphonuclear Neutrophils: 50 per cent; Lymphocytes: 48 per cent; Basophils: 2 per cent. Blood chemistry showed an increased sedimentation rate: 20 mm.; and prolonged prothrombin time: 75 seconds (Stypven method); decreased total proteins: 4.8 Gm.; and normal blood amylase, serum lipase and urea nitrogen. Occult blood in feces (meat-free diet 3 days) positive, gastric analysis showed hyperchlorhydria: free hydrochloric acid: 70; total acid: 86.

X-ray department reported hypertrophic gastric rugae with an ulcer niche on the lesser curvature. The duodenal cap showed spasticity but no evidence of lesion. The patient was given atropine gr. $\frac{1}{200}$ morning and evening by hypodermic; 300 mg. of ascorbic acid by mouth daily and, because of the increased prothrombin time, 6 mg. Vitamin K daily. The diet was a soft convalescent ulcer diet.

Patient showed remarkable improvement twenty days after hospital admission. X-rays taken prior to discharge showed recession of niche.

One week after discharge, patient was readmitted to the hospital with the same symptoms.

Diet at this time consisted of milk and orange juice–jello mixture and the following medication was prescribed: two capsules of Resinat every two hours, atropine gr. $\frac{1}{200}$ by hypodermic, morning and evening. Three days later, the patient showed considerable improvement and twelve days later she was discharged, completely asymptomatic. Eight days after discharge, patient had x-rays taken, which showed no evidence of ulcer. Patient has been followed up for the past seven months and has had no recurrence of symptoms. X-rays taken recently are negative.

The patient has followed a soft diet, with Resinat capsules four times a day. Her blood count is within normal range, and there is no occult blood in the feces. Patient has recovered her original weight and feels very well. When interviewed 15 Feb. 1949, she was well, asymptomatic and had gained considerable weight. Occasionally, she takes Resinat capsules.

Case 2

T.M., fifty-year-old Japanese dentist, was admitted to the hospital, April 12, 1948, complained of epigastric pain which occurred one hour after eating. The pain lasted for two to three hours and was relieved by milk or alkalis. This pain started three weeks ago and would occasionally wake him from sleep. Also, the patient complained of heartburn, feeling of fullness, and had lost approximately five pounds during the three week period. Patient was pale, undernourished, slightly dehydrated and chronically ill. There was no evidence of tarry stools, or jaundice. Physical examination disclosed a normal blood pressure, pulse and temperature. There was tenderness upon pressure in midepigastrium, but no masses were felt in the abdomen.

Routine urine analysis was negative—Hemoglobin was 85 per cent; Red Blood Cells: 4,320,000; White Blood Cells: 6,200—Differential: Polymorphonuclear Neutrophils: 71 per cent; Lymphocytes: 28 per cent; Basophils: 1 per cent. Three-day meat-free-stool was positive for occult blood, gastric analysis showed free hydrochloric acid 62; total acid: 87; Blood: positive. Blood chemistry showed a slightly increased sedimentation rate: 18 mm.; and prolonged prothrombin time: 46 seconds (Stypven method). Blood sugar: 87 mg.; total proteins: 6.05 Gm.; urea nitrogen: 15 mg.

X-ray films taken four days before hospital admission showed a large cone-shaped ulcer niche on the lesser curvature approximately 1½ cm.; the duodenal cap was normal.

Patient was kept on duodenal feedings for ten days with a special formula of protolysate mixture—4 oz. every 2 hours, two Resinat capsules every two hours, and B-complex and Vitamin C—300 mg. Also he was given gr. ½₀₀ atropine by hypodermic, morning and evening.

After ten days, he was given milk and orange juice–jello mixture, which was continued until his discharge.

X-rays taken on April 27th, fifteen days after hospital admission, showed no evidence of niche seen on previous films—only slight irregularity of the antrum due to antral gastritis. Gastric analysis was: free hydrochloric acid 28, total acid 45; for occult blood: negative.

Patient was discharged completely asymptomatic nineteen days after his admission. He was advised to follow the convalescent ulcer diet, rest two weeks at home and then to reduce his working hours and take two capsules of Resinat two or three times daily for twenty days each month.

X-ray of patient, October 6, 1948, 6 months after admission to the hospital and approximately 4½ months after previous x-rays, showed no evidence of ulcer niche. Feels well and is asymptomatic.

Case 3

M.B., a thirty-six-year-old white male, had had intermittent epigastric pain for ten years, relieved by food and particularly milk. Due to excessive milk intake, he had gained 100 pounds in the previous two years. In the six weeks prior to his first visit, his pain had become constant and severe, and he had been drinking up to 6 quarts of milk daily.

Abdominal distention and fingertip tenderness in the midepigastrium were observed on examination. X-ray revealed a niche at the lesser curvature in the prepyloric region with mucosal swelling and a duodenal cap with a tendency to hammerhead deformity.

He was treated for six weeks with conventional antacids and diet without relief. He continued to drink up to 6 quarts of milk daily, and his weight rose to 300 pounds.

On September 29, 1947, Resinat, 0.5 Gm. every two hours, was prescribed with no benefit. The dose of Resinat powder was then increased to 3 Gm. every two hours, day and night. On this dosage of 36 Gm. daily he obtained rapid relief of symptoms.

At the present writing, the patient is on a maintenance dose of 3 Gm. three times daily and has lost 100 pounds as a result of the prescribed diet. X-ray on April 29, 1948, showed the niche in the prepyloric region still present. A subsequent x-ray on January 1, 1949, did not show the prepyloric ulcer previously visualized. The hammerhead deformity of the duodenal cap persisted.

Case 4

W.B., a well-developed and well-nourished, twenty-six-year-old white male, complained of intermittent upper abdominal pain of seven years duration, with exacerbations lasting one to one and one-half months and remissions of four to five months. The pain was described as "hunger" pain and occurred about one hour after meals and at two or three o'clock in the morning. The pain was aggravated by fried or spicy foods and relieved by milk, sodium bicarbonate, and Amphojel.

Physical examination revealed marked point tenderness in the abdomen 3 inches above the umbilicus in the midline. X-rays on October 16, 1948, revealed a persistently deformed duodenal bulb which failed to fill completely with barium. Resinat powder, 1 Gm., was prescribed after each meal and at bedtime and antispasmodic tablets before meals and at bedtime. One week after therapy was begun the patient was asymptomatic.

X-rays after three months of therapy showed that the duodenal cap filled much more completely than in the first films, although persistent filling defects were still noted. The patient continued treatment and remained asymptomatic despite many violations of his dietary regimen. When x-rayed again after five months of treatment, the films showed that the duodenal cap now filled completely

While confirming in general the efficacy of anion exchange resins in the treatment of peptic ulcer, Bargen (1950) emphasized the value of this therapy in cases having a combination of duodenal ulcer and ulcerative colitis. Symptomatically, he found that both the typical discomfort of the peptic ulcer and the severe abdominal cramps associated with the colitis were relieved by proper use of resins.

In 1948, Cummins *et al.* proposed the determination of the time of healing of a peptic ulcer as a baseline for the evaluation of any given therapeutic regimen. Healing time was defined as the interval between original visualization of the ulcer crater and the disappearance of the crater following initiation of treatment. Hall and Hornisher (1950) adopted this criterion in making a direct comparison of the merits of colloidal aluminum hydroxide and anion exchange resins. Comparing average healing times for 33 peptic ulcer patients on resins and 17 on aluminum hydroxide, they found that the values were 19 and 33.7 days respectively. This means that the resin-treated group "healed" in 14.7 days less time than the group on aluminum hydroxide. The figure of 33.7 days to disappearance of ulcer crater compares closely with the figure of 37 days given by Cummins *et al.* (1948) for a comparable group of patients.

TABLE 18

Comparison of a Group of Ambulatory Ulcer Patients Treated with an Anion Exchange Resin and a Group Treated with Aluminum Hydroxide Gel

(From Wirts, C. W., *et al.*, *Gastroenterology*, **15**: 1, 1950)

	Anion exchange resin	Aluminum hydroxide gel
Number of patients	24	20
Males	20	16
Females	4	4
Pain relief		
Good	19	13
Poor	5	7
Constipation	2	10
Ulcer healed	21	16
Ulcer not healed	3	4
Recurrence	6	5
Complications	2	2

The study of Hall and Hornisher (1950) involved two groups of patients whose treatment varied only in that one received an anion exchange resin while the second received colloidal aluminum hydroxide. The age grouping was comparable, and all of the patients in the entire series showed craters in the first part of the duodenum. The only point of variance was in the duration of symptoms, which for the resin group was 4.16 years and for the aluminum hydroxide group 2.33 years. This would if anything have presented a more refractory group for treatment with the exchangers.

Wirts and Rehfuss (1950) and Wirts *et al.* (1950), in addition to subdividing each group into aluminum hydroxide-treated and resin-treated, carried their studies through a series of ambulant and semi-ambulant patients. The semiambulant patients were all hospitalized and therefore subject to detailed study.

Figures for the ambulant group in this study are given in Table 18. Eighty per cent of their patients were relieved of pain and 90 per cent

TABLE 19

Cumulative Per Cent of Patients Well Calculated from the Number from Each Group Symptom-free

(From Moseley, V., and W. G. Coker, Jr., *South. M. J.*, 44: 610, 1951)

Antacid	Hospital cases (wks.)				Outpatient cases (wks.)			
	1st	*2nd*	*3rd*	*4th+*	*1st*	*2nd*	*3rd*	*4th+*
Resin								
Total 33	46.6%	86.6%	93.3%		22.2%	55.5%	72.2%	
Hosp. 15								
OPD 18								
Actual no.								
cases symp-								
tom-free	7	6	1	1	4	6	3	5
Magnesium								
trisilicate								
Total 23	23.7%	61.5%	84.6%		60%	70%	90%	
Hosp. 13								
OPD 10								
Actual no.								
cases symp-								
tom-free	3	5	3	2	6	1	2	1
Aluminum								
hydroxide								
Total 44	51.7%	79.3%	93.1%		0%	20%	33.3%	
Hosp. 29								
OPD 15								
Actual no.								
cases symp-								
tom-free	15	8	4	2	0	3	2	10

healed in the sense of ulcer crater disappearance. The corresponding figures for the aluminum hydroxide–treated group were 65 per cent and 80 per cent respectively. The recurrence rate was 25 per cent in the aluminum hydroxide and resin groups.

In the semiambulant group, there were 13 resin-treated and 11 aluminum hydroxide gel-treated patients. Elapsed time to relief of symptoms was 10 days for the resin and 14 days for the gel. Similarly, time to crater disappearance was 30.1 days for resin-treated and 33.3 days for gel-treated patients. While the authors conclude that these figures indicate approximately the same rate in both groups, it would seem that the resin proved definitely superior to the gel in both spheres.

The results of Segal *et al.* (1950) add little to the general picture. In patients with recurrent peptic ulcer, 17 of 26 experienced clinical remissions and 3 had temporary relief. Patients with complications showed relief of symptoms in 5 out of 15 cases, but there were no clinical remissions. As Segal *et al.* point out, it is hardly to be expected that

TABLE 20
Results of Follow-up X-Ray Studies

(From Moseley, V., and W. G. Coker, Jr., *South. M. J.*, **44:** 610, 1951)

			Healed 7 wks. or less		No change	
Antacid	X-rayed	Not x-rayed	No.	%	No.	%
Resin	15	18	15	100	0	0
Aluminum hydroxide	25	19	22	88	3	12
Magnesium trisilicate	10	13	9	90	1	10
Total	50	50	46	92	4	8

where peptic ulcers occur with complications, an antacid would produce clinical remissions. Based upon the report of Wirts and Rehfuss (1950), Segal *et al.* (1950) indicate their belief that the resins might fail to raise gastric pH and still aid in keeping the pH of the duodenal area above the critical range.

Mosely and Coker (1951) made a direct comparison of the therapeutic efficacy of aluminum hydroxide, magnesium trisilicate and anion exchange resins in a series of approximately 100 peptic ulcer patients. Tables 19 and 20, from their paper, summarize the findings. From these tables, it is seen that the figures for duration of symptoms after starting treatment are 14.8 days for the resin group, 13.4 days for the magnesium trisilicate group, and 25.9 days for the aluminum hydroxide group. Figures for percentage healed within seven weeks showed 100 per cent for the resin, 88 per cent for the aluminum hydroxide, and 90 per cent for the magnesium trisilicate groups. The authors conclude that both anion exchange resins and magnesium trisilicate are superior to aluminum hydroxide in therapeutic efficacy.

Dosage Regimen

Typical dosage schedules in the cases reported by Spears and Pfeiffer (1947) were 6.4 Gm. (2 tablespoonfuls) ½ hour after meals and at bedtime, or 0.5 Gm. (2 capsules) every hour and from 1.5 to 2.0 Gm. (6 to 8 capsules) at bedtime. In their series, the dose range was from 0.5 to 102 Gm. per day; 6.4 Gm. of the resin powder was the maximum well-tolerated dose. Beyond this, the patient was apt to gag or experience a feeling of fullness.

Kraemer (1948) relied upon a multiple approach to ulcer therapy, employing his special diets, which are modified in accordance with the patient's status—hospitalized, ambulant or quiescent. In all regimens, however, he recommends the ingestion of 0.75 Gm. of resin at intervals equally spaced, to give a total of 4.5 to 6.0 Gm. daily. In addition, 0.3 mg. of atropine sulfate and 15.0 mg. of phenobarbital are given four times daily (before each meal and on retiring).

Dosage of any antacid will vary markedly with the patient, and the anion exchange resins are not excepted. Kraemer (1948) and Spears and Pfeiffer (1947) used doses which were large compared to those employed by Peters (1948), who gave 0.25 to 0.5 Gm. of resin after meals and at bedtime. Similarly, Weiss (1948) used 0.25 Gm. of the resin every hour during the waking period and about 1.5 Gm. at bedtime. Peters recommended the use of antispasmodics with the resin; Weiss did not.

The extreme in the adoption of the multiple approach to therapy of peptic ulcers was reported by Martin (1949), who gave 15 drops of tincture of belladonna and 30 mg. of phenobarbital three times daily along with milk, amino acids and a modified diet. Such a plethora of medicaments would raise the question of the possibility of ascribing any specific effect to any single medication, were it not for the fact that all of these patients had been on a regimen involving the use of aluminum hydroxide and this regimen was subsequently modified only through the change from the aluminum preparation to the anion exchange resin. All other factors remained constant.

The regimen employed by Weiss *et al.* (1949*a*) was multiphasic and involved the use of resins in doses of 0.5 Gm. given hourly for 1 or 2 weeks, followed by 0.25 to 0.5 Gm. every 2 or 3 hours during the day. If the patient could not take capsule or powder a duodenal tube was passed, and, following aspiration and lavage with plain water, approximately 5 Gm. of anion exchange resin powder were placed in 4 oz. of water and permitted to drip slowly through the tube. During the period, the patient was told to change his position to permit a more thorough coating of the mucosal surfaces. Repetition of this once or twice weekly was the practice until relief was obtained.

Hall and Hornisher (1950) employed the general principles of the Sippy regimen and in addition gave 0.25 Gm. of resin every 2 hours from 7 A.M. to 9 P.M., totaling about 2 Gm. daily.

A dosage regimen which seems in general to reflect the consensus is that of Wirts *et al.* (1950), who started by giving 8 oz. of milk, or milk and cream, every 2 hours from 8 A.M. to 9 P.M. At each alternate 2-hour period, 1 Gm. of resin powder was given. In addition, 15 drops of tincture of belladonna and 15 mg. of phenobarbital were given at spaced intervals four times daily. When the pain was under control, the sedative and antispasmodic were withdrawn; the antacid was continued.

Segal and his associates (1950) express the opinion that 1 Gm. of resin does not represent an adequate dose. They propose the use of 2-Gm. doses given at intervals of 2 hours with or without milk.

Effect on Free Acid, Gastric pH and Enzymatic Activity

The first recorded studies of gastric acidity as affected by anion exchange resins were those of Spears and Pfeiffer (1947), who studied a series of 25 fasting adult patients following the ingestion of an Ewald test meal. The stomach tube was permitted to remain *in situ* and resin was administered. Subsequent examination of the samples showed that 0.25 Gm. of resin reduced the free acidity, but only for a short period (5 to 10 minutes). In their series, a dose of 6.4 Gm. repeated twice (30-minute interval) was necessary to reduce the free acid value to zero for an hour or more.

Lowered acid formation after histamine stimulation was reported by Lentini *et al.* (1950) following the administration of 15 to 20 Gm. of anion exchange resins daily. The work of these investigators, however, is of a preliminary nature only and therefore cannot be regarded as more than indicative.

The extensive and detailed investigations of Wirts and Rehfuss (1950) covered every phase of gastrointestinal physiology and bio-chemistry concerned in the application of anion exchange resins in the treatment of peptic ulcer. Their goal was that of simulating the most difficult conditions arising clinically for which the resin would be ap-plied. Further, a direct comparison was made involving Sippy powder (0.6 Gm.), aluminum hydroxide (0.6 Gm.) and anion exchange resin (3.2 Gm.).

The first phase of their work involved a study of the effect of these materials following histamine stimulation. Each patient served as his own control in that a series of determinations for acid and peptic activity were made without an antacid and again following the ad-ministration of each of the three antacid materials under consideration. A group of ulcer patients (20) and a group of normal persons (21) were included in each of the experimental series. The results of these experiments are partially summarized in Figure 15. The second phase of the experiments involved insulin stimulation of gastric secretion in ulcer (15) and nonulcer (15) patients. Figure 16 partially summar-izes the results of this experiment.

The general conclusion to be drawn from the reported results is that the anion exchange resin neutralizes acid and inactivates pepsin in the gastric juice of both ulcer and nonulcer patients. The effect is similar whether the stimulation to secretion is from histamine or insulin. Wirts and Rehfuss (1950) used both procedures, as histamine is known to produce the greatest acid secretion and insulin a gastric juice higher in pepsin. In general, the effects of the aluminum hydroxide and Sippy powder paralleled those of the anion exchange resins. Minor variations were noted but regarded by the investigators as lacking significance.

Using a double-lumened tube, Wirts and Rehfuss (1950) studied the pH, free acid and pepsin in samples taken simultaneously from the stomach and the duodenum. In the ulcer patients, the average fast-ing pH value was somewhat lower than in the normal (4.5 compared to 5.5). There was no direct correlation among pH, free acid and pep-sin values in stomach and duodenum. Following the administration of resin, the free acid and pepsin levels in the duodenum dropped while the pH rose. Figure 17 presents average values for free acid, pepsin and pH in gastric and duodenal juices obtained by simultaneous sampling and subsequent analysis.

Segal *et al.* (1950) reported that 1 Gm. of anion exchange resin was not consistently effective in modifying gastric pH; however, 2 Gm.

FIGURE 15
Average Free Acid and Pepsin Curves Following
Histamine Stimulation (Repeated Dose),
Comparing the Effect of Antacids During the
Second Hour in Ulcer Patients

H represents histamine administration and A represents antacid administration.

(From Wirts, C. W., and M. E. Rehfuss, *J. Clin.
Investigation*, 29: 37, 1950)

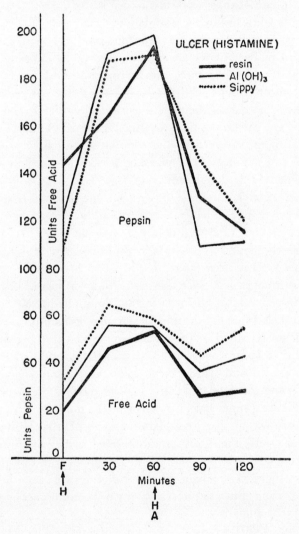

FIGURE 16
Average Free Acid and Pepsin Curves, Comparing the Effect of Insulin Stimulation with Antacids (Resin, Aluminum Hydroxide and Sippy) and Without (Plain) in Ulcer Patients

I represents insulin administration.

(From Wirts, C. W., and M. E. Rehfuss, *J. Clin. Investigation*, 29: 37, 1950)

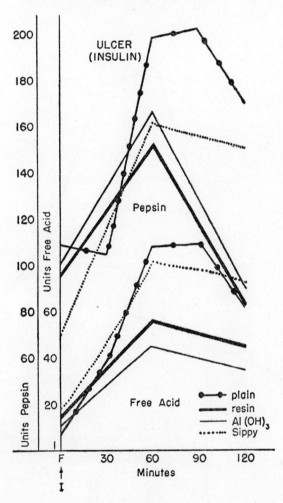

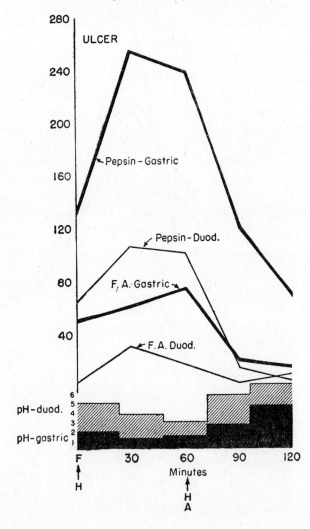

FIGURE 17
Average Free Acid, Pepsin and pH Values Found
in Gastric and Duodenal Juice Obtained
Simultaneously in Ulcer Subjects
Histamine (H) stimulation was given after the fasting contents were removed and again at 60 minutes. The resin (A) was also given at 60 minutes.

(From Wirts, C. W., and M. E. Rehfuss, *J. Clin. Investigation,* **29:** 37, 1950) were practically constant in raising the pH from 1 to around 5 or 6. Total acid and free acid were markedly reduced by the 2-Gm. dose.

Comparative studies are always of great significance in permitting evaluation of medications. Moseley and Coker (1951) have studied the effect of antispasmodics and antacids on gastric pH. The antispasmodics (Banthine and atropine) failed to affect gastric pH following an alcohol test meal; 100 ml. of milk and cream mixture adequately raised pH for a period of 1 hour. This effect was not aided by adding 15 Gm. of protein digests to the milk-cream mixture. These researchers therefore determined to investigate the potentialities of adding various antacids to the milk-cream mixture and found that the standard ones (aluminum hydroxide, magnesium trisilicate and anion exchange resins) were indicated as additions to the procedure, as they extended the period of elevation of gastric pH.

It will be recalled that Moss and Martin (1948) failed to observe any significant capacity of anion exchange resins to inhibit lysozyme at a pH comparable to that of gastric juice, even of gastric juice as modified by resin therapy. Greenblatt *et al.* (1951) state that one such resin, Deacidite, does in fact inhibit lysozyme; however, their studies were carried out at pH values above 6.6 and this pH is rarely if ever attained in the stomach. Furthermore, tests conducted by Moss and Martin (1948) demonstrated that Deacidite did not differ in any respect from other anion exchangers relative to capacity for lysozyme inhibition.

Miscellaneous

There is an added value to the use of anion exchange resins in combination with antispasmodics; this had been under investigation for many years by Sullivan and Martin (1950). These workers found that both anion and cation exchange resins adsorbed or absorbed atropine and similar antispasmodic materials (Sullivan and Martin, 1951). *In vivo,* the acute toxicity of atropine sulfate was markedly reduced when given with the anion exchange resin, indicating a slow release of the toxic chemical with consequent prevention of accumulation in lethal amounts at a given time in the blood stream.

Clinically, Kraemer (1948) had implied the value of such an approach in his suggestion that a more even absorption of alkaloids from the digestive tract would follow when these were combined with resins. The validity of this position has been established by Martin (1950), who found the combined therapy superior in efficacy to the use of either antispasmodics or resins alone.

Side Effects

While Spears and Pfeiffer (1947) reported that 25 per cent of their patients showed gagging, and 7 per cent nausea, it must be recalled that these investigators were dealing with the first resin offered for clinical trial and that subsequent findings demonstrated the trace contaminants and led to their removal. They reported diarrhea in a single case and no instance of constipation. This is a point of tremendous importance, as the popular antacids of the aluminum type are without exception markedly constipating.

These investigators noted no effect of the resin on removal of phosphate and chloride ions from the body fluids and did not observe any acid rebound.

Kraemer (1948) re-emphasized the lack of patient complaints regarding constipation and diarrhea in his series of 100. Further, there was freedom from bloating and gas. Another feature of great importance was the absence of any effect on acid-base balance. The importance of side effects was underscored by Kraemer and Siegel (1947) in their listing of the disadvantages of the more commonly used antacids:

1. The salts of aluminum, bismuth and calcium are constipating.
2. The salts of magnesium are laxative and cause perianal burning.
3. Sodium bicarbonate is absorbed and predisposes to alkalosis and the formation of kidney stones.
4. All of the carbonates bring on belching as their carbon dioxide is released by hydrochloric acid.
5. The aluminum salts have an astringent taste, are expensive, and since they appear to exert their best influence in liquid suspension, they must be taken in large amounts.

Undesirable side effects of anion resins were listed by Peters (1948) as gagging, nausea and fullness in the stomach. No percentage figures were given, but the statement was made that these were "not common." Weiss (1948) observed no single instance of diarrhea or constipation in his series of 44 patients. Confirmation of the findings of Weiss on the point of the complete absence of side effects came with the report of Marks (1949), who found no complications developing in his series of 30 cases.

As most gastroenterologists find aluminum preparations constipating in some degree, it is interesting to note that Martin (1949) found that the vast majority of patients who had experienced constipation on the previous medication were restored to normality after taking the resin.

FIGURE 18
Average Curves of Free Acid, Comparing the Effect
of Antacids Without Gastric Stimulation
The antacids were given immediately after the fasting samples were taken.

(From Wirts, C. W., and M. E. Rehfuss, *J. Clin. Investigation,* **29:** 37, 1950)

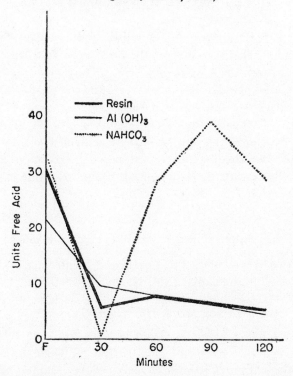

Detailed studies of blood, urine and bile chemistry carried out by Weiss *et al.* (1949*a*) failed to reveal any changes. While of their 120 patients, 8 manifested nausea or constipation, it was felt by these research clinicians that this was coincidental and not due to the use of the resins.

Among the serious complications of the use of soluble alkalis in the treatment of peptic ulcer is the acid rebound. In order to evaluate this factor following use of sodium bicarbonate, aluminum hydroxide and anion exchange resins, Wirts and Rehfuss (1950) compared average values for free acid in 14 patients after administration of these agents and found that no acid rebound occurred with resin or with aluminum hydroxide. Figure 18 shows clearly the marked acid rebound following the administration of sodium bicarbonate and the absence of this complication with the two other antacids employed.

Another unpleasant side effect of many antacids is their tendency to prolong gastric emptying time, thereby disturbing normality of gastrointestinal function. Using a radio-opaque meal and continuous fluoroscopic examination, Wirts and Rehfuss (1950) demonstrated that anion exchange resins have no significant effect on gastric emptying time.

Wirts *et al.* (1950) treated hospitalized and ambulant patients and reported a remarkable record for the resins relative to aluminum hydroxide gels from the standpoint of constipation. For example, of 24 patients in the ambulant group treated with resins, some 17 started out with marked constipation, a complaint overcome in all but 2. By contrast, of 20 patients on an aluminum hydroxide group, 15 were constipated at the outset and 10 of these remained so throughout the experiment. Constipation due to aluminum preparations was also a serious problem with the hospitalized group, requiring laxatives for correction.

Other Clinical Applications of Anion Exchange Resins

One of the groups studied by Spears and Pfeiffer (1947) comprised 23 patients with abdominal pain due to one of the following conditions: gastritis, hyperchlorhydria, carcinoma, sarcoma, allergy, spasm, renal or gallbladder disease. Of this group, 11 were relieved of their pain at least temporarily. As would be expected, pain relief did not preclude the necessity for individual treatment. These authors suggest that the mechanism of pain induction in those instances wherein the resin had a nonspecific pain-relieving effect might be the same as in peptic ulcer.

In 1949, Gounelle and Teulon reported on a group of 21 patients suffering from gastralgias (apparently acute gastritis) which were treated by anion exchange resins. These patients showed no evidence of organic lesions as seen radiologically, and had generally been treated with belladonna, choleretics and similar material prior to the use of resins. In the dose used (5 to 15 Gm. daily), the resin caused a disappearance of pain in 16 cases (76 per cent). It also suppressed dyspeptic disorders, flatulence, nausea and vomiting. In a single case, a nettle rash of alimentary origin was cleared up. Generally, the first ingestion of the resin was completely effective. A point of importance lies in the efficacy of the resins in patients with normal gastric acid, which strongly suggests unknown factors in the action of resins. A potential use of resin to increase patient tolerance of medications such as salicylates and p-aminosalicylic acid is advanced by these investigators.

Weiss *et al.* (1949a) greatly extended the sphere of application of anion exchange resins by utilizing these agents in chronic hypertrophic gastritis, simple hyperacidity, heartburn, cholecystic conditions with dyspepsia and in some forms of colitis. In heartburn due to gastric hyperacidity or in gallbladder disease, the patient was directed to take 0.25 to 1.0 Gm. at intervals, dependent upon the severity of the symptoms. In some instances, a duodenal tube was passed using the same procedure as in peptic ulcer (see section on dosage regimen), with the exception that the patient was instructed to use the powder through an open drip.

One clinical application of resins of the anionic type is in the control of the skin irritation around an enteroabdominal fistula (Bargen, 1950). This condition develops as a result of the continuous flow of digestive juices onto the skin surrounding the fistula and is extremely difficult to control, with resultant marked discomfort to the patient. Bargen recommends sprinkling the resin onto the skin or patting it on in a thick layer and states that this procedure results in "greater comfort to the patient than many of the substances in common use." In his experience, the pleasant effect was attributed to the absorbing of irritating fractions of the excreta and to the fact that none of the unpleasant side effects commonly seen following ointments and other powders resulted.

Kasdon (1948) applied the anion exchange resin in the treatment of heartburn during pregnancy. The rationale was based upon the concept that the etiology of heartburn is regurgitation of gastric contents into the distal end of the esophagus, which irritates the sensitive neural endings. The controls were treated with Prostigmine (15-mg. tablets) and the experimental resin series received one or two doses of 250 mg. each of the anion exchanger. Thirty-one out of 35 patients on the resin were relieved. This compares favorably with the results

TABLE 21

Anion Exchange Resins in Peptic Ulcer Therapy

No. Patients	Dose	% Pain relief	% Radiologically healed	Average time to radiological cure	Reference
30	0.5 Gm. every hr. and 3 or 4 Gm. at bedtime	96.7%	70%	Not determined	Spears and Pfeiffer, 1947
100					
18 hospitalized 82 ambulant	0.75 Gm. each 2nd hr. (4.5–6.0 Gm. daily)	85% 92%	Not determined	—	Kraemer, 1948
44	0.25 Gm. every hr., 1.2–2.0 Gm. at night	91%	88%	10–14 days	Weiss, 1948
25	0.25–0.5 Gm. after meals and at bedtime	Satisfactory progress 88% in 4 days	Not determined	—	Peters, 1948
30	0.5–1.0 Gm. every 2 hrs.	83.2%, 76.6% in 5 days	—	—	Marks, 1949
100 61 psychiatrically normal 39 psychiatric	0.5 Gm. after meals and 1 Gm. at bedtime	96.5% in 3 days, 48% in 3 days	87% 30%	—	Martin, 1949

No.	Dosage	Response	%	Duration	Reference
120	0.5 Gm. each hr. for 1–2 weeks, then 0.25–0.5 Gm. each 2–3 hrs.	Excess of 90% in 48–72 hrs.	Excess 80%	2–4 wks.	Weiss, *et al.*, 1949
33	0.25 Gm. each 2 hrs. (2 Gm. daily)	100% in 5.8 days, limited 14 cases	100%	19 days	Hall and Hornisher, 1950
10	1–3 Gm. at mealtime and bedtime	100%	Not stated	—	Bergen and Greenberg, 1950
37 24 ambulant 13 semiambulant	1 Gm. every 2 hrs. (7–8 Gm. daily)	80–87% in 10 days	Ambulant 90% Semiambulant 100%*	1–3 mos. 30.1 days	Wirts et al., 1950
26	2.0 Gm. every 2 hrs. (14 Gm. daily)	77%	Not stated	—	Segal et al., 1950
33	0.5 Gm. every hr.	85% in 14.8 days	15 included 100%	7 wks. or less	Moseley and Coker, 1951
30	3 Gm. before each meal and 3–5 Gm. evening (20 Gm. daily)	86% in 48 hrs.	73%	2–6 wks.	Greenblatt *et al.,* 1951

* Not specifically stated.

obtained with Prostigmine. In fact, in Kasdon's patients if no relief was obtained with resin none was obtained with Prostigmine. The elapsed time to full relief was generally about 10 minutes.

Safety

Twelve patients in the Spears and Pfeiffer (1947) series received an average of 1 to 2 Gm. of the resin daily for a period of 12 months with no adverse effects. One patient had received 32 Gm. of the resin daily for the period and showed no loss in weight, change in blood count, urinalysis, sedimentation rate or fecal examination findings. Doses as high as 102 Gm. were given daily for a limited period without complications. Kraemer and Lehman (1947) also studied blood and urine of patients on anion exchange resins without finding any evidence of toxicity; further, there were no sensitivity reactions.

The possibility that anion exchange resins might damage the gastric mucosa was eliminated by the observations of Kraemer (1947) and Weiss (1948), who examined the mucosa of patients gastroscopically and following resection. All of these patients had been on resin therapy for several months.

All other investigators (Peters, 1948; Weiss, 1948; Weiss *et al.*, 1949*a*; Bergen and Greenberg, 1950; Hall and Hornisher, 1950) attest to the nontoxicity and lack of sensitivity effects of the anion exchange resins.

RECAPITULATION AND COMMENT

The major clinical indication for anion exchange resins is in the field of peptic ulcer management. Doses vary widely, but average 0.25 to 0.5 Gm. every hour from 8 A.M. to 9 P.M., a total of from 3 to 6 Gm. in a 24-hour period. It is difficult to understand why McChesney *et al.* (1951) gave the figure of 25 Gm. daily as the recommended dose. In general, the clinicians have used a multiphasic approach including an antispasmodic, a barbiturate and a modified diet. There can be little question of the logic of this procedure. (See Table 21.)

The superiority of the anion exchange resins over the colloidal aluminum hydroxide composition lies in the absence of side effects. Constipation almost precludes the continued use of aluminum preparations, but continuing treatment is specifically indicated for the prevention of the recurrence of ulcers. Many clinical men recommend continuation of antacid treatment for a period of 1 year following disappearance of the ulcer crater. Such conservative treatment seems to offer some insurance against recurrence and ultimate surgery. The same case holds for the antispasmodics when used as the sole therapeutic factor; namely, side effects are severe and the speed of healing and relief of pain are not significantly superior. From the available clinical evidence there seems little question but that the anion exchange resins represent the agent of choice in the treatment of peptic ulcer.

The capacity of the anion exchange resins can probably be increased by a factor of two. Further, the way seems open to liquid forms of these resins, and it is probable that such forms will improve patient acceptability for all ion exchangers even in large doses. Although we do not at present have the ideal resin for the purpose, we do utilize the best available, the polyamine formaldehyde types.

Another possibility for the future lies in the application of anion exchange resins with antispasmodics adsorbed upon their surfaces. The result will be a slow liberation of the antispasmodic, preventing side effects and yet permitting full antacid and antipepsin activity on the part of the resinous materials. The multiphasic approach may indicate the adsorption in a similar manner of barbiturates, providing a three-pronged attack upon a problem of complex nature.

The chances are that even the use of antacids, antispasmodics, barbiturates and modified diets would not constitute a therapeutic regimen of sufficiently broad spectrum to approach the optimal. The healing of an ulcer must involve strong and healthy capillaries, and this depends upon many factors, key among which are the bioflavonoids and vitamin C. Further, availability of amino acids and proteosynthetic enzymes is important and can be improved by proper supplementation with intact proteins or high protein diets.

REFERENCES

ALPERT, S., and G. J. MARTIN. *Am. J. Dig. Dis.*, 16: 10, 1949.

ALPERT, S., and G. J. MARTIN. *Rev. Gastroenterol.*, 17: 251, 1950.

BARGEN, J. A. *Gastroenterology*, 16: 507, 1950.

BERGEN, O. M., and A. GREENBERG. *New York State J. Med.*, 50: 1495, 1950.

CUMMINS, G. M., M. I. GROSSMAN, and A. C. IVY. *Gastroenterology*, 10: 714, 1948.

DEMOLE, M. G., MILHAUD, and B. WISSMER. *Helvet. med. acta*, 17: 460, 1950.

DEMOLE, M., and B. WISSMER. *Rev. méd. Suisse Rom.,* 69: 591, 1949.

DRAGSTEDT, L. R. *Arch. Surg.,* 44: 438, 1942.

DRIVER, R. L., R. H. CHAPPELL, and E. B. CARMICHAEL. *Am. J. Dig. Dis.,* 12: 166, 1945.

GOUNELLE, H., and H. TEULON. *Bull. mém. Soc. méd. hôp. Paris,* 65: 319, 1949.

GOUNELLE, H., and H. TEULON. *Presse méd.,* 58: 1254, 1950.

GRACE, W. J., P. H. SETON, S. WOLF, and H. G. WOLFF. *Am. J. M. Sc.,* 217: 241, 1949.

GRACE, W. J., S. WOLF, and H. G. WOLFF. *Gastroenterology,* 14: 93, 1950.

GREENBLATT, I. J., M. JACOBI, and T. D. COHEN. *Am. J. Dig. Dis.,* 18: 362, 1951.

HALL, A. A., and C. J. HORNISHER. *Gastroenterology,* 16: 181, 1950.

HAY, L. J., R. L. VARCO, C. F. CODE, and O. H. WANGENSTEEN. *Surg., Gynec. Obst.,* 75: 170, 1942.

HERRIOTT, R. M. *J. Gen. Physiol.,* 24: 325, 1941.

JERZY GLASS, G. B., B. L. PUGH, W. J. GRACE, and S. WOLF. *J. Clin. Investigation,* 29: 12, 1950.

JORDAN, S. M. *Gastroenterology,* 9: 237, 1947.

KANTOR, J. L. *J.A.M.A.,* 120: 254, 1942.

KASDON, S. C. *New England J. Med.,* 239: 575, 1948.

KRAEMER, M. *Postgrad. Med.,* 2: 431, 1947.

KRAEMER, M. *Connecticut M. J.,* 12: 305, 1948.

KRAEMER, M., and D. J. LEHMAN, JR. *Gastroenterology,* 8: 202, 1947.

KRAEMER, M., and L. H. SIEGEL. 96th Annual Session, A. M. A., Atlantic City, N. J., June 9–13, 1947.

LENTINI, S., U. GIANGRANDI, and G. PAMPANELLI. *Minerva Med.,* 41: 1024, 1950.

LEVEEN, H. H. *Proc. Soc. Exper. Biol. Med.,* 63: 254, 1946.

LEVEEN, H. H. *Gastroenterology,* 8: 648, 1947.

LEVEEN, H. H., and L. HALLINGER. *J. Clin. Investigation,* 26: 761, 1947.

MCCHESNEY, E. W., F. C. NACHOD, and M. L. TAINTER. *J. Am. Pharm. A. (Scient. Ed.)* 40: 193, 1951.

MANN, F. C., and J. L. BOLLMAN. *J.A.M.A.,* 99: 1576, 1932.

MARKS, J. A. *Rev. Gastroenterol.,* 16: 82, 1949.

MARTIN, C. L. Unpublished data, 1949.

MARTIN, C. L. Unpublished data, 1950.

MARTIN, G. J. *Am. Druggist,* 116: 84, 1947.

MARTIN, G. J. *Am. J. Dig. Dis.,* 18: 16, 1951.

MARTIN, G. J., and J. WILKINSON. *Gastroenterology,* 6: 315, 1946.

MATZNER, M. J., C. WINDWER, A. E. SOBEL, and S. H. POLAYES, *Proc. Soc. Exper. Biol. Med.,* 34: 243, 1936.

MEYER, K., A. GELLHORN, J. F. PRUDDEN, W. L. LEHMAN, and A. STEINBERG. *Am. J. Med.,* 5: 482, 1948a.

MEYER, K., A. GELLHORN, J. F. PRUDDEN, W. L. LEHMAN, and A. STEINBERG. *Am. J. Med.,* 5: 496, 1948b.

MOELLER, H. C., H. C. MARSHALL, and J. B. KIRSNER. *Proc. Soc. Exper. Biol. Med.,* 76: 159, 1951.

MOSELEY, V., and W. G. COKER, JR. *South. M. J.,* 44: 610, 1951.

MOSS, J. N., and G. J. MARTIN. *Am. J. Dig. Dis.,* 15: 412, 1948.

PATTERSON, W. B., and DE WITT STETTEN, JR. *Science,* 109: 256, 1949.

PETERS, A. G. *Acta Gastroenterol. Belg.,* 11: 136, 1948.

REIFENSTEIN, R. W., S. J. Gray, H. M. SPIRO, C. G. YOUNG, and E. P. CONNOLLY. *Gastroenterology,* 16: 387, 1950.

SCHIFFRIN, M. J., and A. A. WARREN. *Am. J. Dig. Dis.,* 9: 205, 1942.

SEGAL, H. L., H. A. FRIEDMAN, E. E. ELLIS, and J. S. WATSON, JR. *Am. J. Dig. Dis.,* 17: 293, 1950.

SEGAL, H. L., H. HODGE, J. S. WATSON, JR., and W. J. M. SCOTT. *Gastroenterology,* 4: 484, 1945.

SPEARS, M. M., and M. C. J. PFEIFFER. *Gastroenterology,* 8: 191, 1947.

SULLIVAN, M. J., and G. J. MARTIN. *Am. J. Pharm.,* 122: 48, 1950.

SULLIVAN, M. J., and G. J. MARTIN. U.S. Patent 2,554,072, May 22, 1951.

VANZANT, F. R., A. E. OSTERBERG, W. C. ALVAREZ, and A. B. RIVERS. *J. Clin. Investigation,* 12: 557, 1933.

WEISS, J. *Rev. Gastroenterol.,* 15: 826, 1948.

WEISS, S., R. B. ESPINAL, and J. WEISS. *Rev. Gastroenterol.,* 16: 501, 1949a.

WEISS, S., R. B. ESPINAL, and J. WEISS. *Rev. Gastroenterol.,* 16: 336, 1949b.

WILKINSON, J., and G. J. MARTIN. *Arch. Biochem.,* 10: 205, 1946.

WIRTS, C. W., and M. E. REHFUSS. *J. Clin. Investigation,* 29: 37, 1950.

WIRTS, C. W., B. H. SULLIVAN, and W. C. HAMMERLY. *Gastroenterology,* 15: 1, 1950.

CHAPTER 6

Medical Applications of
Cation Exchange Materials

SYMPTOMATIC of various disorders, edema is associated with fluid increase in extracellular spaces. Any such increase is undesirable and may, with the appearance of "pitting edema," become dangerous. In general, a sudden weight gain not otherwise accounted for may be ascribed to water imbalance arising from some basic pathologic alteration.

Although many conditions are associated with edema (such as increased capillary pressure, diminished colloid osmotic pressure of the blood, increased osmotic pressure in the tissues, and increased capillary permeability), we are concerned here only with those related in origin to sodium retention: e.g., edema of congestive heart failure, hypertension and cirrhosis. What underlies the altered physiological state responsible for sodium retention is not clear. There are renal factors, including diminished filtration and increased reabsorption, and there are many other correlatives, including general cationic and anionic composition of the cellular and blood milieu. Whatever the primary cause, retention of sodium is synonymous with edema, and it was recognition of this fact which led to the adoption of the low sodium diet and to the use of mercurial diuretics.

Of all diuretics, the mercurials alone have so far become of importance in the control of edematous states, due to the peculiar ability to alter renal physiology so as to prevent reabsorption of sodium from the tubule, with consequent excretion. But valuable though they are, we must concede certain drawbacks in the unavoidable toxicity and the recognized difficulty of administration. The low sodium diet, because of its monotony, is not readily followed by the patient. These limitations have made imperative the discovery of a more adaptable procedure.

In 1944, our laboratories undertook the study of ion exchange resins. The anion exchange resins found their natural application in the removal of hydrochloric acid from gastric content and in the treatment of peptic ulcer. The cation exchange resins seemed to offer the potential for sodium removal, and study was initiated.

The chemistry of the cation exchange resins is considered in detail in Chapter 3. In summary, in the formation of a cation exchange resin, substituted benzoic acid molecules may be condensed with formaldehyde, forming long chains of carbon-to-carbon units. At intervals, depending upon the conditions of the reaction, cross-linkages occur. These cross-linkages unite one chain to another and actually form the insoluble resinous macromolecule. Exchange occurs through the pores of the gel-like structure, and involves the carboxyl groups or other similar acidic radicals. The ionic character of the group is the same in the resin as it is in a simple organic compound. If we consider benzoic acid as the prototype, the reactions of the carboxylic radical of benzoic acid parallel exactly and obey the same law of mass action as do the carboxyl groups of the complex resin unit.

Cation exchange resins possess constant powers of exchange for different cations when such cations are simple metallic ions. Divalent cations are bound more strongly than the univalent, and in each series the strength of binding by the exchanger increases as the atomic weight increases. In other words, exchange is not selective but dependent upon atomic weight, valence, concentration and other physicochemical factors.

IN VIVO LABORATORY STUDIES

The first researches undertaken *in vivo* were those of Dock (1946), who reported results of balance studies in animals. He found that fecal sodium loss varied from 3.3 to 5.1 mg. per kilogram per day. By adding a cation exchanger, the values were raised to from 34 to 64 mg. per kilogram daily. The sodium uptake on the resins used, which were of the sulfonic type, was 20 to 30 mg. per gram of resin. Most of the sulfonic types of resins have a maximum exchange capacity of 5 mEq. per gram, which is approximately 115 mg. per gram of resin.

Dock apparently did not feel optimistic about the potentialities of cation exchange resins, and so for a period of three years and until others took up the line of approach no further work was published. Then, in 1949, Crismon presented his findings. He used a sulfonated polystyrene resin, fed at a 10 per cent level, and reported that the capacity of the resin to reduce sodium absorption was from 96 to 70 per cent when the animals were on a high sodium diet and from 96 to 34 per cent when on a low sodium diet. Somewhat similar figures were given for potassium balance. Plasma sodium and potassium values were essentially normal, but the corresponding figures for muscle showed a reduction.

By 1950, the potentialities of the field had been recognized and several detailed balance studies were published. Ch'en and Freeman (1950) used three sulfonic-type resins (Nalcite, Duolite C-3 and Amberlite IR-100H), with *in vitro* capacities ranging from 2.25 to 4.01 mEq. per gram. The affinity of any one of these resins decreased from calcium, to potassium, to sodium. Further, these workers observed that the uptake of an individual cation was more of a function of its affinity for the resin than of its ionic concentration.

For their *in vivo* experiments, they employed three diets varying in salt content; the high sodium diet contained 27.5 mEq. of sodium per 100 grams of diet, the low sodium diet contained 8.98, and the salt-free diet contained no sodium. The experimental design involved the use of conditioning periods during which adjustment could be made by the rat to a new diet, and each period had corresponding control and experimental diets. For purposes of comparison, the data are assembled

TABLE 22
Cation Removal by Sulfonic Resins (All Values per 100 Gm. of Ingested Diet or of Diet)

(Modified from Ch'en, J. S., and S. Freeman, *J. Lab. Clin. Med.*, 35: 99, 1950)

Diets	Cations	*Millimoles of fecal cation*			*Millimoles of dietary cation*		
		A Control	B Duolite	C Amberlite	A Control	B Duolite	C Amberlite
High salt diet	Na	3.72	11.32	7.44	27.55	28.05	27.71
	K	3.59	8.36	5.89	17.71	17.73	17.74
	Ca	16.65	16.08	16.33	17.71	17.81	17.84
	Total	23.96	35.76	29.66	—	—	—
Low salt diet	Na	0.95	5.31	3.84	8.98	9.49	9.14
	K	3.45	7.10	5.50	17.71	17.73	17.74
	Ca	14.83	13.72	14.40	17.71	17.81	17.84
	Total	19.23	26.13	23.78	—	—	—
Salt-free diet	Na	0.18	4.75	4.46	0.0	0.51	0.16
	K	0.69	10.00	9.32	0.0	0.02	0.03
	Ca	1.29	3.90	3.71	0.56	0.59	0.64
	Total	2.16	18.65	17.49	—	—	—

in Table 22, which is a modified form of the presentation used by Ch'en and Freeman (1950).

From the table it is seen that cation excretion via the feces is increased by the hydrogen cycle resin whether the diet is high in sodium or low. While a similar situation holds for the potassium balance, it does not seem to follow for calcium. As Ch'en and Freeman indicate, calcium balance is somewhat difficult to ascertain, since the major portion of ingested calcium is not normally absorbed but rather remains in the tract in the form of insoluble phosphate combinations. One point of great interest is the observation that calcium content of the diet markedly modifies the capacity of the resin to remove mono-valent cations such as potassium. This is striking in the case of potas-sium fecal excretion and is marked for sodium excretion, conclusions reached from a comparison of the fecal sodium and potassium figures for the low salt diet and for the salt-free diet. In the latter, the calcium content is lowered to about 3 per cent, and in spite of essential absence of potassium and sodium from the diet the fecal sodium and potassium either remain the same or, for potassium, are actually elevated. This is significant in reference to the work of Martin *et al.* (1953), who demonstrated that the chelation of calcium and other polyvalent ca-tions increased the capacity of a resinous cation exchanger for mono-valent cations.

Several additional points are made by Ch'en and Freeman from an analysis of their data. One of these is that hydrogen cycle cation ex-changers of the sulfonic type do not modify phosphorus metabolism; another refers to the fact that resins *in vivo* do not manifest more than a fraction of their *in vitro* capacity. For Duolite, the *in vivo* capacity was 1.44 millimoles, as contrasted to an *in vitro* capacity of 3.5. This would indicate that about 40 per cent of the potential capacity had been utilized. Of the *in vivo* total capacity of 1.44 millimoles, 0.24 millimole was taken up by calcium. If calcium could be eliminated as a factor, the efficiency of the resin would be increased by about 20 per cent. This analysis is made for future reference related to the use of chelators for polyvalent cation removal. If the total exchange capacity could be directed toward sodium alone, for Duolite the amount of sodium removed by 1 Gm. of resin would be 3.5 millimoles; whereas in fact the amount is 0.46 millimole or only about 14 per cent.

It is desired to underscore this point, as it is abundantly clear that the future line of research should be toward increase in the *in vivo* efficiency of resins and not the *in vitro* capacity. The latter may be of some importance, but comparatively speaking it is not the key.

Also in 1950, the results of McChesney and McAuliff were pub-lished. They used sulfonic and carboxylic types of cation exchange resins and varied the dietary content from 5 to 15 per cent. This range of resin content of the diet did not modify the cation uptake per gram of resin administered. For the carboxylic type resin (Amberlite XE-64), they reported *in vivo* capacity as 1.3 mEq. for sodium, 0.6 mEq. for potassium, and 0.6 mEq. for calcium; the corresponding figures for the sulfonic type (Win 3,000) were 0.65, 0.30 and 0.0

mEq. This would give the carboxylic type a decided advantage over the sulfonics, had not McChesney *et al.* (1951) indicated that these figures were found to be inaccurate by their subsequent investigations.

These investigations presented some evidence indicating that the sulfonic type of resin lost less of its capacity than did the carboxylic when both were employed with a low sodium diet. This aspect, if established, would be of importance to the clinical use of such resins; however, more extensive studies would be essential to the establishment of the point. Furthermore, clinical evidence would not seem to substantiate this position. One point does seem clear from this and subsequent work, and it is that negative sodium balance cannot be induced through the use of cation exchange resins. After 21 days on a low sodium diet containing 10 per cent resin, the blood levels of sodium and potassium were normal; however, muscle content of sodium was below normal.

Hegsted *et al.* (1951) agree only in part with the findings of McChesney and McAuliff (1950) and those of Crismon (1949). The major point made is that results of resin testing will vary as the diet employed varies. They conclude that with the sulfonic resins the cations bound are primarily, and in fact almost exclusively, those of exogenous origin. Further, the binding of these dietary cations in the upper intestinal tract does not permit subsequent establishment of an equilibrium with the cation composition of the digestive fluids. In the view of the present author, this does not seem a sound position because the kinetics of ion exchange would almost ensure the establishment of an equilibrium in the lower bowel. This should be particularly true of a strong-acid ion exchanger of the sulfonic type. One point made by Hegsted *et al.* (1951), to the effect that the sulfonic type binds cations in the acid gastric juice, seems unquestionable. Theoretically, this would differentiate the weak-acid and the strong-acid types, in that the strong-acid type would bind in the gastric juice, whereas the weak-acid carboxylic type would not begin to exchange until the pH had shifted toward the alkaline side and had in fact reached a pH of approximately 8.0. Strangely enough, the potentiality suggested by these facts, that combinations of sulfonic and carboxylic resins would be superior in capacity, has not been borne out by clinical observation (see clinical section of this chapter).

Selective removal of sodium or at least the aspect of differential selectivity proposed by McChesney and McAuliff (1950) is not confirmed by the results of Hegsted *et al.* (1951), who conclude that the ratio of sodium to potassium in the feces of resin-fed rats is essentially the ratio of these two cations in the diet.

One novel feature of the work of Hegsted *et al.* (1951) concerned the induction of weight loss when resin was added to a diet relatively low in sodium and minerals in general. The addition to this regimen of any given cation in sufficient amount counteracted the weight loss. In this connection, sodium, potassium, calcium and magnesium were tried and all proved effective; the two monovalent cations were, however, quantitatively more effective than the divalent cations tested.

As indicated above, there should be a marked contrast between the point of prime exchange activity of a carboxylic cation exchanger and a strong-acid type such as the sulfonic. The work of McChesney and McAuliff (1950) and of Hegsted *et al.* (1951) establishes the initial exchange point for the sulfonics as the gastric juice in the stomach. These investigators indicate that the cation removed is primarily that of exogenous origin. By contrast, Heming and Flanagan (1951) observed that the binding capacity of a carboxylic resin is negligible in the stomach and in the first 3 feet of the intestine of the dog. They concluded that the sodium carried out in the feces by this type of resin must be from the intestinal secretions rather than from dietary sources. Confirmation of binding of dietary cations by the sulfonic resins was offered.

Attempts to establish quantitative comparisons of efficacy of cation exchange resins are of value only if marked differences occur, as the experimental techniques involved are for quantitative purposes lacking in sensitivity. McChesney (1952*a*) has undertaken a comparison of sulfonic and carboxylic types, reporting that the total extra fecal cation following the use of the sulfonic resin is 2.4 mEq. per gram and that the corresponding value for the carboxylic is 1.8 mEq. In this paper McChesney concludes that cation exchange is not limited to the upper part of the intestinal tract, a conclusion based upon the finding that the ratio of sodium and potassium must be about 5 to 2 in order to account for the ratios of sodium and potassium removed by the resins. The position is also taken that the dietary ratio of these ions is not necessarily correlated with their concentration on the resins.

Relative to the binding of divalent cations by resin, McChesney's figures would indicate that about 0.5 mEq. of calcium is bound by either resin and that significant amounts of magnesium are also fixed on the resins, the actual amount of magnesium being somewhat lower than the corresponding values for calcium. The single other polyvalent cation studied was iron, and the amount bound, while detectable, was stated to be very small. The significance of the binding of iron or of any other polyvalent cation would depend upon the ionic composition of the diet of the animal or patient. If a marginal iron intake is the problem, it is probable that the feeding of resins could precipitate a deficiency of this element, and this has in fact been reported to occur in patients receiving resin therapy (Lippman, 1951).

The potentiality that resins would remove organic cations is very great, but with regard to certain of these functioning as food elements this does not seem to be the case. In the experiments of McChesney (1951) there was no loss of amino acids, thiamin, or riboflavin. This is in conformity with the results of Flanagan *et al.* (1951*a, b*), whose acute and chronic toxicity studies revealed the complete nontoxicity of carboxylic resins either in the ammonium cycle or in the ammonium-potassium form as reflected in growth rate, hematological examination, reproduction records, tissue electrolyte content, and gross and histo-pathology. These experiments were conducted with rats and dogs and involved both normal and low salt diets. It is most interesting that the addition of a resin to a salt-free diet does not modify the effect. The conclusion is that equilibration in the instance of the salt-free diet is such as to cause the retention by the resin of virtually no cations. This point is of importance in considering the possible effects of cation exchange resins administered to patients on low salt or salt-free diets. From the results of Flanagan *et al.* (1951*b*) it would seem probable that no hyponatremia could be induced by resinous exchangers. This probability has been borne out by subsequent extensive clinical trials.

The studies of Flanagan *et al.* (1951*a, b*) with the carboxylic resins have been in large measure paralleled using the sulfonic type of resin (McChesney, 1952*a*). The results indicate that the nontoxicity of the resin is at levels below 15 per cent of the diet. Confirmation of prior clinical findings relative to the resin-induced marked increase of phosphate absorption from the gut was presented by McChesney (1952*d*).

In the experiments of Flanagan *et al.* (1951*b*) with dogs, the carboxylic cation exchange resins were given at levels of 3 to 5 Gm. per kilogram daily for periods of from 1 week to 6 months. The resin used was the ammonium cycle form of the carboxylic cation exchanger. Similar studies conducted by Danowski *et al.* (1951*a*), using a straight hydrogen cycle carboxylic cation exchange resin at levels of 30 to 60 Gm. per day (probably 3 to 6 Gm. per kilogram per day) for a period of 7 to 11 days, gave evidence of decreased serum sodium, rise in serum chloride, and a metabolic acidosis characterized by a fall in serum carbon dioxide content and pH. Other changes induced by feeding of resin included increased urinary volumes, lowered sodium in the chloride space, and in general a negative potassium balance, both external and cellular. It is hard to account for the variation of results reported by these two groups of investigators; probably it is an example of the difficulty of conducting comparable experimental procedures. The effects of modifications of diet have in the broader sense not been investigated, but wherever an attempt has been made to study this aspect it has been observed that dietary changes do markedly modify the efficacy of resin therapy. In the experiments discussed above, the fact that one resin under study was in the hydrogen cycle and the other in the ammonium cycle should make no essential difference except in the sense that disposal of the ammonium ions might raise stress conditions in the kidney.

One highly significant finding reported by Danowski *et al.* (1951*b*) was that the feeding of cation exchange resins did not alter the external balance of sodium. The increased stool sodium was in large measure compensated for by decreased urinary sodium, with resultant stability of external balance; however, these researchers indicated that their studies involved diets high in sodium, and this of course could entirely cloud the potential induction of salt depletion in diets of lower salt content.

One of the obvious potential complications of using cation exchange resins in medical practice lies in the danger of inducing potassium deficiency. From the outset this has been clearly recognized, and when the first resins were marketed the products contained enough of the resin in the potassium cycle to prevent the development of hypokalemia. McChesney (1951), from *in vivo* studies with rats, concluded that the optimal potassium content of both carboxylic and sulfonic types of resins was between 1 and 2 mEq. per gram. At this level, the potassium lost in the feces would be compensated for by that portion of the ingested resin in the potassium cycle. The suggestion was made that if a slight degree of compensated acidosis was desired the resin should be closer to the value of 1 mEq. of potassium per gram of resin. He cautioned that even the level of 2 mEq. of potassium per gram of resin would not entirely prevent acidosis, and recommended that the daily intake for a patient be 12.5 Gm. of potassium cycle form and 37.5 Gm. of hydrogen or ammonium cycle resin. This ratio would, according to

McChesney, assure a positive potassium balance, little modification in acid-base balance, and yet result in the removal of approximately 1 Gm. of sodium via the intestine. In general, the cation exchange resin products marketed do fall roughly in this range, from the standpoint of potassium cycle form contained.

The danger of inducing an uncompensated acidosis in patients through the use of cation exchangers is remote but nevertheless real. As mentioned above, combination of fixed-base cycle resin with hydrogen cycle tends to minimize this problem, which is rendered of even less significance by virtue of the fact that a mild compensated acidosis is indicated for the induction of a diuresis, with its resultant beneficial effect on the edematous patient. Recently, McChesney (1952b) has reported in detail on the neutrality-regulating mechanisms in rats receiving cation exchange resins of the sulfonic type. From balance studies he found that the net fecal loss of alkali resulting from resin ingestion under the conditions of the experiment was 2.4 mEq. per gram. This conclusion was reached by feeding a resin containing 2.4 mEq. per gram of alkali and noting no change in the urinary excretion of sodium or potassium. Compensation for alkali loss in animals receiving primarily hydrogen cycle resins is by the increased excretion in the urine of acid phosphate and ammonia; however, this mechanism is not adequate to compensate for the alkali loss and the result is a compensated acidosis. If the alkali content of the ingested resin is raised, a point is reached at which there is no effect on acid-base balance. Accompanying the various metabolic shifts is that of increased phosphate absorption from the gut, which has been credited by various investigators to the binding of calcium and magnesium by the resin, thus freeing the phosphate for absorption.

Several clinicians have subscribed to the idea that combination of anion and cation exchange resins increases the capacity of the cation exchangers and in general decreases the tendency toward the development of acidosis. In the animal experiments of McChesney (1952c), combinations exhibited no properties which would indicate their clinical usefulness. The only modification of the balance pattern observed was in the increased absorption of phosphate which results from the ingestion of cation exchangers, and the tendency toward nullification of this action resulting from the use of anion exchangers. The conclusion of McChesney (1952c) was that "the use of mixed anion-cation exchangers in edema appears to offer no clear-cut advantage."

While it is true that cation exchange resins of the carboxylic and sulfonic types have found wide application in medical practice, a major deterrent to a still broader use is the bulk of such agents required for therapeutic efficacy. The present author postulated that capacity would be augmented through the removal of polyvalent cations by chelating agents, leaving only the monovalent cations for exchange with the resin. Clearly, if this ideal state could be even approximated, improvement would ensue. Ethylenediamine tetra-acetic acid or any similar agent will chelate only with polyvalent cations, and it is these ions which possess the greater affinity for cation exchange resins and therefore reduce *in vivo* capacity. Table 23 illustrates the results obtained from an investigation of the foregoing premise.

Martin *et al.* (1953) found that ethylenediamine tetra-acetic acid (EDTA) given alone does not modify sodium, potassium or chloride content but does reduce the calcium content of feces. The chelator tends to increase urinary calcium and chloride, with no modification in sodium or potassium. In explanation, it is proposed that calcium, as a result of its chelation, is removed from insoluble salts normally present in the intestine and rendered soluble, with resultant absorption and subsequent excretion via the kidney. The facilitation of chloride absorption caused by the EDTA, as reflected in increased urinary excretion, results from reduction by it of calcium cation concentration normally restricting some chloride ions to the intestinal tract.

The combination of EDTA with the cation exchange resin compared to resin alone results in a marked increase in the capacity of the resin for sodium and potassium removal. Calcium excretion in the feces is decreased by the concomitant administration of EDTA with the resin. The proposed explanation of these findings is that calcium is chelated as when EDTA is given alone, and as a result is absorbed and rendered inactive. This frees the full capacity of the resin for exchange with monovalent cations, and the result is increased capacity. The degree of this effect will be associated with the relative abundance of polyvalent and monovalent cations in the intestinal content; the higher the relative polyvalent ion concentration, the more marked will be the potentiation manifested by the EDTA.

EDTA given alone does not modify fecal chloride but does increase urinary chloride. Given with the resin, it modifies the resin effect by reducing urinary chloride and increasing fecal chloride. It will be recalled that anion exchange resins modify the altered anion excretion caused by cation exchangers in that urinary chloride excretion is decreased and fecal chloride excretion is increased (Martz *et al.,* 1950,

TABLE 23
Effect of Ethylenediamine Tetra-acetic Acid on In Vivo Capacity of Cation Exchange Resin (All Values in Milligrams per 100 Gm. of Ingested Food)*

(From Martin, G. J., *et al.*, *Proc. Soc. Exper. Biol. Med.*, **82:** 373, 1953)

Value Determined	EDTA	Carboxylic cation ex- change resin		Combined resin + EDTA		Controls
Fecal Na	86 (4)	127	(5)	346 (2)		75 (20)
	—	123	(10)	176 (10)		51 (19)
	—	175	(7)	245 (7)		67 (20)
	—	164	(7)	211 (7)		—
Urinary Na	536 (4)	388	(5)	476 (2)		458 (20)
	—	312	(10)	202 (10)		350 (19)
	—	249	(7)	189 (7)		309 (20)
	—	244	(7)	194 (7)		—
Fecal K	110 (4)	138	(5)	409 (2)		114 (20)
	—	124	(10)	234 (10)		84 (19)
	—	139	(7)	273 (7)		81 (20)
	—	127	(7)	221 (7)		—
Urinary K	593 (4)	674	(5)	823 (2)		595 (20)
	—	571	(10)	405 (10)		436 (19)
	—	478	(7)	398 (7)		438 (20)
	—	503	(7)	460 (7)		—
Fecal Ca	487 (4)	639	(5)	899 (2)		741 (20)
	—	729	(10)	529 (10)		641 (19)
	—	584	(7)	541 (7)		705 (20)
	—	638	(7)	462 (7)		—
Urinary Ca	44 (4)	21	(5)	38 (2)		14 (20)
	—	16	(10)	18 (10)		27 (19)
	—	14	(7)	15 (7)		29 (20)
	—	17	(7)	22 (7)		—
Fecal Cl	103 (4)	102	(5)	194 (2)		118 (20)
	—	57.8	(10)	179 (10)		61 (19)
	—	113	(7)	189 (7)		104 (20)
	—	92	(7)	152 (7)		—
Urinary Cl	954 (4)	716	(5)	903 (2)		815 (20)
	—	626	(10)	552 (10)		630 (19)
	—	463	(7)	490 (7)		532 (20)
	—	626	(7)	604 (7)		—

* Figures in parentheses represent number of pairs of rats in each experiment leading to average value stated.

TABLE 24
Modification of Mineral Balance in the Rat Caused by Ingestion of a Phosphonic Resin (All Values in Milligrams per 100 Gm. of Food Ingested)*

(From Sullivan, M. J., *et al.*, *J. Am. Pharm. A.* [*Scient. Ed.*], **42**: 357, 1953)

Value determined	No.	Control	Phosphonic cation exchange resin		Carboxylic cation exchange resin	
Sodium, feces	1	50 (10)	(5)	42 (10)	(5)	123 (10)
	2	39 (10)	(5)	41 (9)	(5)	191 (10)
	3		(5)	55 (9)	(5)	175 (7)
	4		(5)	59 (10)	(5)	164 (7)
	5		(10)	101 (6)	(10)	335 (9)
	6		(10)	64 (7)		
Sodium, urine	1	378 (10)	(5)	255 (10)	(5)	312 (10)
	2	342 (10)	(5)	294 (9)	(5)	272 (10)
	3		(5)	587 (9)	(5)	249 (7)
	4		(5)	447 (10)	(5)	244 (7)
	5		(10)	202 (6)	(10)	184 (9)
	6		(10)	243 (7)		
Potassium, feces	1	85 (10)	(5)	63 (10)	(5)	138 (5)
	2	33 (10)	(5)	53 (9)	(5)	124 (10)
	3		(5)	59 (9)	(5)	139 (7)
	4		(5)	74 (10)	(5)	127 (7)
	5		(10)	121 (6)	(10)	276 (10)
	6		(10)	81 (7)		
Potassium, urine	1	493 (10)	(5)	445 (10)	(5)	674 (5)
	2	518 (10)	(5)	450 (9)	(5)	571 (10)
	3		(5)	426 (9)	(5)	478 (7)
	4		(5)	447 (10)	(5)	503 (7)
	5		(10)	342 (6)	(10)	702 (10)
	6		(10)	398 (7)		
Calcium, feces	1	574 (10)	(5)	587 (10)	(5)	639 (5)
	2	1114 (10)	(5)	603 (9)	(5)	729 (10)
	3		(5)	582 (9)	(5)	584 (7)
	4		(5)	616 (10)	(5)	638 (7)
	5		(10)	453 (6)	(10)	672 (10)
	6		(10)	424 (7)		

TABLE 24 (*Continued*)

Value determined	No.	Control	Phosphonic cation exchange resin		Carboxylic cation exchange resin	
Calcium, urine	1	9.2 (10)	(5)	12.7 (10)	(5)	21 (5)
	2	16 (10)	(5)	18.6 (9)	(5)	16 (10)
	3		(5)	22.0 (9)	(5)	14 (7)
	4		(5)	21.2 (10)	(5)	17 (7)
	5		(10)	14.1 (6)	(10)	719 (10)
	6		(10)	19.6 (7)		
Chloride, feces	1	34 (9)	(5)	16.9 (10)	(5)	102 (5)
	2	33 (10)	(5)	16.0 (9)	(5)	58 (10)
	3		(5)	5.1 (9)	(5)	113 (7)
	4		(5)	7.3 (10)	(5)	92 (7)
	5	104 (20)	(10)	104 (6)	(10)	61 (10)
	6		(10)	79 (7)		
Chloride, urine	1	606 (10)	(5)	526 (10)	(5)	715 (5)
	2	645 (10)	(5)	561 (9)	(5)	626 (10)
	3		(5)	720 (9)	(5)	463 (7)
	4		(5)	815 (10)	(5)	626 (7)
	5		(10)	482 (6)	(10)	687 (10)
	6		(10)	625 (7)		
Phosphate, feces	1	287 (6)	(5)	173 (6)	(5)	176 (7)
	2	282 (14)	(10)	382 (7)	(5)	173 (7)
	3		(10)	418 (7)		
	4					
	5					
	6					
Phosphate, urine	1	80 (6)	(5)	117 (6)	(5)	181 (7)
	2	121 (14)	(10)	211 (7)	(5)	180 (7)
	3		(10)	245 (7)		
	4					
	5					
	6					

* Figures in parentheses on left of each experimental value give per cent of resin in diet; figures in parentheses on right of each experimental value give number of pairs of rats used.

1952). Whether or not **EDTA** reduces the hyperchloremia resulting from cation exchange resin administration has not yet been investigated. There is also the possibility that the combination will reduce the tendency toward the development of acidosis associated with the use of resins.

The search for improvement is constant, and therefore with the appearance of phosphonic resins these too were checked for their *in vivo* capacity. Fed at 10 per cent level in the diet of rats, this new type of resin showed a minimal effect, increasing the fecal content of sodium by only 0.2 mEq. per gram (*in vitro* capacity about 8.45 mEq. per gram). Table 24 gives the results obtained by Sullivan *et al.* (1953).

No explanation is offered for these results, which are entirely anomalous viewed in terms of the sulfonic and carboxylic resin effects. It is a point of interest that the sulfonic and carboxylic groups are monobasic, while the phosphonic type is dibasic.

$$
\begin{array}{ccc}
\overset{\textstyle O}{\underset{\textstyle O}{\overset{\|}{\underset{\|}{R\!-\!S\!-\!OH}}}} & \overset{\textstyle O}{\overset{\|}{R\!-\!C\!-\!OH}} & R\!-\!O\!-\!P\diagup\!\!\overset{OH}{\diagdown}\!\!\overset{}{=}O \\
\text{Sulfonic Type} & \text{Carboxylic Type} & \text{Phosphonic Type}
\end{array}
$$

The key to the difference in *in vivo* capacity must lie in the exchange grouping. In the sulfonic and phosphonic types the acid radical is attached to an aromatic nucleus; by contrast the carboxylic radical is attached to an aliphatic unit. If this aspect of structure were of importance to *in vivo* capacity, the sulfonic and phosphonic resins would parallel, and they do not. In the case of both the sulfonic and the carboxylic, the linkage is sulfur to carbon or carbon to carbon, while with the phosphonic resin the linkage is phosphorus to oxygen to carbon. This may confer upon the molecule modified resonance.

The carboxylic resins possess the highest total capacity (10 mEq. per gram) and are weak acids, dissociating maximally at pH 10. The sulfonic resins possess the lowest total capacity (4.5 mEq. per gram) and are comparatively strong acids, dissociating entirely at pH 3 or above. The third type, the phosphonic resin, possesses an intermediate *in vitro* capacity (8.46 mEq. per gram) and has a pK_1 of 2.5 and a pK_2 of about 8. From these physical chemical factors, it is not possible to explain the major differences seen among these resins *in vivo*. The first two behave in large measure in accordance with expectation, but the phosphonic resin does not. The point of consideration would seem to be the dibasic nature of the phosphonic form, and it is from that point that one is led to consideration of the potential chelating power of this organic phosphate molecule. Certain inorganic phosphates such as sodium hexametaphosphate possess exceptional powers as chelating agents (Smith, 1934). Further, organic phosphorus compounds such as adenosine triphosphate are capable of forming complexes with cations such as potassium (Melchoir, 1952). As a hypothesis it is proposed that the exchange power of the phosphonic group is blocked in some manner as a result of chelate ring formation with some organic material or with some cation of valence exceeding two.

CLINICAL STUDIES

Congestive Heart Failure

Introduction. The first clinical studies to be reported involving the use of cation exchange resins were published in 1948 by Greenblatt and Gilwood. Using a sulfonic type of exchanger, they gave some 17 Gm. of the material before and after each meal. This would mean a total of some 102 Gm. daily per patient, but they succeeded in keeping about 19 hospitalized persons on this regimen. Of these, 11, or about 58 per cent, showed increased fecal excretion of sodium, but the other 8 failed to respond even when the dosage was elevated to 200 Gm. daily. Casts were observed in the urine of these patients.

Cobbey and his associates (1949) administered a carboxylic cation exchanger (75 Gm. daily) to a patient with cardiac edema and to a normal person. The excreta were collected for several 4-day periods and analyzed. During the first 4-day period, the resin removed approximately 2 mEq. of sodium per gram of resin; for the second 4-day period, the value dropped to about 0.5 mEq.; subsequently, the resin seemed to exert no significant effect on cation balance. This is most unusual and at variance with the reports of many other investigators. The probability exists that some experimental error in cation determination occurred after the first two periods of the experiment.

Also in 1949, Irwin and his group presented their findings involving the use of cation exchange resins in a variety of clinical states. In summary, the sodium and potassium were diverted from their customary channels of excretion via the urine and increased in the feces by an amount indicating that 1 Gm. of resin was removing about 1.5 mEq. of sodium and 1.2 mEq. of potassium. After the first 10 to 12 days on the regimen, a profuse diuresis occurred, accompanied by a restoration of the sodium and potassium excretion via the kidney and a compensated metabolic acidosis. The acidosis was to have been anticipated, as a sulfonic type of cation exchange resin in the hydrogen cycle was used. High blood levels of chloride were concomitant findings. In patients with edema of cardiac or cirrhotic origin, a level of resin ingestion could be obtained at which gradual decline in body weight occurred. Further, when the resin was removed from the diet the weight increased, indicating storage of body water and coincident return or accentuation of edema.

Reviewing the literature on the use of cation exchangers in medical practice led the author to the belief that major papers should be considered individually and subsequently collectively relative to a specific phase of resin action. This plan of approach has been followed and it is believed offers adequate detail to permit adoption of the regimens used by specific clinicians, as well as summation for group opinion.

Cardiac Patients, General. Those patients with cardiac decompensation and edema failing to respond to mercurials and digitalization were selected by Kleiber and Pickar (1951) for study of the efficacy of cation exchange resins. During the first series treated the carboxylic resin used was in the hydrogen cycle and toleration of the dosage employed was not good; however, with those patients who could tolerate the resin the results were favorable. Of particular importance was the finding that the spacing of mercurial injection could be extended. This is well illustrated in Figure 19.

These investigators permitted their patients a diet moderately restricted in salt content. By this they mean a diet in which the patient is allowed ordinary milk, bakery bread and ordinary butter, but is not permitted salty foods or the use of the salt shaker. Kleiber and Pickar emphasize that the use of resins does not eliminate the necessity for other therapeutic measures such as mercurials, but state that the spacing of mercurial injections at greater intervals "avoids the necessity for further impairing a normal function [tubular reabsorption] by the toxic effects of mercury."

These clinicians conclude that resin therapy is particularly indicated in patients with irreversible congestive failure which no longer responds to other drugs, in patients having recurrent free fluid in pleural or abdominal cavities, and in those unable to adhere to a low sodium diet.

Control of edema, either partial or complete, over prolonged periods has been reported by Emerson and his associates (1951). They also remark upon the fact that mercurial injections could be eliminated, and upon patient reaction, which was more favorable to the slow and continuous weight loss in contrast to the rapid fluctuation in water balance induced by mercury. Mercury seemed constantly to give as side effects feelings of weakness, lassitude and depression. In general, these workers did not increase the salt content of the diet above 2 Gm.,

FIGURE 19
Cation Exchange Resins and Mercurials
Case 3. A 57-year-old hypertensive patient with known congestive heart failure for approximately 2½ years and known ascites for 9 months.

(From Kleiber, E. E., and G. Pickar, *Ann. Int., Med.,* 34: 407, 1951)

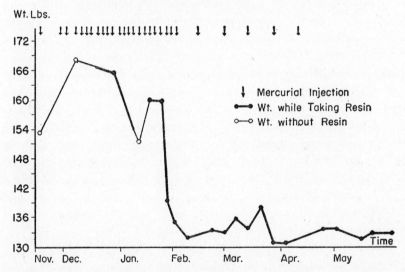

as they felt that this was the maximum practicable over prolonged periods. The conclusion reached was that resin therapy should be regarded as an adjunct to other approaches, and this seems to represent the consensus.

The capacity of cation exchangers is limited, and therefore the amounts which must be ingested are in a comparative sense high. To be sure, studies are constantly under way attempting to improve the efficiency of cation exchangers, and such efforts may succeed beyond expectation, but for the present certainly the conservative conclusion of the adjunct role of resins is valid. Resin therapy should be viewed in the light of the fact that the removal of limited amounts of sodium is better than no removal. Emerson and his associates suggest that a low salt diet be maintained with the initial phases of resin therapy and that the ingestion of salt may be increased cautiously until the patient begins to show signs of water retention. They further suggest that if larger amounts of salt are desired the joint use of resin and mercurial is indicated.

Voyles and Orgain (1951) selected for their studies of carboxylic resins 3 ambulatory patients with long-standing chronic cardiac decompensation uncontrolled by rest, rigid dietary sodium restriction, digitalization and mercurial diuretics. These patients were on a diet containing 500 mg. of sodium and on a regimen of rest, digitalis and diuretics prior to the administration of the resin; then they were instructed to take the resin mixed with milk or fruit juice in 15-Gm. doses three times daily with meals. Supplements of calcium lactate (5 Gm. daily) or 16 oz. of milk were provided to protect against possible hypocalcemia. The 3 patients who had had recurring periods of cardiac failure requiring hospitalization became relatively free of these episodes. The exercise tolerance of all was improved and 2 became and remained free of edema; the third was improved in this respect. Mercurial injections could either be eliminated or spaced at much greater intervals. Voyles and Orgain (1951) emphasize the potentiation of the action of mercurial diuretics by cation exchange resins. Figures listed by these investigators indicate that resin-treated patients ingesting 3.0 to 4.0 Gm. of sodium (7 to 10 Gm. of salt) will show removal by the resin of 2 mEq. of sodium per gram. If the amount of sodium ingested is 0.5 Gm. (22 mEq.), the corresponding figure for sodium removal is 0.5 mEq.

Wood *et al.* (1952) stress the fact that resin therapy is not a cure-all but rather an adjunct to be used with other measures. The proposal is made that patients responding to rest, digitalis and moderate restriction of sodium do not need resins. Beyond question this is true, but it does not necessarily represent the whole truth. If moderate sodium restriction is indicated in such patients, might it not be wise to bring this about by resin ingestion or perhaps bring about a portion of the sodium restriction by means of resins? These investigators indicate that resins are of value in the patient with heart failure and edema unable to attain a suitable level of sodium restriction, and particularly in those patients with long-standing chronic congestion, refractory to mercurials. They state, "in brief, the more severe and more refractory cases of congestive heart failure appear to be the ones to whom this principle [resin therapy] may be properly applied." The present author feels that this is putting the resins to the ultimate acid test, that it is delaying the use of a weapon in the therapeutic armamentarium of the physician which might prevent the onset of such refractory states, and that it is subjecting the patient to a therapeutic regimen which if properly balanced by the use of resins might make life far more bearable. The use of even small amounts of resins would seem logical for sodium restriction in any clinical situation requiring such practice.

These investigators (Wood *et al.*, 1952) used a dietary regimen of 1.0 Gm. of sodium (2.5 grams of salt) intake combined with 15 Gm. of resin taken three times daily. It was their feeling that augmentation of intake to possibly 60 Gm. resulted in no additional benefit to the patient. At the 45-Gm. level, the resin possesses a capacity for sodium removal of 40 to 100 mEq. An innovation introduced by Wood and his associates is that of alternate periods of resin administration, 4 days on resin and 3 days off. The rationale of this approach is their finding that following discontinuation of resin feedings the restriction of sodium absorption continues for a lag period averaging 3 days. Further, these workers propose a reduction in resin intake following elimination of edema to a lower feasible level, 30 Gm. daily.

Of 22 cardiovascular patients with edema, 15 showed clinical improvement directly attributable to the resin; 7 showed striking results, having failed to respond to digitalis, ammonium chloride and mercury. Diuresis occurred in 16 of these patients. The latter action was attributed to the ammonium chloride formed and absorbed systemically from the exchange reactions of the ammonium cycle resin. In any event, whether or not this was the explanation of the result, the diuresis induced by mercurials was markedly potentiated by the resins. The probability is greater that the mechanism was the induction of a compensated acidosis, which might result from the ammonium chloride formed as described above, or from other causes. It seems of value to include one case history as given by Wood *et al.* (1952):

D.D.M. . . . was admitted with rheumatic heart disease, mitral stenosis, auricular fibrillation and advanced congestive heart failure, marked edema and ascites. Heart failure had occurred four and one-half months before, while edema and ascites had increased in spite of rest in bed, digitalization and dietary salt restriction. Repeated mercurial injections had become progressively ineffective. Diuresis and loss of edema began with resin alone, and marked potentiation of mercury reappeared. Progressive loss of edema proceeded with a zero urinary excretion of sodium, but a continued urinary potassium excretion and adequate serum potassium levels. Early intermittent [carboxylic resin] dosage gave way to smaller [15 Gm. twice daily] dosage, with absence of edema despite resumption of activity. Plasma chloride levels were well maintained except after marked mercurial diuresis on the 20th day, but resumption of resin therapy was followed by normal plasma chloride levels.

It is of great importance that they record the development of 2 cases of low salt syndrome in the series under study (about 35 patients). One of these patients was not eating well, and the group attributes the hyponatremia to this factor superimposed upon continued use of the resin. Response to intravenous isotonic sodium chloride and to potassium chloride by mouth was immediate, with restoration of normal blood urea levels and a return of appetite. These investigators emphasize the dangers of resin administration when patients are not eating and when there is renal insufficiency.

Realizing that resin therapy would become general, Wood and his associates listed their concept of "Minimal Precautions," which included:

1. If nitrogen retention is found, indicating renal insufficiency, the resins should not in general be used.
2. Daily weight recordings should be taken.
3. Reasonably good appetite.
4. Reasonably good flow of urine.
5. Administration of a mercurial without ensuing diuresis should be regarded as a danger sign, indicative of renal failure or the low salt syndrome or both.
6. Hyperpnea, nausea and vomiting should be signs for the discontinuance of resin usage until blood analysis has clarified the picture.

In the series of Feinberg and Rosenberg (1951), of 6 patients with congestive heart failure treated with a carboxylic resin in the ammonium-potassium cycle, 5 were benefited. Once again, the aspect of marked reduction in the number of mercurial injections necessary to maintain the patients free of edema was emphasized. Another aspect of the resin regimen regarded by these investigators as worthy of emphasis was the necessity for increased vigilance if the patient's appetite were very poor and particularly if food ingestion stopped entirely. To this situation, dangerous because of the potential development of hyponatremia, they added one equally ominous, the risk of the use of resins in extremely hot weather where loss of sodium through sweating might be a major factor. They regarded a fall in carbon dioxide–combining power to a figure below 20 mEq. per liter as the first change associated with impending development of untoward reactions. The patients were all ambulant and had been studied for periods ranging from 6 weeks to over a year. In every instance they were seen at weekly intervals and checks were made on their blood chemistry until such time as a baseline could be established; then the visits were spaced at 2- and 3-week intervals.

Callahan and his associates (1952) used two types of resins in their studies, one of the carboxylic type (22 per cent in the potassium and 78 per cent in the ammonium cycle) and one of the sulfonic variety in the ammonium cycle. Of 22 patients on the carboxylic resin, all with congestive heart failure, 7 were maintained for periods of from 5 to 38 weeks. Fifteen of the patients were taken off resin therapy after periods varying from 1 day to 12 weeks, due to toxic reactions or failure to respond. Of the series, 3 showed improvement characterized by edema reduction and weight loss; 9 showed no significant change in the congestive heart failure. This indicates the value of resin therapy in 12 of the 22 patients under study. The authors remarked that these patients were eating more liberal sodium diets and that they required less in the way of other drugs such as mercurials. It is also to be held in mind that this series were all ambulant and therefore comparatively difficult to control from the standpoint of actual knowledge of salt intake. Analysis of these results was rendered difficult because of salt intake modification, but one feature was striking and that was the reduction in the frequency of mercurial injections. Table 25 lists the results.

The group treated by Callahan *et al.* (1952) with an ammonium cycle sulfonic resin consisted of 15 hospitalized and 7 ambulant patients. The hospitalized patients could be properly controlled, and in this group diuresis occurred, usually on the second day of therapy, accompanied by a weight loss of 1 to 2 lbs. daily until a stabilized weight was attained. The sodium chloride content of the diet was 6 Gm. and the dose of resin varied from 28 to 96 Gm. Seven patients in this series of 22 did not improve with resin administration.

Analysis of the work of Callahan *et al.* (1952) is difficult if one desires to compare the efficacy of carboxylic with that of sulfonic resins, as the series on the carboxylic resin were all outpatients permitted to modify salt intake, and 15 of the 22 in the series on sulfonic were hospitalized and kept on a diet containing a constant amount of salt. Further, the sulfonic resin was used in the ammonium cycle, and this is not the sound approach, as all resins must be given partially in the potassium cycle to prevent the development of hypokalemia. Difficulty encountered in an attempted analysis of the results relative to therapeutic efficacy is similarly found in any study of the findings on inci-

TABLE 25

The Diagnosis and Effect on Mercurial Requirements of 22
Patients Treated with Carboxylic Resin*

(From Callahan, E. J., *et al.*, *Am. J. M. Sc.*, **223**: 117, 1952)

				Rate of mercurial injections	
Patient	Age	Sex	Diagnosis†	Before resin	During resin
1	74	M	ASHD	Every 7 days	None
2	63	M	HCVD	" 5 "	"
3	36	M	RHD	" 2 "	"
4	51	F	HCVD	" 7 "	"
5	50	F	RHD	" 4 "	Every 5 wks.
6	65	F	RHD	" 2 "	" 9 days
7	49	F	RHD	" 2 "	" 2 "
8	51	F	HCVD	" 2–4 "	" 7 "
9	53	F	HCVD, ASHD	" 7 "	" 5 wks.
10	60	M	RHD	" 3 "	None
11	66	M	ASHD	" 7 "	"
12	47	F	RHD	" 2 "	Every 7 days
13	46	F	RHD	" 7 "	" 5 wks.
14	47	M	RHD	" 2–3 "	" 3 days
15	68	M	ASHD	" 7 "	None
16	34	F	RHD	" 3 "	" 7 days
17	48	F	RHD	" 7 "	None
18	58	M	ASHD	" 7 "	"
19	58	F	RHD	" 7 "	"
20	49	F	RHD	" 7 "	Every 3–4 wks.
21	64	M	ASHD	" 2–3 "	" 5 days
22	46	M	RHD	" 4–7 "	" 10 "

* All patients were maintained on digitalis and low salt diets before resin therapy.
† ASHD—arteriosclerotic heart disease; HCVD—hypertensive cardiovascular disease; RHD—rheumatic heart disease.

dence of side effects with the two resin types. The only conclusion that can be reached from this study is that both types of resins possess therapeutic merit and that both precipitate certain undesirable side effects.

One conclusion reached by this group is of great importance in the practical use of resins. This conclusion is: "All the toxic effects that occurred with the carboxylic resin used in this study were manifest clinically with the exception of minor electrocardiographic changes. Consequently, we do not feel that elaborate laboratory studies are necessary to follow these patients." In other words, the clinician may with confidence take the view that costly laboratory determinations are not essential to the proper control of patients receiving resins, as clinical manifestations are clear guideposts to impending side effects. They recommend pretreatment evaluation with a check for impaired renal function and evidence of previous digitalis toxicity, and consider a baseline electrocardiogram along with determination of serum sodium, potassium and calcium as useful but not necessary. Subsequent checks should be spaced at weekly intervals for the first 6 weeks. Modification in digitalis intake may be indicated if signs of toxicity occur. Pulse changes are regarded as most helpful in detecting excessive digitalis effect. The spacing of mercurial diuretic administration may be extended as adjustment to the regimen occurs.

The sulfonic type of cation exchange resin was used by Barker and McKay (1951) in 2 patients with congestive cardiac failure. The resin was given at a level of 100 Gm. daily, and while the initial effect was good, there was a gradual decline in the response of both patients, attributed by the authors to lowered sodium content of the intestinal juices. The capacity of the resin for sodium removal, determined by a method based upon changes occurring in urinary chloride-sodium excretion differences, was given at 0.21 to 0.86 mEq. per gram of resin (averaging 0.5 mEq. per gram).

Lefken *et al.* (1952), using carboxylic resins in 8 patients with cardiac decompensation and edema, found that 6 of those treated were able to tolerate diets with a more liberal salt content and that in general the effect of mercurials was increased. Similar results are reported by Bonner (1952), who found that he could induce negative sodium balance by the use of resins and low sodium diets. A point of great practical importance emphasized by Bonner is that resins not only increase the efficacy of mercurial diuretics but render refractory patients once again responsive. Additional substantiation of the power of resin therapy to potentiate the action of mercurials and even to initiate such action on the kidney has been presented by Elkinton *et al.* (1952).

Klingensmith and Elkinton (1952) studied the clinical efficacy of a combined ammonium-potassium cycle resin in 27 patients with edema due to chronic congestive heart failure. The edematous state was eliminated in refractory cases, and it was possible in some 23 cases to prevent the reaccumulation of edema during the period of decreased use of mercurials and following liberalization of low salt regimens. While gastrointestinal complications were rather common, occurring in 20 of the 34 patients studied, these investigators observed no evidence of depletion of sodium or potassium, no potassium intoxication, no severe chloride acidosis and no calcium depletion. They concluded that if the patients are carefully selected, resin therapy is a useful and safe adjunct to the treatment of chronic congestive failure over prolonged periods of time. Of the 34 patients comprising the group studied, 27 were maintained for periods up to 62 weeks; the average was 26.4 weeks.

A series of 12 patients with severe congestive heart failure and edema were studied by Greenman *et al.* (1953a) over a period up to 15 months on resin therapy. These patients were selected, in that none had renal disease. The regimen prior to resin therapy was continued without change, but with cessation of treatment with ammonium chloride and mercurials. The resin used was 80 per cent in the hydrogen and 20 per cent in the potassium cycle. All patients in the series were outpatients and were seen at 1- or 2-week intervals during the first months and subsequently at monthly intervals. In this group, edema was controlled without additional diuretics in all but 2. Particularly striking is the fact that in 5 of the patients edema had disappeared within 1 week; in 2 more within 2 weeks; and in yet another 2 within 4 weeks. Four of the edema-free patients were taken off resins and within a few days the edema recurred.

An attempt to liberalize the salt intake in these patients who had been on mercurials and ammonium chloride and were subsequently transferred to resin did not meet with success. In specific instances where the sodium intake was increased from 0.3 to 0.5 Gm., from 0.3 Gm. to a diet without salt shaker, or from a diet which omitted extra salt to one utilizing small amounts, immediate gains in weight and redevelopment of edema were noted. This, of course, does not mean that increased salt intake could not have been managed through the combined use of resin and mercurials. It is particularly interesting to note the reaction of the patients to resin therapy. As stated by Greenman *et al.* (1953a): "All the patients who had been receiving mercurials previously said they preferred resin therapy to mercurial diuresis. The latter frequently left them feeling weak and tired. In addition, they objected to the reaccumulation of fluid which occurred before the next injection. They preferred the relatively even control of edema achieved by resin ingestion."

No resin form can be given in the straight hydrogen or ammonium cyclic without serious side effects. Studies of a sulfonic resin in the ammonium cycle led Kraus (1950) to the conclusion that such resin could not be employed clinically. He did observe diuresis and weight loss within 2 or 3 days.

The proposal has been made that combinations of anion and cation exchange resins possess merit exceeding that of the cation exchangers alone. The proposal is based upon the contention that such combinations have greater capacity for sodium removal, lowered tendency to cause acidosis and the power to prevent anion shift to the kidney from the gut (Martz *et al.*, 1952). These points are considered in detail in sections devoted to such phases. The mixture used by Martz *et al.* (1952) consisted of 12 per cent anion exchange resin, 29 per cent potassium cycle cation exchange resin and 59 per cent hydrogen cycle cation exchange resin, and was given to 42 patients with congestive heart failure and 14 with cirrhosis of the liver with ascites. In all but 6 of these patients, the desired therapeutic effect was achieved. Four of the 6 could not tolerate adequate quantities of the resin, due to factors fundamentally associated with their disease. This means that therapeutic success was noted in a high percentage of these patients on a diet containing 1.5 Gm. of sodium and receiving 30 to 60 Gm. of resin. These investigators recommend the intermittent use of mercurial diuretics in those patients with a severe grade of sodium retention, rather than very large doses of resin and markedly restricted sodium intake. They noted a significant potentiation of the effect of the mercurial due to resin ingestion.

Efficacy of an ammonium cycle cation exchange resin given in doses ranging from 30 to 120 Gm. was reported by Currens *et al.* (1950) in 4 patients with cardiac edema. Clinical improvement in the signs of congestive circulatory failure was observed in all patients. The major complications observed were potassium loss and chloride retention. The first of these would be expected from a straight ammonium cycle resin.

Combined anion-cation therapy was employed by Aaron and Weston (1952) in 8 cardiacs with edema who had failed to respond to other types of therapy. Satisfactory clinical results were obtained in all cases. As with other forms of cation exchange therapy, this combined form

tended to reduce or even to permit the elimination of the use of mercurial diuretics. Two patients of the group were able to return to a
normal, active life, tolerating an unrestricted diet. The impression given
by the patients was that they felt so much better generally that they
refused to discontinue the resin, despite moderate gastrointestinal
irritation. These investigators emphasize the need for proper control of
patients receiving cation exchange resins and compare such therapeutic
practice with the use of insulin, digitalis or mercurials and the associated potentialities for harmful effects. The need for individualized
schedules is emphasized, as the rational approach will vary with the
patient. Serum carbon dioxide and chloride levels are recommended,
and the statement is made that such chemical control permits avoidance of any hazards. From the work of this group, it would seem that
the incidence of acidosis is essentially parallel when either anion-cation
combinations or straight cationic forms are used.

The use of combinations of anion and cation exchange resins has
been studied by Best (1952a), who concluded that the synergism observed between mercurials and ammonium chloride or other acidifying
salts is essentially parallel to that seen between mercurials and cation
exchange resins. The striking efficacy of cation exchange resins in
restoring responsiveness to mercurials has been generally observed, and
the proposed parallelism may offer the proper perspective for mechanism of action. Two factors are regarded as aiding mercurial diuresis—
compensated acidosis and normal or elevated plasma chloride level
—and there is little question but that cation exchange resins induce
both states of modified systemic biochemistry. In this study of 8 patients,
Best makes no direct comparisons between resin preparations containing no anion exchange resins and similar products incorporating such
resins. Certainly there is no conclusion offered on the relative tendency
to acidosis caused by both product forms. He does state that cation
exchange resins may be safer and more effective in patients with renal
disease and incapacitating edema. Once again, emphasis is placed on
proper control and observation of patients, with oliguria, anorexia,
mental confusion or muscular weakness to be used as danger signs. As
with the straight cation exchange resin products, with the combination
form it is recommended that periodic laboratory checks be made particularly on sodium, potassium, chloride and carbon dioxide–combining
power of the plasma, as acidosis and sodium or potassium depletion
can and do occur.

In the studies of Chapman *et al.* (1951) combinations of anion and cation exchangers were used. Unfortunately no direct comparisons were made in this investigation between the acidotic tendency of cation exchangers when used alone and when used in combination with the anion exchange resins. Very little acidosis was observed whether the group received hydrogen-potassium cycle resins alone or in combination. In this study as in virtually all others, reactivity to mercurial diuretics was increased by the concomitant administration of resins. Dosage regimen consisted of four 12-Gm. units given at spaced intervals throughout the day—after each meal and at bedtime. Carbon dioxide and urea nitrogen determinations at intervals of 10 days to 2 weeks were regarded as adequate for proper control of the patient.

Summary. Cation exchange resin therapy is in general to be considered as an adjunct to other modes of therapy in cardiac cases (Emerson *et al.*, 1951; Kleiber and Pickar, 1951; Klingensmith and Elkinton, 1952; Wood *et al.*, 1952; Greenman *et al.*, 1953a), but has been in many instances the sole and successful therapeutic approach (Wood *et al.*, 1952; Greenman *et al.*, 1953a).

Use of resin therapy is generally recommended in conjunction with a restricted sodium intake: a diet from which the effects of the salt shaker are eliminated, or one containing approximately 2 Gm. or less of salt (Emerson *et al.*, 1951; Kleiber and Pickar, 1951; Voyles and Orgain, 1951; Martz *et al.*, 1952; Wood *et al.*, 1952; Greenman *et al.*, 1953a, b). Doses recommended vary from 30 to 120 Gm. taken in divided quantities, these quantities of resin removing from 0.5 mEq. to 1.5 mEq. of sodium (equivalent to 0.03 to 0.09 Gm. of sodium chloride) per gram of resin ingested (Currens *et al.*, 1950; Barker and McKay, 1951; Chapman *et al.*, 1951; Emerson *et al.*, 1951; Kleiber and Pickar, 1951; Voyles and Orgain, 1951; Callahan *et al.*, 1952; Martz *et al.*, 1952; Wood *et al.*, 1952). Alternate periods of resin therapy, generally 4 days on and 3 days off, have been recommended (Wood *et al.*, 1952).

Control of edema with diuresis is either markedly facilitated or complete (Currens *et al.*, 1950; Barker and McKay, 1951; Emerson *et al.*, 1951; Feinberg and Rosenberg, 1951; Kleiber and Pickar, 1951; Aaron and Weston, 1952; Bonner, 1952; Callahan *et al.*, 1952; Klingensmith and Elkinton, 1952; Lefken *et al.*, 1952; Martz *et al.*, 1952; Wood *et al.*, 1952; Greenman *et al.*, 1953a).

There is a general agreement on the beneficial effects of cation exchange resin therapy. All investigators report that the use of resins extends the intervals between required mercurial diuretic injections or permits elimination of such therapy (Chapman *et al.*, 1951; Emerson *et al.*, 1951; Feinberg and Rosenberg, 1951; Kleiber and Pickar, 1951; Aaron and Weston, 1952; Best, 1952*a*; Bonner, 1952; Callahan *et al.*, 1952; Elkinton *et al.*, 1952; Klingensmith and Elkinton, 1952; Lefken *et al.*, 1952; Martz *et al.*, 1952; Wood *et al.*, 1952); and further that tolerance to such diuretics is eliminated (Best, 1952*a*; Bonner, 1952; Elkinton *et al.*, 1952; Wood *et al.*, 1952). Another jointly held opinion is that mercurial diuretics are both toxic and difficult to use properly (Emerson *et al.*, 1951; Kleiber and Pickar, 1951).

Sodium. Electrolyte balance studies are extremely difficult to carry out quantitatively even with animals, and when such studies involve patients the complications are infinitely greater. It is therefore necessary to view all results as semiquantitative and under no conditions to apply them to a specific case.

Emerson *et al.* (1951) emphasized the aspect of variations in sodium balance which occurred from period to period in the same patient and concluded that differences between patients were of such magnitude that they virtually precluded comparison. This is a most important aspect. Reasons offered in explanation include: variation in sodium and other ion intake; variation in the amount of sodium and other ions secreted into the intestine; variation in the ionic milieu resulting from additive effects of ingestion and secretion of ions; pH factors varying with the dietary, with the intestinal flora, etc.; availability of the various ions, a factor primarily but not exclusively affecting the multivalent ions which may be chelated or present in some insoluble form; variation in the speed with which the intestinal content moves through the gut; variations in hormone balance modifying electrolyte exchange, e.g., desoxycorticosterone and its action on sodium excretion and retention; and other factors.

There is general agreement that cation exchange resins increase fecal excretion of sodium (Emerson *et al.*, 1951; Feinberg and Rosenberg, 1951; Aaron and Weston, 1952; Elkinton *et al.*, 1952; Martz *et al.*, 1952; Greenman *et al.*, 1953*b*) and some similarity of data indicating the capacity of resins for sodium removal; thus Emerson *et al.* (1951), using both sulfonic and carboxylic resins, gave values of 0.25 to 0.8 mEq. per gram of resin, figures which compare well with those of Greenman *et al.* (1953*a*), who report values of 0.75 to 1.3 mEq.

per gram. Expressing the values given by Emerson *et al.* (1951) in terms of total sodium removed by 40 to 60 Gm. of resin per day, the figures are 7.9 to 36.1 mEq., or from 0.91 to 2.1 Gm. of sodium calculated as sodium chloride. Table 26, from Emerson *et al.* (1951),

TABLE 26
Change in Fecal Excretion of Cations Induced by Oral Administration of Cation Exchange Resins*

(From Emerson, K., Jr., *et al., Arch. Int. Med.,* **88:** 605, 1951)

Patient	Resin†	Dose (Gm./ day)	No. of days	Sodium		Potassium		Calcium	Magnesium
				Total (mEq./ day)	mEq./ Gm. resin	Total (mEq./ day)	mEq./ Gm. resin	Total (mEq./ day)	Total (mEq./ day)
M.L.	Permutit Z	40	3	+16.0	+0.25	+24.0	+0.60	—	—
		60	9	+22.0	+0.37	+12.1	+0.21	—	—
	Amberlite (1)	45	9	+36.1	+0.80	+83.3	+1.85	−10.0	+0.54
	Amberlite (2)	60	7	+33.0	+0.55	+72.0	+1.20	− 1.0	—
	Amberlite (2)	80	9	+27.7	+0.35	+96.0	+1.20	+ 0.2	—
F.C.	Amberlite (3)	25	9	+ 7.9	+0.32	+54.0	+2.16	+ 1.0	—
	Amberlite (3)	50	6	+15.0	+0.30	+78.0	+1.56	+ 5.0	—
H.A.	Amberlite (1)	45	9	+33.9	+0.75	+12.0	+0.27	− 3.0	+3.0
G.D.	Amberlite (2)	40	6	+20.8	+0.52	+92.8	+2.32	± 0.0	—
C.T.	Amberlite (4)	60	6	+15.6	+0.26	+73.1	+1.22	—	—

* The values represent the increase (+) or decrease (−) in cation excretion during resin therapy as compared with excretion during a prior control period with approximately the same dietary intake.

† Amberlite (1) was composed of approximately two-thirds of the ammonium form and one-third of the potassium form (potassium equaled 5.2 per cent). This was Resodec. Amberlite (2) contained equal parts of ammonium and potassium forms (potassium equaled 9.4 per cent). Amberlite (3) was the potassium form (potassium equaled 18.7 per cent). Amberlite (4) was the ammonium form.

would tend to indicate the superiority of the carboxylic resin over the sulfonic from a capacity standpoint.

Hyponatremia does develop as a result of resin administration, as indicated by results such as those of Greenman *et al.* (1953*a*), in which sodium levels below 134 mEq. were noted in 5 of 12 patients. In almost all such cases the patients involved either are not eating well at the time of development of the hyponatremia (Feinberg and

Rosenberg, 1951; Greenman *et al.*, 1953*a*), are exposed to extremely hot weather and are perspiring excessively, thus losing sodium (Feinberg and Rosenberg, 1951), or are on very low salt diets (Aaron and Weston, 1952). Critical hyponatremia due to resin treatment alone seems most improbable in view of the findings of Elkinton *et al.* (1952) and Greenman *et al.* (1953*a*), who noted reduced capacity figures for resins as the sodium intake was reduced. At a level of 200 mg. for sodium intake, the capacity of the resin was reduced to 0.3 mEq. per gram. This may in some measure be due to a changed ratio of monovalent to polyvalent cations, and if so would be corrected by the use of chelating agents, a procedure magnifying the danger of hyponatremia.

Clinical indications of the onset of hyponatremia include nausea, vomiting, weakness, apathy, mental changes, lethargy, dehydration and anorexia (Aaron and Weston, 1952; Greenman *et al.*, 1953*a*). Laboratory data where possible should include serum sodium determinations, but lacking proper facilities, an estimate can be reached by taking the sum of serum carbon dioxide and chloride concentration plus ten (milliequivalents per liter) (Aaron and Weston, 1952). The limitations of this practice are reviewed by Hald *et al.* (1947) and Greenman *et al.* (1953*a*), both groups indicating that there is no substitute for direct determination of sodium itself.

The determination of the existence of a state of hyponatremia by means of laboratory findings does not indicate clinical manifestations, as these have occurred in only 1 of 5 patients with low serum sodium values (Greenman *et al.*, 1953*b*). Further recovery has followed in all patients within 4 to 9 days after the withdrawal of the resin and the addition of salt to the diet (Greenman *et al.*, 1953*b*). In no single instance was there a typical low sodium syndrome.

There is some difference of opinion on the relative merits of the several resin forms. Comparisons of sulfonic and carboxylic resins tend to indicate close parallel in capacity, although Emerson *et al.* (1951) present data supporting the contention that the carboxylic types are superior. Another phase of this problem relates to the efficacy of various cycles of a given resin. Here there is general agreement that metallic cation forms are of lower capacity than the hydrogen. For example, Elkinton *et al.* (1952) compared the ammonium with the potassium-ammonium types and found the latter less efficacious in terms of sodium removal. Finally, the question of augmented capacity due to combined anion-cation resin administration has been raised by Martz *et al.* (1952). These workers give figures indicating such increase in studies conducted on 5 patients. In one of these receiving 60 Gm. of cation resin, the fecal sodium was 138 mEq., and with the addition of 8 Gm. of anion exchange resin this figure rose to 150 mEq. This would indicate that a 13.3 per cent increase in total weight of resin given caused a 9 per cent increase in fecal sodium. Clearly this would represent a net loss per unit weight of resin ingested, although there would be an increase in the amount of sodium removed per unit weight of cation exchanger. There would be no advantage in this, as a similar increase in cation exchanger ingested would increase fecal sodium by an amount in excess of that caused by the anion-cation combination.

Several investigators have proposed that the effect of cation exchange resins is not due solely to sodium removal. For instance, Dock and Frank (1950) noted, in the early phases of resin administration, a weight loss occurring at a rate greater than that which would result if fecal loss of sodium were the only factor. They consider this as due in part to a rise rather than the usual fall in urinary sodium caused by the compensated acidosis, but due in a major sense to the shift of sodium into muscle to replace potassium losses.

Acidosis. Acidosis is frequently cited as a major deterrent to the use of cation exchange resins. It is therefore important to consider this side effect in some detail, for its incidence, severity and significance have been unduly emphasized, with the result that clinicians are inclined to view the hazards of resin therapy in a disproportionate sense. Initially, it is well to review compensated and uncompensated acidosis. The compensated form of acidosis is characterized by a modified alkali reserve as reflected in the carbon dioxide–combining power of the plasma, but it causes neither symptoms nor pathological changes; it is in direct contrast to an uncompensated acidosis, which is dangerous and does produce symptomatic manifestations such as hyperventilation. A compensated acidosis is beneficial for edema reduction, as we shall show.

Impaired renal function is generally regarded as a contraindication to resin therapy (Irwin *et al.*, 1949; Danowski *et al.*, 1951*b*; Emerson *et al.*, 1951; Feinberg and Rosenberg, 1951; Kattus, 1952; Kleiber and Pickar, 1951; Voyles and Orgain, 1951; Greenman *et al.*, 1953*a*), since reduced ammonia formation by the diseased kidney would facilitate development of an uncompensated acidosis. The increased loss of base via the intestinal tract caused by the use of resin requires a compensatory increase in ammonia and acid in the urine; a damaged kidney reduces the natural biological compensatory mechanism. To the present author, the statement of Emerson *et al.* (1951), to the effect that the potential danger of development of an uncompensated acidosis is the limiting factor in the therapeutic use of resin in patients with renal involvement, seems more logical. In other words, resin therapy is not contraindicated in patients with renal damage but does constitute a limiting factor, due to the greater probability for the development of an uncompensated acidosis. Renal damage is the signal for increased vigilance but not necessarily for cessation of resin therapy. The danger signals as given by Emerson *et al.* (1951) are absence of increased urinary ammonia excretion during the early period of resin therapy and/or decreased carbon dioxide–combining power of the plasma.

These investigators (Emerson *et al.*, 1951) cite the example of a patient with nephrosis, showing normal renal function except for proteinuria, who developed no acidosis after 3 months of continuous resin therapy, manifesting a tenfold increase in urinary ammonia. By contrast, a patient with glomerulonephritis immediately developed an acidosis, necessitating cessation of resin therapy.

The actual incidence of uncompensated acidosis among patients on resin therapy is very low. Thus Kleiber and Pickar (1951) observed no instances in their studies. The first report of Voyles and Orgain (1951) substantiated this finding. In fact, they reported no acidosis in their chronic decompensated cardiacs during periods of 8 and 9 months of resin therapy, this despite the fact that some of the patients had renal involvement. A few additional references will serve to substantiate the statement that uncompensated acidosis, while possible, is of rare occurrence. Wood *et al.* (1952) record the development of a mild compensated acidosis in 10 of 14 patients with cardiac decompensation. Of their entire series of 23, some 15 showed a carbon dioxide combining power below 20 mEq. per liter. They concluded that this represents only a moderate hazard and that in patients whose plasma bicarbonate falls slightly to moderately, recovery to normal levels will occur with continuation of resin therapy. To quote from their paper, "in no instance has the acidosis appeared to be a clinical hazard where adequate renal function was present."

When uncompensated acidosis does occur, the dangers are not great. Feinberg and Rosenberg (1951) noted the development of an uncompensated acidosis in 1 of their 7 patients. In this instance, the carbon dioxide–combining power fell to 11 mEq. per liter, and concomitantly symptoms such as apathy, weakness, stupor and anorexia developed. These patients showed kidney impairment, but despite this responded quickly to therapy with salt, alkali and fluids.

Presentation of such detail with reference to acidosis is deemed logical by the present author, as it is believed that this side effect of resin therapy is in fact not serious and that the induction of a compensated acidosis is even desirable. Further, the development of an uncompensated acidosis, while a matter for immediate attention, is not of vital importance; in very few instances has it been reported that such uncompensated acidosis had serious consequences.

Three proposals have been made with respect to resin dosage forms and the incidence of acidosis, compensated or uncompensated. The first of these, involving the inclusion in the dosage form of a potassium cycle fraction, has been universally accepted. The studies of Callahan *et al.* (1952) are of importance in consideration of this problem. Of 22 patients treated with a carboxylic resin in the ammonium-potassium cycle, 1 patient developed acidosis, showing a carbon dioxide–combining power of the serum of 37 volumes per cent and manifesting related symptoms. Further, he was the sole patient of the group with evidence of renal damage. All patients receiving an ammonium cycle sulfonic resin developed acidosis.

The difference lies largely in the absence of potassium cycle form in the sulfonic composition. This would restrict fixed base intake. The conclusion to be drawn from this study is that in the absence of renal damage uncompensated acidosis associated with resin administration is a rare thing, and further, such absence of acidosis is a reflection in large measure of the presence in the form administered of a proper portion in the potassium cycle.

Danowski and his associates (1951*b*) were able to produce a decrease in serum carbon dioxide content within 3 or more days in all patients given straight ammonium or hydrogen cycle resins. When the same resins were given in the sodium, potassium or calcium cycles, no acidosis or hyperchloremia occurred. The goal according to this group (Greenman *et al.*, 1953*a*) is the production of a compensated but prevention of an uncompensated acidosis, and this was achieved in patients receiving hydrogen-potassium cycle forms. The position is taken that the clinical efficacy of resin therapy depends partially on sodium removal and partially or even mainly on the acidifying effects of the resins. In no single instance did the biochemical findings reflect themselves in clinical symptoms. In other words, when the resin form containing potassium was used (20 per cent potassium cycle), a compensated acidosis essential to the production of a diuresis occurred, but in no instance did this pass over into an uncompensated acidosis. These investigators recommend vigilance on the part of the clinician against potential uncompensated acidosis, and the employment of precautions paralleling those observed in the continued use of ammonium chloride. It is to be emphasized that in this group of 12 cardiacs, none of whom had renal involvement, not a single case of uncompensated acidosis occurred.

Dock and Frank (1950) had presented the biochemical basis for the induction of acidosis by hydrogen cycle resin and had simultaneously offered the rationale for the inclusion of potassium cycle forms. They indicated that exchange would entail the displacement of hydrogen ions by mono- or polyvalent fixed-base cations, thus tending to acidify via the liberation of the hydrogen ions, and at the same time removing from the body fixed base ordinarily utilized by the kidney for pairing with anion and for subsequent excretion. The result of hydrogen cycle resin ingestion would be greater production by the kidney of ammonium ions to be paired with anions in replacement of the fixed base normally so utilized. With continued administration the plasma carbon dioxide–combining power falls, a state designated as compensated acidosis; however, if kidney function is impaired, this state of compensated acidosis can pass over into an uncompensated state and clinical acidosis ensue, with apathy, anorexia and hyperventilation. This, however, should not be interpreted to indicate an advantage with ammonium cycle forms, as the nephrotic patient of Kattus (1952) was given a sulfonic resin of this type and developed an uncompensated acidosis on the tenth day.

Voyles and Orgain (1952) had raised this issue in stressing the dangers of acidosis related to the use of hydrogen-potassium cycle resins as contrasted to ammonium-potassium cycle forms. Repeated tests have shown that there is no difference. For example, Holley (1952) states: "We have not noted any significant difference between the hydrogen and ammonium forms as far as acid-base balance is concerned." The second of the proposals made relative to acidosis incidence and dosage forms contended that ammonium cycle types were superior; this can be disposed of immediately, as there is no difference between the hydrogen and the ammonium cycle forms.

The third proposal concerning dosage forms suggested that combined use of anion and cation exchangers reduced the degree and incidence of acidosis. This is probably academic, in view of the position of Danowski *et al.* (1951*a*) that the therapeutic efficacy of cation exchange resins is in large measure due to the precipitation of a compensated acidosis. However, Martz *et al.* (1952) contend that the use of combinations of anion and cation exchange resins produces this effect. The conclusion seems to be based upon 1 patient who developed acidosis while on a cation exchange resin alone, and who, when placed on a combination of anion-cation resin, did not redevelop an acidosis. They assert that this reduced tendency to acidosis follows because the addition of an anion exchange resin tends to reverse the shift of anion from feces to urine. In substantiation of the latter point, the balance figures for 2 patients are given. They indicate that while reversal did occur, the fecal excretion of anions caused by the addition of the anion exchange resin to the cation form did not equal that of the normal period. In other words, there remained a residual tendency toward acidosis.

Again, Aaron and Weston (1952) report incidence of acidosis following the use of anion-cation exchange resin combinations paralleling that observed with ammonium chloride. Prime danger of uncompensated acidosis occurred in patients with impaired kidney function and in older age groups. They regard a serum carbon dioxide value of 20 mEq. per liter or above as satisfactory for the continuation of resin therapy.

Best (1952*b*) and Chapman *et al.* (1951) have studied anion-cation exchange resin combinations, but in neither report was any direct comparison made of the acidosis-inducing power of the forms with and without added anion exchanger.

Conclusions. Uncompensated and compensated acidosis occur when patients are given straight hydrogen or ammonium cycle resins. When resins are ingested partially in the potassium cycle, it is doubtful that uncompensated acidosis occurs. In any event, it is rare. A compensated acidosis will develop, and this seems essential to the induction of diuresis and therefore to the proper function of the resin.

Renal involvement is a danger signal. It does not necessarily contraindicate the use of resins but does call for vigilance. Ammonia excretion in the urine and serum carbon dioxide content can be used as signals for the logical cessation of resin therapy if abnormalities ensue.

There is no difference relative to acidosis incidence between hydrogen-potassium cycle and ammonium-potassium cycle forms. Further, it is doubtful that the inclusion of an anion exchange resin will significantly modify the production of compensated acidosis. In addition, if such action did occur, it would materially reduce the therapeutic efficacy of the regimen.

From the literature, one can only conclude that there has been an uncalled-for emphasis on the dangers of acidosis associated with resin therapy. That caution is indicated is unquestioned, but this is equally true of the use of cortisone, sulfonamides, penicillin or even aspirin. There can be no absolute assurance against uncompensated acidosis, but even if it does occur, the symptomatic signs are clear and correction can be made immediately.

Anorexia with reduced food intake, or any other state involving abnormal electrolyte balance, is a signal for added caution in the use of resins. If resin therapy is continued during such periods, the probability of precipitating side effects, including acidosis, is markedly increased.

Potassium. Cation exchange resins are not selective in their action, and therefore it was to have been assumed that such agents would remove potassium (Dock and Frank, 1950; Hay and Wood, 1950; Emerson *et al.*, 1951; Feinberg and Rosenberg, 1951; Aaron and Weston, 1952; Callahan *et al.*, 1952; Greenman *et al.*, 1953a). Not only do resins remove potassium, but they actually possess a greater affinity for this element than for sodium (Dock and Frank, 1950; Emerson *et al.*, 1951).

Dock and Frank (1950) found the ratio of sodium to potassium in the diet to be the determinant in the degree of potassium removal during resin therapy. When the diet had a normal salt content (over 2 Gm. per day), the ratio of sodium to potassium removed was roughly 1 to 1 or 1 to 1.5, but if the diet contained less than 1 Gm. of salt, the ratio was shifted to 1 to 5. Since five times as much potassium was removed as sodium, they estimate that 100 Gm. of resin might remove as much as 6 Gm. of potassium daily. When patients are on low sodium diets, the potentialities for the development of hypokalemia are magnified. This would be true even with the resin forms in which a portion is in the potassium cycle. Correlation of salt intake with potential potassium removal does not represent a major obstacle to the use of resins, as supplemental potassium salts can be given. Generally, the amount of potassium cycle resin included in the presently available commercial preparations is adequate to prevent hypokalemia but does not provide for all contingencies. The findings of Emerson *et al.* (1951) are in agreement with those of Dock and Frank (1950) and place the range of change or increased fecal potassium excretion at 0.21 to 2.32 mEq. per gram.

Hypokalemia can and does occur following the administration of resins (Hay and Wood, 1950; Feinberg and Rosenberg, 1951; Callahan *et al.*, 1952; Greenman *et al.*, 1953*a, b*). These agents given in the hydrogen cycle are almost certain to cause hypokalemia, but the incidence is low when hydrogen-potassium or ammonium-potassium forms are used. For example, Hay and Wood (1950) precipitated hypokalemia in a patient with ammonium cycle forms, but in their experience no evidence of hypokalemia occurred when resins containing potassium cycle forms were given. Again, Feinberg and Rosenberg (1951) report 4 cases in which a moderate fall of serum potassium occurred but in only 1 of the 4 was the fall of clinical significance. Their results were obtained with a resin in the ammonium-potassium cycle containing about 20 mEq. of potassium per each 15 Gm. of resin. Finally, of 12 cardiacs receiving a hydrogen-potassium cycle resin, 4 developed hypokalemia (serum potassium below 3.5 mEq. per liter) (Greenman *et al.*, 1953). In each instance the patient had not been eating well. An additional 3 patients showed serum potassium decreases of 0.6 to 1.3 mEq. per liter but no hypokalemia.

The most common complaint of patients with abnormally low serum potassium is that of weakness (Greenman *et al.*, 1953*a*) or vomiting and severe diarrhea (Aaron and Weston, 1952). A case report is given by Greenman *et al.* (1953*a*) of a patient who had shifted from hydrogen-potassium cycle resin to straight hydrogen cycle and developed hypokalemia. The first signs of complications were marked muscle weakness and lethargy, resulting in difficulty of movement of arms and legs and a tendency to fall when walking was attempted. Electrocardiographic changes developed with premature beats but no arrhythmias such as are described as being the only diagnostic criteria of hypokalemia. The hypokalemia was corrected by the administration of 0.6 Gm. of potassium chloride given with meals and at bedtime. Subsequently, the patient was given hydrogen-potassium cycle resin without resultant recurrence of hypokalemia. It is emphasized by these workers that available hydrogen-potassium or ammonium-potassium cycle resins provide adequate potassium under conditions of normal dietary intake but not in the event of decreased food intake, vomiting, or other conditions tending in themselves to reduce body potassium.

A point of major importance in any consideration of hypokalemia induced by resins is the increased sensitivity this causes to digitalis (Hay and Wood, 1950; Feinberg and Rosenberg, 1951; Callahan *et al.*, 1952). Signs of digitalis intoxication were used by Hay and Wood (1950) as being indicative of hypokalemia. Support of this contention came from the work of Feinberg and Rosenberg (1951) and was later studied in detail by Callahan and his associates (1952). The latter group reports 8 of 20 cases on ammonium-potassium cycle carboxylic resins manifesting evidence of digitalis toxicity, including ventricular premature beats in 3, multiple ventricular premature beats producing bigeminy in 3, and ventricular rates below 60 in the presence of auricular fibrillation in 2 patients. Two others showed increased digitalis effect as reflected by T wave and S-T segment alteration in the electrocardiogram. Correction of the toxic manifestation resulted from decreased dosage of either digitalis or of resin. As was to have been anticipated, the digitalis toxicity was correlated with decrease in serum potassium levels of more than 0.5 mEq. per liter in 4 of these patients. It is of importance to consider that serum potassium levels do not necessarily reflect the potassium content of heart muscle, which is the direct correlative of increased sensitivity to digitalis. In another patient of the series, serum potassium levels fell below 3.5 mEq. per liter, but such a drastic decrease did not occur in the group of patients manifesting symptoms of digitalis intoxication. In the series receiving the sulfonic type of resin in the ammonium cycle, 3 gave evidence of increased sensitivity to digitalis and in 2 of these the potassium levels in the serum were known to have fallen below 3.0 mEq. per liter. This fall in serum potassium was general in this group, occurring in some 13 patients of the 14 on whom determinations were made. Once again, comparisons cannot be made between these two groups, as the experimental structure was not of a nature permitting comparison. Certainly the latter series clearly indicates the necessity of supplying any cation exchanger partially in the potassium cycle to avoid the dangers of hypokalemia.

Callahan and his associates (1952) emphasize that danger of hyperkalemia exists, if the ammonium-potassium cycle resins are used in patients with kidney damage impairing ability to excrete potassium. From these reports it is clear that patients receiving digitalis to whose regimen resins are to be added must be carefully watched. The best approach is that of dropping the digitalis dose to approximately 50 per cent and then increasing it after electrolyte stability has been achieved.

All resin forms seem about equal with respect to the induction of hypokalemia. Thus, the sulfonic and carboxylic forms are essentially parallel (Emerson *et al.*, 1951), and when these results are compared to those of Aaron and Weston (1952) it is seen that the anion-cation combinations fall into the same general category. The latter workers recommend the drinking of two glasses of orange juice daily (supplying about 20 mEq. of potassium) as a preventive.

Calcium and Magnesium. Divalent and multivalent cations are generally more capable of forming nonionizable complexes than are the monovalent cations, with the result that the pool of these ions available in the gut for exchange with the resins is comparatively small. Despite this, and due to the great affinity of the polyvalent cations for exchange groups, both calcium and magnesium are removed by resins. The degree is indicated to be about 0.1 mEq. per gram of resin for both calcium and magnesium (total 0.2 mEq. for both divalent cations) (Emerson *et al.*, 1951). Another group of investigators (Martz *et al.*, 1952) found that fecal calcium increased by 9.8 mEq. per day during the period of administration of a combination anion-cation resin form.

The problem presented is that of the induction of hypocalcemia by resin therapy, and on this point findings vary but tend to indicate that on prolonged administration low blood calcium levels do occur. Several groups of investigators (Hay and Wood, 1950; Martz *et al.*, 1952) have reported that resin administration even for periods of 9 months did not modify serum calcium values. On the other hand, hypocalcemia was observed in several patients by Greenblatt and Gilwood (1948); by Emerson *et al.* (1951); by Feinberg and Rosenberg (1951) in 2 of 7 patients; by Dock and Frank (1950); and by Greenman *et al.* (1953*a*) in 4 of 12 cardiacs. In general, clinical reflections of lowered blood calcium levels have not been noted, but isolated cases of tetany (total, 3) have been reported by Greenblatt and Gilwood (1948) and by Dock and Frank (1950). Greenman *et al.* (1953*a*), while they observed no clinical evidence of hypocalcemia, list possible dangers thereof as being neuromuscular sensitivity, tetany, cataract formation, osteomalacia and susceptibility to fractures.

Several reports support the contention that polyvalent cations materially reduce the capacity of resins for monovalent ions. For example, Danowski *et al.* (1951*b*) found no significantly increased sodium or potassium content of stools following the administration of a calcium cycle resin. The affinity of the calcium for the exchange sites exceeds that of the monovalent cations, with the result that little if any exchange occurs. Further, when supplemental forms of calcium are given to prevent hypocalcemia, the efficacy of the resin for monovalent cations is reduced markedly (Callahan *et al.*, 1952).

It is highly probable that the stronger-acid exchanger, the sulfonic type, will have a greater tendency to induce hypocalcemia. Callahan and his associates (1952) found no evidence of hypocalcemia in a series of 22 patients receiving a carboxylic resin of the ammonium-potassium form. On the other hand, in a series receiving a sulfonic resin in the ammonium cycle, depression of calcium levels was general by the end of the first week. In 6 of the 14 patients in this group, serum calcium values of 7.5 mg. per 100 ml. were noted after the second week. One specific example given by these workers is that of a patient who showed a serum calcium level of 7.5 mg. per 100 ml. on the ammonium cycle sulfonic resin, and subsequently when placed on the carboxylic resin showed normal serum calcium even after 33 weeks on the regimen. Similar findings were recorded by Emerson *et al.* (1951), who observed hypocalcemia in a patient receiving a sulfonic resin over a period of 6 weeks, but found no parallel side effect with the carboxyl forms.

Greenman *et al.* (1953*a*) conclude that calcium depletion in human beings is a concomitant of long-continued use of resins, and offer three possible solutions: first, intravenous injection of calcium as the gluconate or the citrate; second, intermittent administration of the resin; and third, supplementation with oral calcium salts. Election of the first carries with it the impracticality of continued parenteral therapy; of the second, the danger of recurrence of edema; and of the third, decreased efficacy of the resin for monovalent cations.

There is a fourth possible approach to the problem not indicated by Greenman *et al.* (1953*a*), and this is through the concomitant use of chelating agents such as ethylenediamine tetra-acetic acid which would bind the calcium preferentially in the gut, preventing its fixation on the resin, but which in the blood stream would liberate the captive calcium, providing adequate supplies of this essential ion. Certainly the problem is real, and as indicated by Greenman *et al.* (1953*a*) will become more and more acute as with the passage of time uninterrupted resin therapy over prolonged periods becomes common practice. The immediate solutions are given above; the final solution, it is believed, will come by way of the use of chelators.

The practical aspects of selection of the third approach discussed above are easily resolved. Emerson *et al.* (1951) recommend the daily administration of 0.5 Gm. of dicalcium phosphate. This figure approximates that of Hay and Wood (1950), which is 18 mEq. of calcium to be given during the day. Any parallel regimen can be employed, but it should be held in mind that the efficacy of the resin is thereby reduced.

Chloride. It is generally agreed that elevation of plasma chlorides follows the administration of resins (Danowski *et al.*, 1951*a*; Wood *et al.*, 1952; Greenman *et al.*, 1953*a*). The incidence of such elevation is high, occurring in some 15 of 16 patients receiving 45 Gm. daily of an ammonium-potassium cycle resin (Wood *et al.*, 1952), and in 11 of 12 patients receiving a resin in the hydrogen-potassium cycle (Greenman *et al.*, 1953*a*). In general, hyperchloremia develops within 3 days or shortly thereafter (Danowski *et al.*, 1951*a*).

Miscellaneous Usage. The broader aspects of the application of cation exchange resins have not been explored. Several proposals have appeared, supported by clinical results, indicating use in the control of obesity (Emerson *et al.*, 1951), in the treatment of premenstrual tension (Emerson *et al.*, 1951; Voyles and Orgain, 1952), for edema associated with constrictive pericarditis (Hay and Wood, 1950), and for arteriosclerotic heart disease (Bonner, 1952).

In the control of obesity, Emerson *et al.* (1951) cite 1 case in which a 10- to 15-lb. weight loss was induced after an 800-calorie diet had failed. Premenstrual tension was susceptible to treatment with resins in those cases showing weight gain in the immediate premenstrual period (Emerson *et al.*, 1951; Voyles and Orgain, 1952).

Bonner (1952) studied 4 patients with hypertensive arteriosclerotic heart diseases, 3 with arteriosclerotic heart disease, 1 with Laennec's cirrhosis, 1 with carcinomatosis of the peritoneum, and 1 with heart disease due to myxedema; all showed various degrees of water retention. Of the group, 8 responded with weight loss ranging from 8 lbs. in 3 days to 26 lbs. in 10 days after having been placed on sulfonic types of resins in doses of 60 Gm. daily.

Restriction of electrolyte intake by the use of resins offers vast potentialities for the treatment of disease. Ion balance and ion ratios have been neglected in recent years in favor of more spectacular and less fundamental aspects of medical science, but it would seem that there has already been a shift back to consideration of electrolyte balance, and such study offers vast possibilities. Selective removal of ions will become more important with the passage of time, and resins alone can accomplish this.

Modes of Taking Resins. Callahan *et al.* (1952) recommend 15-Gm. doses three times daily at mealtime in coffee, tea, water, fruit juice or ginger ale. Another and similar recommendation is made by Feinberg and Rosenberg (1951), who propose water or salt-free tomato juice. Voyles and Orgain (1952) gave three 15-Gm. doses daily mixed with cold fruit juice, water or in some cases with foods such as mashed potatoes or apple sauce.

Yet another approach is proposed by Greenman *et al.* (1953a), who noted that the majority of patients preferred to mix the resin with water and drink the suspension as rapidly as possible. Some patients seemed to prefer cold grapefruit juice or carbonated beverages.

Prolonged Chronic Use. There have been comparatively few studies on the prolonged use of cation exchange resins, and of those reported the results are found to be at variance. This is not unexpected when one considers that diet would be a significant factor, and it would vary from group to group. The predominance of opinion expressed is that with care resins can be used for periods of 1 to 2 years.

Emerson and his associates (1951) were among those employing supplemental daily administration of potassium chloride (1.5 Gm.). In their series, when a resin partially in the potassium cycle was used, after 2 years there was no hyponatremia and only a mild degree of intracellular hypokalemia. The resin was well tolerated and clinical efficacy was maintained throughout. Similarly, Voyles and Orgain (1952) in their studies of 7 cardiacs, which extended over periods of 7 to 14 months, encountered only 1 patient who developed a severe electrolyte disturbance. In this case, the precipitating factor was a failure to ingest food during a period when the patient had an attack of gallbladder colic. Clinical acidosis and hypokalemia were observed. Certainly in any case subject to factors modifying the electrolyte balance picture materially, such as sweating or failure to ingest food, resin therapy should either be withdrawn or dosage reduced.

The conclusion reached by Greenman and his associates (1953*a*) was that the biochemical findings reported in their series of 12 cardiacs treated for periods up to 12 months probably preclude continuous long-term therapy with resins. In 7 of the group there was abnormally low serum concentration of either sodium, potassium or calcium; further, in many instances, these abnormalities were multiple. Again, this group emphasized the dangers of resin therapy in subjects who do not eat, who are vomiting or are experiencing other conditions which in themselves tend to reduce sodium and potassium. They observed the development of hyponatremia between the ninety-first and the four hundred and ninth days; of hypokalemia between the one hundred and twenty-seventh and two hundred and sixty-sixth days; and of hypocalcemia between the one hundred and seventy-ninth and four hundred and ninth days. They concluded from this that: "These resins provide a relatively safe supplement to the basic therapy for approximately six months," but after this period potentialities for the development of excessive demineralization mount.

There are several means of circumventing demineralization and thus safely extending the period of resin treatment. These have been discussed but are repeated here for emphasis. The first involves intermittent therapy (4 days on resin and 3 off); the second centers around supplementation with calcium and potassium salts; and the third involves the use of chelating agents. The last procedure has not yet been worked out clinically but looks most hopeful; the first two can be employed now, as full clinical information is available.

Additional Side Effects. The chances are good that constipation and other gastrointestinal side effects associated with resin therapy are the result of the concomitant regimen rather than the resin itself. There will be exceptions to this, but in general if such side effects were directly attributable to the resins a larger percentage of authors would so indicate; furthermore, animal studies would have reflected the defect, and neither situation holds. There is yet another factor which the present author feels supports the contention that cation exchange resins in themselves are not constipating, and it is the number of reports listing both constipation and diarrhea as side effects of the use of resin. Generally, when both diarrhea and constipation are recorded as resulting from a given agent, the true cause lies elsewhere.

The reported incidence of constipation varies, as can be seen from Table 27. The basis of the variation doubtless lies in the mode of administration of the resin and in the dietary regimen adopted. Correction of the constipation can be brought about by the use of laxatives and increased fluid intake (Voyles and Orgain, 1951; Aaron and Weston, 1952), or by slowly increasing the resin ingestion until the full therapeutic level is reached. Aaron and Weston (1952) report the latter procedure successful in eliminating or reducing such side effects. Dock and Frank (1950) are the only investigators to report that fecal impaction may occur, but they give no statistics in support of the statement.

Palatability is another problem directly related to the regimen employed. There are many ways of administering resins, and the most effective will vary with the patient. Alternate modes of administration should be proposed to the patient, permitting a choice. Small individual dosage units properly spaced throughout the day and arranged to the patient's taste will doubtless reduce this problem to a minimum.

There seems little reason to believe that various resin forms or cycles differ materially with respect to side effect causation. The results of Callahan *et al.* (1952) would seem on superficial examination to constitute an indictment of the carboxylic resin used in their trials, but the experimental design is such as to preclude all comparisons, e.g., the first series were ambulant and the majority of the second (on the sulfonic resin) were hospitalized. By contrast, Dock and Frank (1950) state, "Digestive disturbance is less with the carboxylic than with the sulfonic types of resin." Further, the anion-cation exchanger combinations induce approximately the same incidence of side effects (Aaron and Weston, 1952).

Danowski and his associates (1951*b*) found alterations in bowel habits were minimal following the administration of potassium-hydrogen cycle carboxylic resins. Most patients objected to the grittiness and bulk of the resin during the first weeks of treatment (Greenman *et al.*, 1953*a*) and generally experienced gastric irritation and eructation immediately following ingestion of the resin. In all cases these complaints subsided. These authors conclude that gastrointestinal symptoms are not an insurmountable obstacle to continued treatment even over a period extending from 150 to 451 days.

Proper construction of the therapeutic regimen adopted will minimize the incidence of gastrointestinal symptoms. The patient must be instructed in ways and means of preparing the resin for ingestion.

TABLE 27

Gastrointestinal Symptoms Attributed to Resin Therapy

Palatability	Anorexia	Side effects					Resin type	Reference
		Constipation	Diarrhea	Nausea	Vomiting	Other		
2-7						Burning in stomach 1-7	Carboxylic H+	Kleiber and Pickar, 1951
		1-3					Carboxylic K+, NH4+	Voyles and Orgain, 1951
		Majority					Carboxylic K+, NH4+	Voyles and Orgain, 1952
Majority		Majority					Carboxylic K+, NH4+	Hay and Wood, 1950
			Occurred	4-35	4-35	Rectal irritation	Carboxylic K+, NH4+	Wood et al., 1952
	10-22	6-22	4-22	11-22	8-22		Carboxylic K+, NH4+	Callahan et al., 1952
	2-22	5-22	4-22	4-22			Sulfonic NH4+	Callahan et al., 1952
		Majority fecal impaction 20-34	Majority	Majority			Sulfonic H+	Dock and Frank, 1950
							Carboxylic K+, NH4+	Klingensmith and Elkinton, 1952
Majority	3-12	6-12	1-12	7-12	3-12		Carboxylic K+, H+	Danowski et al., 1951 a, b Greenman et al., 1953
	Common	Common		Common			Anion Cation	Aaron and Weston, 1952

Above all, he must be given a choice of regimen and adjusted psychologically to it. If these precautions are taken, gastrointestinal side effects of resin therapy will be largely eliminated.

Special Aspects. For some time, it has been known that the decreased cardiac output associated with heart failure leads to venous congestion of the liver and in turn to a reduced power of the liver to inactivate those cortical hormones acting on the kidney to cause retention of sodium. While this was generally recognized, the impact of these corticosteroids on the excretion of sodium into the lumen of the gut was not known. The first evidence of control of sodium transfer into the gut by steroids was presented by Berger *et al.* (1951). These investigators, using cation exchange resins to trap the intestinal sodium of rats, found that desoxycorticosterone markedly reduced the intestinal sodium content without significantly altering the potassium concentration. This conclusion was deduced from the approximately 40 per cent reduction in the amount of sodium in the feces of the resin-fed animals. Results paralleling those observed in the rat were obtained in 3 patients. From these results, Berger and his associates (1951) properly concluded that descoxycorticosterone controls not only the transfer of sodium from the blood stream to the lumen of the kidney tubule but similarly controls such transfer in the intestine, and in the sweat and salivary glands. In each instance, the net effect is limitation of the escape of sodium from the body.

Extending this line of approach to the general problem of edema, this same group (Berger *et al.,* 1951) found again by employing cation exchange resins as sodium traps that the colon of the edematous patient retains sodium to a greater degree than does the colon of the normal subject. They conclude that edema in association with cardiac failure and in cirrhosis of the liver is in some measure the result of disturbed hormonal control of sodium transfer.

This line of research leads automatically to consideration of the potentialities of increasing the capacity of cation exchange resins through the use of steroid hormones counteracting or blocking the action of desoxycorticosterone, or of possible steroid factors which would in a positive sense increase the transfer of sodium into the gut, thereby rendering it available in greater concentration to the exchange action of the cation exchange resin. Such studies are at the present time being conducted in our own laboratories, and are mentioned here simply to call attention to the complexity of the mosaic of mineral balance and to emphasize the magnitude of the problems not yet resolved but of prime importance to this field.

Edema in Cirrhosis of the Liver

Irwin *et al.* (1949) first reported the clinical efficacy of cation exchange resins in the control of edema associated with cirrhosis of the liver. The resin was of the sulfonic type, hydrogen cycle. Generally, the biochemical findings reported coincide with those seen following the use of such resins in the treament of other clinical states, e.g., increased fecal sodium and potassium, serum chloride increase, serum carbon dioxide fall, urinary sodium and potassium decrease and so forth. The efficacy of the resin in control of edema was clearly demonstrated by alternating periods with and without the therapy, with notation of returning edema during the control period.

In controlling edema associated with cirrhosis through the use of cation exchange resins, the development of acidosis is a problem, and for the resolution of this difficulty Martz and his associates (1952) have proposed the use of combinations of anion and cation exchange resins. They conclude that the tendency to acidosis is reduced through use of these combinations (see section on acidosis in this chapter). While their clinical results were good, they emphasize that the factor of hypoproteinemia can and does complicate the picture. If hypoproteinemia is present, electrolyte concentration of body fluids can be in the hypotonic range without eliminating the edema. According to these workers, 2 deaths had been reported to them as having occurred in patients receiving the resins. These were far-advanced cases of cirrhosis with marked ascites, in which all other methods of control had failed. Serum protein was low and the picture was further complicated by anorexia and diarrhea, the latter two conditions tending to magnify cation withdrawal by the resins as a result of decreased intake.

Among the early groups of workers studying the effects of cation exchange resins for the control of edema in cirrhosis of the liver were Moser and his associates (1951). They employed a combination anion-cation exchange product in a study of 8 cirrhotic patients. A 1.5-Gm. sodium diet with supplemental protein (salt-free) was administered, and after a control period during which it was observed that this regimen failed to relieve the ascites, resin therapy was instituted at a level of 30 to 50 Gm. In 5 of the patients this resulted in control of the ascites; with the other 3, sodium intake was either elevated or lowered, with ultimate success in ascites control. Figure 20, from this paper, illustrates well the rather striking effect of resin therapy in ascites. In this case ascites and pedal edema disappeared completely in 28 days on resin therapy and reappeared almost immediately upon discontinuance. A second resin regimen once again induced complete clinical control of the edema.

FIGURE 20
The Effect of Resins on Body Weight and the Urinary Excretion of Sodium and Potassium

(From Moser, R. H., *et al., Gastroenterology,* **19**: 336, 1951)

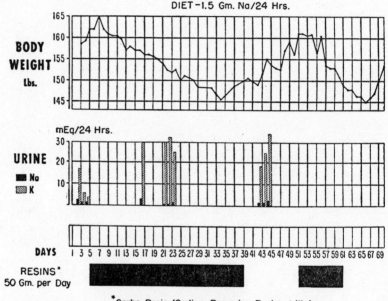

When this series of cirrhotics with ascites was extended to include some 24 patients, the results continued essentially parallel, as seen from Table 28, taken from the investigators' paper (Rosenak *et al.,* 1952). Two important contributions are made in this second report. The first establishes plasma carbon dioxide, sodium and potassium determinations as completely adequate for proper laboratory control of the cirrhotic liver patient with ascites. The carbon dioxide determinations can at the outset be made at weekly intervals. As knowledge of the patient's reaction to resin therapy increases, the interval between such determinations can be extended. Potassium determinations are stated to be desirable but not essential, as the symptomatology of hypokalemia is easily recognized and electrocardiographic evidence of lowered potassium is generally available. Again, sodium determinations are not considered essential but should be immediately available should the question arise. These authors recommend discontinuation of resin therapy and salt administration in all doubtful cases. From Table 28

TABLE 28
Results of Treatment in 24 Cases

(From Rosenak, B. D., *et al.*, *Gastroenterology*, **22**: 575, 1952)

Result	No. of cases	Complications	No. of cases
Good—absence of ascites and edema	17	Hypokalemia	
Fair—persistence of some ascites and/or edema with continued paracentesis	4	Mild—responded to oral K salts. Resin resumed	3
		Severe—associated with hyponatremia. Resin stopped. Parenteral Na & K	1
Poor—no response or drug not tolerated	3	Acidosis	
	Total cases 24	Mild, transient—dose of resin reduced	2
		Nausea and vomiting	
		Drug stopped	1
		Dose reduced	1
		Total cases 8	
		Resin stopped 2	

it is noted that only 1 instance of hyponatremia occurred in their series of 24 cases. From their discussion it is clear that lowered food intake should be regarded as a serious complication of resin therapy in the sense that reduced cation ingestion may upset ion balance and precipitate a condition such as hyponatremia. If this factor is taken into consideration and watched carefully, it is doubtful that hyponatremia would ever occur.

The second important thought advanced by Rosenak *et al.* (1952) is that of intermittent therapy as originally proposed by Hay and Wood

(1950). They suggest that resin administration be continued until such time as the ascites and edema are brought under control, and that at this time the resin therapy be discontinued for 1 or 2 days or until the time of reappearance of water retention; such intermittent administration of resin should, according to these authors, markedly increase the safety of resin administration without reducing the therapeutic efficacy. This approach seems to offer the final answer to the mode of administration of resins: markedly increased safety without reduction in therapeutic effect, combined with lowered cost to the patient and greater general acceptability. By this procedure, four of the major problems of the use of resins are resolved.

Combinations of anion and cation exchange resins were used by Best (1952b) in his studies of 9 patients with portal cirrhosis and marked ascites. In each case, the patient had required mercurial diuretics and paracentesis for at least 6 months prior to the initiation of resin therapy. On a regimen involving ingestion of 60 to 70 Gm. of the resin combination with an unrestricted diet (only alcohol being forbidden), 2 patients died (esophageal and postoperative hemorrhage), 4 remained free of ascites (without paracentesis or mercurial) over a period of 8 to 11 months provided the resin was continually administered, and 2 remained free of ascites for 6 months or more following discontinuance of the regimen. In only 1 patient was it found necessary to continue the mercurial in order to control the ascites. Mild acidosis developed in these patients but was not accompanied by clinical symptoms. In general, the biochemical findings reported by Best (1952b) parallel those seen following the use of cation exchange resins in whatever form.

Irwin *et al.* (1949) first reported the clinical use of sulfonic-type resins in the control of edema associated with cirrhosis. It is of importance in each clinical entity under study to consider a resin type in its own light; cation exchange resins should not be considered as a class; a sulfonic resin is not necessarily the equivalent of a carboxylic. Each resin type, and for that matter each resin form (cycle variations), must be reviewed independently. Cation exchange resins cannot be regarded as a class with respect to medical application. Following the work of Irwin *et al.* (1949) with the sulfonic type as used in the treatment of edema of cirrhotic origin, McHardy and his associates (1951, 1952) used this resin type in 36 patients with hepatic diseases complicated by edema and ascites. Their results in the broader aspects tend to indicate the equivalence of sulfonic and carboxylic resin types in this application. They did not make a direct comparison, but the final tabulation of efficacy leads to this conclusion. Of the 36 patients, 8 did not respond, but the other 28 were effectively controlled without untoward side effects. In 9 instances, the duration of therapy exceeded 12 months, and during that period no recurrence of ascites was noted. This is one of the few groups of clinicians to suggest that prognostic benefit follows the use of resins. They state: "In those patients responding favorably to resin there has been improvement in all serial liver function studies other than sulfobromophthalein excretion." By this, these workers do not imply that the progress of the disease is modified in any major degree; rather they underscore the fact that during the 3-year period of the study, 17 patients of the group died. Of importance is their observation that all patients receiving the ammonium cycle sulfonic resin developed cylindruria, which they feel was due to the irritation of the kidney incident to increased ammonium chloride excretion.

One of the most pessimistic reports relative to cation exchange resins is that of Gabuzda *et al.* (1952). These workers were critical primarily of ammonium cycle resins, whether of the carboxylic or of the sulfonic types. While the clinical results relative to the relief of edema were satisfactory (10 of 12 responding with diuresis and consequent reduction of ascites and edema), neurological disturbances were noted in 6 of the 8 patients receiving ammonium cycle resins. The 4 patients who received hydrogen cycle cation exchange resin did not develop the neurological symptoms, but as would be expected from the use of straight hydrogen cycle forms they did show acidosis and hypokalemia.

The neurological symptoms developing as a result of the ammonium cycle resin therapy paralleled those seen in hepatic stupor and coma, e.g., mental dullness and apathy, disorientation, generalized flapping tremor. These manifestations of nerve disorder could not be correlated with biochemical findings and were found to disappear with discontinuance of the ammonium cycle resin. In explanation, Gabuzda and his associates (1952) state that the ammonium ion is released in amount equivalent to 9 Gm. of ammonium chloride, and that following absorption this large amount of ammonium ion must be converted into urea by the liver. This added burden to an already diseased liver precipitates an ammonium intoxication. It is of particular interest to note that a resin form partially in the ammonium and partially in the potassium cycle also gave the neurological manifestations; this side effect of ammonium cycle resins was not reported by McHardy *et al.*

TABLE 29

Laboratory Data on Patients with Cirrhosis of the Liver and Ascites Treated with Cation Exchange Resins

(From Gabuzda, G. J., Jr., et al., New England J. Med., **246**: 124, 1952)

Patient	Sodium (mEq./l.)			Potassium (mEq./l.)			Carbon dioxide (mM./l.)			Chloride (mEq./l.)			Calcium (mg./100 cc.)			Diuresis	Untoward reactions
	Control	Last day of resin	3–7 days after resin	Control	Last day of resin	3–7 days after resin	Control	Last day of resin	3–7 days after resin	Control	Last day of resin	3–7 days after resin	Control	Last day of resin	3–7 days after resin		
H. M.*	135.8	142.0	141.0	5.0	3.7	4.8				102	112	106				Good	Disorientation, confusion, inappropriate behavior
	139.0	137.6	139.7	4.4	3.6	4.7				98	112	108		9.0	10.1	Good	Disorientation, confusion, inappropriate behavior, slurring speech
J. L.*	142.0	138.0	134.2	5.8	5.8		29.0	20.0		123	111	92				Good	Constipation, leg cramps
		144.6	152.6					18.6	28.5	92	115	115				Good	Tremor, drowsiness, slurring speech, disorientation, constipation
A. R.*	140.4	142.5	144.0		4.6	4.8				110						Good	None
	141.3	142.5	142.5													Good	Leg cramps
	133.0	133.0	133.0													Good	Leg cramps, anorexia, fecal impaction

Patient	Serum Na	Serum K	NPN / CO₂	Serum Cl	Response	Clinical findings
R.E.*	141.5	3.6, 3.6	21.0, 21.0	114	Fair	Tremor, disorientation, confusion, inappropriate behavior
M.S.†	137.8, 140.7, 140.5	4.1, 4.0, 4.2	4.6, 3.5, 3.3 / 4.6, 4.2, 4.2 / 20.0, 23.4	8.6, 8.0, 8.0 / 8.2, 7.8, 8.1 / 8.2, 8.0	Good, Good, Good	None
N.B.†	137.9, 136.0, 137.0 / 137.0, 134.8, 137.3			105	Good	None / Resin stopped because of massive gastrointestinal bleeding
J.G.†	133.0	4.8, 2.1			None	Hypokalemia, fecal impaction; died of esophageal bleeding
J.C.†	141.0, 139.0	1.5, 3.6	10.7, 21.0	95, 106	Good	Hypokalemia, acidosis, constipation
H.H.‡	133.5, 144.5, 132.5	4.1, 4.0	26.5 / 12.8, 17.6		Good	Drowsiness, slurring speech, epigastric distress, fecal impaction
R.P.‡	130.0, 130.9, 132.5	4.2, 4.0	25.9 / 26.0	102	Poor	Mental change without frank disorientation; tremor
	132.5, 132.0, 130.5	4.2, 4.1	26.0 / 26.0, 23.3	96	Poor	Mental change without frank disorientation; tremor; electroencephalographic changes
A.B.‡	118.5, 132.0, 131.5	3.8, 3.0, 3.3	24.5, 21.5	75, 100, 101	Good	Tremor, drowsiness, slurring speech, mild disorientation
M.H.‡	141.0, 139.5, 136.3	3.5, 3.2, 3.2	17.3, 14.0, 18.7	108, 118, 106	Good	Disorientation, confusion, delirium, tremor, drowsiness

* Ammonium cation exchange resin used.
† Hydrogen cation exchange resin used.
‡ Ammonium-potassium cation exchange resin used.

(1951, 1952). In order to permit individual consideration of the results of Gabuzda *et al.* (1952), Table 29, from their paper, is reproduced here.

As in the case of the decompensated cardiac, with the edematous
cirrhotic the colon tends to retain sodium to a greater degree than
normal (Berger *et al.*, 1951). The phenomenon of sodium retention
in these patients is not only a modification of kidney function but also
of the colon, the sweat glands and the salivary glands. That disturbed
hormonal control of sodium excretion is such a factor in cirrhotics suggests strongly the potentialities of concomitant use of hormone therapy
with resins.

Cation Depletion. As with patients having cardiac decompensation,
with those showing edema related to cirrhosis of the liver, adequate
food intake must be assured to prevent precipitate modifications in intake of sodium or potassium which might result in hyponatremia or
hypokalemia. Moser *et al.* (1951) observed lowered sodium and potassium in the serum of 2 of 8 patients; these 2 patients failed to consume
their full dietary allowance due to poor seasoning. In 1 case an added
factor was an abdominal paracentesis performed 10 days before the
observed decline of serum sodium and potassium.

Martz and his associates (1952) report 2 deaths in advanced
cirrhotic patients receiving resin therapy and manifesting hypoproteinemia. Anorexia with marked reduction in food intake, combined
in 1 case with severe diarrhea, doubtless profoundly reduced sodium
intake. This should have called for immediate modification in resin
dosage, or elimination of the therapy, but due to the severity of the
ascites the same regimen was continued. It is of course questionable
in what measure the resin withdrawal of cation contributed to the fatal
outcome. The probability is excellent that the situation represented no
more than a coincidence, as cation exchange resins will remove little,
if any, sodium when that cation is found in critical levels in the body.
Nevertheless, reduced sodium intake resulting from anorexia or diarrhea should be a signal causing immediate reduction of resin intake or
complete cessation of therapy for a period.

In general, there seems little reason to believe that various resin forms
differ materially in their tendency to bring about excessive ion depletion. McHardy *et al.* (1951, 1952) reported 9 cases continuously
treated with sulfonic-type cation exchangers for periods exceeding 12
months. They observed no evidence of excessive depletion of sodium,

potassium or calcium. In the interests of conservative management, these authors proposed the avoidance of resin therapy in patients with renal insufficiency and emphasized that hypocationemia can and does occur following resin therapy.

Acidosis. Moser *et al.* (1951) observed some compensated acidosis associated with moderately decreased carbon dioxide content of plasma. The tendency toward acidosis varied from patient to patient and at various times with the same patient. It is to be recalled that this group worked with anion-cation resin combinations. The results clearly demonstrate that such combinations do not afford protection against acidosis. In a more extended series (24 patients), Rosenak *et al.* (1952) record the development of a mild transient acidosis in 2 patients. They believe that plasma carbon dioxide determinations at weekly intervals are adequate for control of this potential complication. The proposal is made that therapeutic efficacy can be maintained and safety greatly increased if the resin is given intermittently.

Similarly, Martz and his associates (1952) have proposed that the use of combinations of anion and cation exchange resins reduces the tendency toward the development of compensated or uncompensated acidosis in the cirrhotic as well as in the patient with cardiac decompensation. It should be recalled that compensated acidosis may well be the major key to the clinical efficacy of cation exchange resins, in which event reduction of the tendency toward acidosis would not represent an improvement. Danowski *et al.* (1951*b*) state: "First, it seems reasonable to suggest that the acidosis and hyperchloremia which accompany therapy with the hydrogen or the ammonium form of the resin may facilitate the delivery of edema in patients, exerting effects comparable to those seen with acidifying diuretics. Obviously this change may prove undesirable if it reaches proportions sufficient to produce an uncompensated acidosis or overbreathing. It can be avoided by judicious selection of resins in other cycles, administered alone or in combination."

Evidence presented to date, particularly that of Greenman *et al.* (1953*a*), would seem to support the contention that anion-cation exchange resin combinations do in some measure reduce the incidence of acidosis. It should, however, be emphasized that use of such combinations is by no means a guarantee of the absence of acidosis (Best, 1952*a*); only the incidence of acidosis is reduced. In other words, severe and uncompensated acidosis can and does follow the use of combinations of anion and cation exchange resins. The need for vigilance is not reduced; the necessity for constant observation remains the rule of treatment. Furthermore, the induction of some measure of acidosis is deemed desirable (Danowski *et al.*, 1951*a, b*; Greenman *et al.*, 1953*a*).

Other Side Effects. The 8 patients with cirrhosis of the liver under study by Moser *et al.* (1951) seemed to find the anion-cation exchange resin combination acceptable. Constipation was noted in 1 individual and was easily controlled by laxatives. When this series was extended to 24 (Rosenak *et al.*, 1952), essentially the same incidence of side effects was reported, e.g., occasional constipation controlled by laxatives, and a few instances of nausea and vomiting.

The ammonium cycle sulfonic resins produce cylindruria (McHardy *et al.*, 1951, 1952). This is apparently due to kidney irritation associated with increased excretion of ammonium chloride. While the condition is reversible (vanishing upon resin withdrawal), it indicates that ammonium cycle resins may contribute to renal involvement and should therefore be regarded with caution in patients who might be susceptible to renal disease. Certainly in the case of patients with known renal involvement, the use of ammonium cycle forms would be questionable.

Hypertension

In 1951, Groff reported the efficacy of cation exchange resins for sodium removal in the control of hypertension. While his series comprised but 6 cases, the experimental approach was of such nature as to give great significance to the results. All patients were ambulatory, and attempts were made to cause them to react to the medication in a negative psychological manner. From Table 30 it can be seen that the entire group responded with blood pressure drops, both systolic and diastolic.

Generally, the dosage used by Groff was a tablespoonful (20 Gm.) of the resin (hydrogen cycle, carboxylic type) before meals. While the series consisted of patients with relatively benign and moderately labile types of hypertension, it was concluded that pressure levels could be reduced with increased capacity for work and relief of anginal seizures and exertional dyspnea.

Substantiation of the conclusions reached by Groff (1951) followed with the publications of Craig (1952), Griffith *et al.* (1952) and Gill and Duncan (1952, 1953). Differing in details but agreeing in principle, each of these investigational groups concluded that cation ex-

TABLE 30
Summary of Treatment

(From Groff, D. N., *N.Y. State J. Med.*, **51**: 758, 1951)

Patient	Age	Sex	Blood pressure before resin	Blood pressure during resin	Dose	Comment
J.T.C.	48	M	230/110 180/90	150/100	Tablespoon before meals	Pressure change after 2 weeks of resin treatment
R.G.	55	F	220/110 140/110	140/110	Teaspoon before meals	More tired after work
W.S.	47	M	280/120 140/100	120/90	Tablespoon before meals	Marked relief of exertional dyspnea; continued treatment requested
E.T.	61	M	240/120 170/90	160/90	½ teaspoon before meals	Marked relief of anginal pain and exertional dyspnea
P.W.	53	F	200/110 200/100	160/90 160/85 180/100	Teaspoon before meals	Long-term hypertensive; increased energy, loss of vertigo
H.W.	61	M	220/120 190/110	120/80 140/85	Tablespoon before meals	More energetic

change resins do control hypertension. Craig's series consisted of four groups of hypertensives, totaling 102 cases treated over a 12-month period. In the first group were 8 hospitalized cases of severe cardio-renal disease; in the second, 5 patients with hypertension of nephritic origin; in the third, 26 patients with hypertension associated with arteriosclerosis or aortic atherosclerosis; and in the fourth group were hypertension cases in the climacteric or preclimacteric phases. The results obtained are recorded in Table 31. The conclusion of Craig (1952) is that: "Natrinil [a potassium-hydrogen cycle cation exchanger of the carboxylic type] is a valuable adjunct in the treatment of edema and of hypertension caused by cardiac, renal, vascular or gonadal dysfunction."

Findings paralleling in large measure those of Groff (1951) and of Craig (1952) were given by Griffith *et al.* (1952) for a series of 15 cases of essential hypertension. Therapeutic procedure consisted of placing patients on a 200-mg. sodium diet and giving an anion-cation exchange resin combination. On this regimen, 8 patients were restored to normal blood pressure levels within 2 weeks to 1 month, 2 improved markedly, and 5 failed to respond. Following blood pressure stabilization at an essentially normal level, the patients were placed on a 1.5-Gm. sodium diet with increased consumption of resin to maintain urinary sodium at the same levels. A correlation was established between ability to lower urinary sodium and blood pressure response to the regimen. If the urinary sodium could not be lowered, no beneficial effects were reflected in the blood pressure picture. Manifestations of improvement in the condition of the patients included lowered body weight, decreased transverse cardiac diameter, drop of absolute eosinophils, and an elevation of plasma renin substrate concentration.

By far the most extensive and detailed study of the use of resins in the treatment of hypertension is that of Gill and Duncan (1952, 1953), who studied 38 ambulatory patients receiving 45 Gm. daily of an ammonium-potassium cycle carboxylic resin and a 1- to 3-Gm. sodium diet. The patients all had a diastolic pressure of at least 100 and showed good renal function; none were classified as in the malignant phase of hypertension. Calcium lactate (2 Gm.) and potassium citrate (2 to 3 Gm.) were given daily as supplemental measures.

Gill and Duncan (1952, 1953) found a direct correlation between lowering of urinary sodium excretion and response to the therapeutic procedure. In this respect their findings correlate well with those of Griffith *et al.* (1952). The critical level for sodium excretion in the urine is placed at 0.5 Gm. or less, and if the patient does not show such lowered urinary sodium values the probability is that no blood pressure lowering will ensue. A lag phase is seen in that a period of 4 weeks or more may precede a drop in blood pressure after the proper urinary sodium excretion levels have been reached. In fact, Gill and Duncan

TABLE 31

Cation Exchange Resins in Treatment of Hypertension

(Data from Craig, P. E., *M. Times*, 80: 92, 1952)

Group	Classification	No. of cases	Average blood pressure at start of resin therapy	Average drop in blood pressure		Comment	General treatment
				Systolic	Diastolic		
1	Advanced cardio-renal disease	8	228/112	30	10	Average wt. loss of 18 lbs. Marked diuresis with disappearance of edema. Gradual dilation of retinal vessels	250 mg. sodium diet. Digitoxin, atropine, quinidine, coramine if needed
2	Hypertension of nephritic origin	5	165/95	40	—	Edema disappeared. Renal function improved	Low salt, soft diet. Cortisone every 6 hrs.
3	Hypertension associated arteriosclerosis and aortic atherosclerosis	26	206/105	46	14	Retinal circulation improved. Retinal arteries dilated	Nitrates and sedatives
4	Hypertension associated with climacteric or preclimacteric	64	Not given	Not given		Spasm of retinal vessels disappeared	Hormones, sedatives, thyroid

(1952, 1953) regard a period of 2 months as a reasonable one for judging the patient's reactivity to lowered sodium. This 2-month period is considered to extend from the date at which the 24-hour urinary sodium drops to 0.5 Gm. or below. Table 32, from the paper of Gill and Duncan (1952), shows the results obtained.

From Table 32 it is noted that there is a direct correlation between the degree of lowering of urinary sodium excretion and decrease in diastolic blood pressure. A further finding of Gill and his group was that systolic pressure dropped 25 mm. or more in 22 of the 38 patients. As in other clinical syndromes, resin therapy is an adjuvant in hypertension and cannot replace dietary sodium restriction entirely. It seems

TABLE 32
Results of Cation Exchange Resin and Restriction of Dietary Sodium Therapy in Hypertension

(From Gill, R. J., and G. G. Duncan, *New England J. Med.*, **247**: 271, 1952)

Result	No. of cases
Decrease in diastolic pressure of 20 or more	15 (39%)
Decrease in diastolic pressure to 100 or below	17 (45%)
Combined decrease in diastolic pressure of 20 or more and to 100 or below	9 (24%)
Total	38

highly probable that any reduction in sodium intake caused by resin ingestion will reflect to the benefit of the patient. To be sure, this point cannot be substantiated with clinical findings at present, but as a point of logic it is proposed that there is no "all or nothing" law operative relative to sodium balance. Any reduction in sodium intake is better than none, and by virtue of this fact amounts of resin which do not cause major and spectacular improvements in the patient's condition can nevertheless be doing a great deal of good.

The potentialities of intermittent resin medication are raised by Gill and Duncan (1952, 1953) in the sphere of hypertension therapy with resins. They observed that once blood pressure has been lowered as a result of sodium restriction, the pressure will rise again but only slowly and over a period of days or even weeks. This offers the probability for success with intermittent use of resins, providing rest periods for the patient. As in other clinical spheres for application of resins, intermittent treatment offers four major advantages. The first is greater safety for use, with reduced incidence of side effects—especially those related to excessive ion removal. The second is reduction of the cost of medication to the patient. The third relates to patient acceptability, which is bound to increase with the prospect of treatment-free periods. The fourth is greater therapeutic efficacy by virtue of more rigid adherence to the regimen.

While resin therapy may owe a portion of its efficacy in the control of edema to the production of a systemic compensated acidosis, this could not possibly be a factor in hypertension, where sodium removal and sodium removal alone must play the dominant role. The efficacy of resin therapy in hypertension must remain for future work to decide in a quantitative sense, but clearly in a significant percentage of cases sodium removal through resin therapy is most useful and when properly employed as an adjuvant can mean the difference between success and failure.

In the studies of Craig (1952), 16 of the 102 patients complained of constipation, but in no case was this of such severity as to render necessary discontinuation of the treatment. Similarly, Gill and Duncan (1952, 1953) report constipation, anorexia and a sensation of abdominal fullness as complaints of patients early in the course of resin treatment. In their experience, these symptoms gradually decreased and never represented a threat to the regimen.

Palatability of resins is always a problem, but Gill and Duncan (1952) found that patients who had been on rice diets or on veratrum viride therapy preferred the resin program and did not wish to return to their former treatment.

With hypertensives as with other clinical types amenable to resin therapy, patients should be screened to eliminate those with kidney involvement. Gill and Duncan (1952) feel that a normal urinalysis, combined with a demonstration of normal concentrating power of the kidney or normal blood urea nitrogen, constitutes adequate evidence for normal kidney function. As a follow-up, they recommend interval determinations of blood urea nitrogen and carbon dioxide–combining power.

The probabilities favor the statement that side effects following resin therapy in hypertensives parallel in all respects those seen when resins are used for the treatment of other clinical entities. Little chance for untoward reactions exists if intermittent therapy is employed, or if the regimen is supplemented by the use of calcium and potassium salts.

The Nephrotic Syndrome and Cation Exchange Resins

Virtually all clinical investigators are agreed that cation exchange resin therapy should be used with caution, if at all, in patients with renal disease or insufficiency. The kidney functioning as a controlling mechanism in acid-base balance must perform with some measure of efficiency if the desirable compensated acidosis associated with such therapy is to be prevented from developing into the dangerous uncompensated phase. The commendable caution of the clinician has created a tendency to overemphasize the dangers of cation exchange therapy. In general, the type of patient under treatment is such as to raise question concerning any treatment, and properly so, but comparison of the complications associated with resin therapy with those associated with the administration of mercurial diuretics immediately demonstrates the superiority of the resin. The advocation by numerous clinicians (Hay and Wood, 1950; Lippman, 1951; Gill and Duncan, 1952, 1953; Rosenak *et al.*, 1952) of intermittent resin therapy reduces to the vanishing point the dangers formerly associated therewith. Clearly resin therapy possesses great merit in the control of clinical entities associated with extremely delicate life and death situations.

Friedman *et al.* (1951), while studying the value of resin therapy in a variety of clinical states, noted the development of casts, frequently as many as 100 casts per low-power field of a centrifuged urine specimen. They attributed this cast development to change in the pH of the urine and stated that when the pH was above 6, casts were no longer present. Further, cast development was not regarded as an indication for discontinuation of the resin, as no kidney pathology could be demonstrated in either the patients under treatment or the laboratory animals maintained for periods of 80 days on diet containing large amounts of resins.

The Nephrotic Syndrome. The term nephrotic syndrome refers to any renal disease associated with massive edema and albuminuria. The early investigators were therefore confronted with the dangers of uncompensated acidosis whenever they used cation exchange resins in such patients. Furthermore, the edema of the nephrotic syndrome might well be the result of lowered serum proteins rather than due to sodium retention. During 1951 and early 1952, many groups reported their findings with resin therapy in the nephrotic syndrome; all achieved some measure of success.

The term nephrosis is confused with nephrotic syndrome in that the two are frequently used interchangeably, but in some instances, as in the classification of Fashena and Harrison (1950), nephrosis is distinguished as being not primarily of inflammatory or vascular origin but basically degenerative in nature. It seems reasonable from the viewpoint of consideration of the merit of resin therapy to consider the two as equivalents and to make no attempt to distinguish between them.

Beck and Goodman (1951) and Danowski *et al.* (1951*b*) presented the first evidence of the value of resin therapy. The former reported results with two patients with chronic glomerular nephritis in the nephrotic stage; they used an ammonium cycle sulfonic cation exchange resin and observed the development of acidosis in both patients —compensated in one case and uncompensated in the other—with diuresis in but one. The latter (Danowski *et al.*, 1951*b*) used a number of resin forms alone and in combination on a single patient with nephrosis, reaching no conclusions on the merit of the therapy but inferring that the resin removed ingested rather than endogenous sodium.

Later in 1951, several groups of investigators (Lippman, 1951; Mateer *et al.*, 1951; Payne and Wilkinson, 1951) established quite clearly the merit and limitations of cation exchange resin therapy in the nephrotic syndrome. Each of the three groups doing the most extensive work used hydrogen or ammonium cycle resins of either the sulfonic or carboxylic types. Two groups (Lippman, 1951; Payne and Wilkinson, 1951) used a comparatively coarse-mesh resin (20- to 80-mesh) and the third (Mateer *et al.*, 1951) employed a fine-mesh material (200-mesh). Despite the emphasis placed on a shift from coarse- to fine-mesh material by Lippman (1951), it seems improbable that except from the standpoint of palatability any great difference was noted in capacity.

The therapeutic response noted by the three groups was essentially identical, each observing an increased fecal excretion of sodium and other cations, accompanied by diuresis and in general relief of the edema. As is to be anticipated in the treatment of any disease with any medication, results were not 100 per cent; Payne and Wilkinson (1951) observed reduction of body weight and edema in all 6 of the children in their series but failed to effect modification of ascites where it occurred; Lippman (1951) obtained diuresis in 11 of his series of 14 patients; and Mateer *et al.* (1951) reported success in their patients

(2 in number) who were not kept on low sodium diets. All indicate in their reports that the tendency toward hyperkalemia is materially reduced or eliminated by this treatment. It will be recalled that these investigators were using cation exchange resins in either the ammonium or the hydrogen cycles; most resin preparations available at present are partially in the potassium cycle, and one would immediately question the value of such preparations for use in the nephrotic syndrome. This problem is satisfactorily answered by the reports of Feinberg and Rosenberg (1951), of Best (1952a), and of Wood *et al.* (1952), who used commercially available cation exchange resin preparations in nephrotic syndrome patients without untoward effects and in general with success paralleling that reported for the straight hydrogen or ammonium cycle forms of the resins. In the work of Best (1952a) 2 patients in the nephrotic syndrome associated with glomerulonephritis or intercapillary glomerulosclerosis were relieved of their edema and could be permitted far more liberal sodium-containing diets than prior to the use of the resins. Resin utilization in treatment of such patients must of course be considered as a correlative to other measures, particularly high protein, high caloric diets.

Dosages of resin employed have varied, but within definite limits. Payne and Wilkinson (1951) gave 12 to 20 Gm. of resin to children (30 to 50 lbs. in weight) on diets containing 8 mEq. of sodium daily; Lippman (1951) gave a somewhat larger dose (32 to 48 Gm. daily) to children of similar weight who were apparently (not stated) on a regular hospital diet. Mateer *et al.* (1951) used a low sodium diet (1 to 3 mEq. of sodium per day) with resin doses of 30 to 40 Gm. (actual ingestion approximately 18 Gm. due to lack of patient cooperation). Under these conditions, they were unable to demonstrate any increased fecal sodium resulting from the resin ingestion; further, the speed of reduction of edema and of body weight was not accelerated. When the diet contained considerable amounts of sodium, the stool values for this ion did increase, which fact they interpreted as indicating the merit of resins. Even in the patients on low sodium intake, this group concluded that: "This therapy may have, however, prolonged the diuresis through its acidifying effects." In the adult, Lippman (1951) used a dose of 32 to 48 Gm.

The side effects coincident with use of cation exchange resins in the nephrotic patient seem parallel in all ways to those noted in other clinical states so treated. Acidosis was reported by all investigators (Lippman, 1951; Mateer *et al.,* 1951; Payne and Wilkinson, 1951).

Mateer and his associates (1951) credited to their induction of acidosis some measure of the therapeutic effect of resins. They observed serum carbon dioxide content drops of 4.1 mEq. per liter (9.1 volumes per cent) in patients receiving the resin; these values returned to normal following cessation of therapy. There can be little question but that serial determination of serum carbon dioxide values must be made, and that resin administration should be discontinued if the values drop below a critical level, regarded by Lippman (1951) as being 30 volumes per cent. He feels that intermittent therapy (48-hour intervals between resin periods) reduces the problem of acidosis. This seems to be the consensus and leads to the recommendation that resins may be administered for periods of 4 to 7 days, with resin-free intervals of 2 or 3 days. Under this general type of regimen, the therapeutic benefits are not reduced and there is virtually an elimination of side effects.

Hypokalemia is a common finding (Lippman, 1951; Mateer *et al.*, 1951; Payne and Wilkinson, 1951), regarded in some measure as beneficial in that it reduces the trend toward hypokalemia due to ingestion of potassium cycle resin (Mateer *et al.*, 1951) and is susceptible to correction by the administration of 2 Gm. daily of potassium citrate (Payne and Wilkinson, 1951). Lippman (1951) recommends the administration of 1 Gm. of potassium chloride with each dose of resin in order to prevent the tendency toward hypokalemia. When the condition (hypokalemia) is detected through symptoms of weakness and confusion, electrocardiographic changes, or in serum potassium determinations, potassium chloride can be given intravenously (Lippman, 1951).

Hyponatremia has not been reported. Lippman (1951) is of the opinion that it would not develop until the edema had been completely reduced, and the likelihood of its occurrence under any conditions seems remote, from the findings of Mateer and his associates (1951) to the effect that resins do not increase sodium excretion via the feces when the amount of sodium ingested is low.

With respect to other cations, there seems little potential for the development of side effects. Lippman (1951) indicated that there is a possibility for removal of iron with resultant development of anemia, and recommends iron supplements. This finding was applied only when he was giving resins continuously and not when intermittent courses were employed. Calcium removal does not seem to be a major problem. Hypocalcemia is observed (Mateer *et al.*, 1951) but does not lead to the development of tetany. Mateer and his group (1951) are inclined to attribute the hypocalcemia to the lowered concentrations of serum albumin rather than to the administration of the resin.

Patient acceptability is a problem, particularly with the child. Circumvention of this problem is not impossible, however. Lippman (1951) recommends that the child be separated from the parent during the initiation of the treatment, as nursing care and patience seem imperative to success. Camouflaging with puréed fruit, jelly or syrup is useful, and the resins can even be baked into breads, cakes or candies (Lippman, 1951). The resin used by Payne and Wilkinson (1951) was heat-sensitive, with the result that they incorporated it into various foods in the cold. In the experience of Mateer *et al.* (1951) the resins could be most advantageously administered in capsules. They point out that their patients were on a very low sodium diet and that if the diet is more liberal the patient experiences correspondingly less difficulty in ingesting the resin.

The nephrotic patient's response to resin therapy varies from no effect whatever to the spectacular one described by Lippman (1951), who wrote: "The difference in their clinical condition since the initiation of resin therapy can be compared to the dramatic effects produced by cortisone administration in a patient with severe rheumatoid arthritis." The high degree of therapeutic success following the use of resins in these patients is well illustrated by the case reported by Kattus (1952), which is that of a nephrotic woman showing remarkable weight loss and reduction of edema following the use of resin.

In summary, the use of ammonium or hydrogen cycle and probably other resin forms in patients with the nephrotic syndrome will bring about the following results: decrease in body weight with reduction in edema (Lippman, 1951; Mateer *et al.*, 1951; Payne and Wilkinson, 1951); diuresis within 1 to 4 days following initiation of resin therapy (Payne and Wilkinson, 1951); serum potassium drops as high as 2.5 to 3.3 mEq. per liter (Payne and Wilkinson, 1951) but averaging 1 mEq. per liter (Mateer *et al.*, 1951); plasma carbon dioxide decrease as high as 13 to 16 mEq. per liter (Payne and Wilkinson, 1951) but averaging 4 mEq. per liter (Mateer *et al.*, 1951); elevation of fecal sodium and potassium values (Lippman, 1951; Mateer *et al.*, 1951; Payne and Wilkinson, 1951); drop in urinary sodium and potassium values (same groups); resin capacity per gram for sodium and potassium combined of 1.5 mEq.; fecal chloride not materially modified but with urinary chloride drop (Mateer *et al.*, 1951); elevated nonprotein nitrogen of the blood may be restored to normal (Mateer *et al.*,

1951). On the basis of these studies, the therapeutic merit of cation exchange resins in the control of the nephrotic syndrome is unquestionable. Side effects can and do occur. Prevention of these deleterious actions of resins can be controlled by proper laboratory procedures or they can be to all intent and purpose eliminated by intermittent periods of resin therapy—4 or 5 days on resin, and 2 or 3 days off.

Potassium Retention. As previously mentioned, Mateer and his associates (1951), Payne and Wilkinson (1951), and Lippman (1951) observed reduction in the tendency toward hyperkalemia in their patients with the nephrotic syndrome. The nonselectivity of cation exchange resins causes them to remove all cations, a fact supported by all ion balance studies reported (e.g., Irwin *et al.*, 1949; Kahn and Emerson, 1950; Danowski *et al.*, 1951*b*). The marketed forms of resins are partially in the potassium cycle in order to reduce if not eliminate the tendency toward the induction of hypokalemia, the natural corollary to the desired effect of sodium removal.

Elkinton and his associates (1950) have studied in detail the efficacy of cation exchange resins for potassium removal in 3 patients with severe renal insufficiency associated with oliguria and anuria. Potassium retention with resultant cardiotoxicity has long been recognized as one of the cardinal dangers associated with such pathological changes (Winkler *et al.*, 1941; Keith *et al.*, 1944; Marchand and Finch, 1944) and the work of Elkinton *et al.* (1950) clearly demonstrates that hyperkalemia can be effectively controlled by resin administration.

The resin used was a carboxylic type used in the ammonium cycle and was given either orally in a 7 per cent suspension in milk or by tube, in which case a 17 per cent water suspension proved useful. Although in 1 case with repeated regurgitation of orally administered resin the use of an enema containing 10 per cent resin was effective, these investigators feel that the administration of resins by mouth gives the most reliable results. It is to be emphasized that resin forms other than those partially in the potassium cycle are indicated in these cases. In fact, potassium cycle resin forms are specifically contraindicated. In 1 patient, sodium removal by the resin caused an acidosis necessitating correction by the administration of sodium carbonate. While this complication was not regarded as serious, it does raise the point of use of sodium cycle resins in such cases. The resin would contain sodium in an amount calculated to prevent sodium loss and consequently to re-

FIGURE 21
Potassium Retention and Cation Exchange Resins
(From Elkinton, J. R., *et al., Am. J. M. Sc.,* 220: 547, 1950)

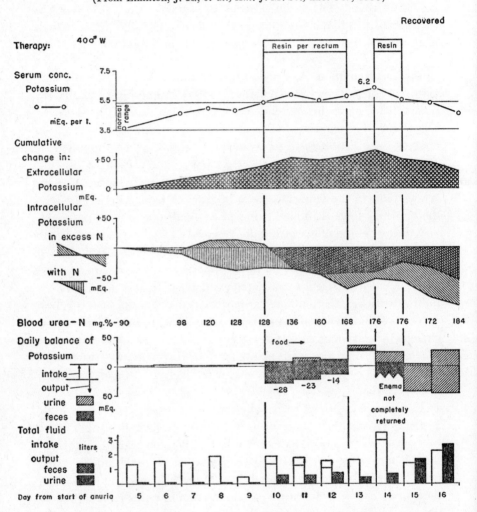

duce any tendency toward acidosis. Other resin cycle forms might also be useful. The point is made with the thought of indicating potentialities for future developments.

In all 3 patients, reduction of serum potassium levels resulted from resin therapy. Two of the patients died of unrelated complications but the third had an uneventful recovery. Figure 21, from the paper of Elkinton *et al.* (1950), gives in some detail the objective findings in.

the last case. These investigators indicate clearly the necessity of employing a regimen involving water restriction, preservation of electrolyte concentrations in body fluids, control of acidosis, use of high caloric diets along with such adjuvants as administration of aluminum hydroxide to control phosphate level, calcium salt injections to guard against the onset of tetany coincident with alkali therapy, and support of the circulatory system. The additional factor of control of potassium accumulation made possible by cation exchange resins should, according to these investigators, "greatly facilitate the ordinary medical treatment of anuria."

The doses of resin employed varied. In one patient with a serum potassium of 7.6 mEq. per liter, 50 Gm. of resin were given during each of the two 24-hour periods (thirteenth and fifteenth days of oliguria), with an intervening resin-free period of 24 hours. In a second patient, 50 Gm. of resin were given by enema on the ninth day of anuria when the serum potassium had reached 7.7 mEq. per liter. The third patient received resin enemas in like amount on the tenth day of anuria and this was continued until the fourteenth day, at which time the serum potassium had dropped to normal. The implication of the work reported is to the effect that resin dosage in such patients must be controlled by the serum potassium levels, but that in general the administration of 50 Gm. of resin for from 2 to 4 days will return such levels to within the normal range.

The merit of cation exchange resins in controlling potassium levels in terminal uremia with hyperkalemia is supported by the observations of Emerson *et al.* (1951), who used similar doses and the same resin given rectally. In one patient, a serum potassium level of 8.5 was reduced to 5.3 mEq. per liter in 3 days; in the second case, an even more dramatic reduction in serum potassium—from 9.0 to 5.8 mEq. per liter—occurred. Clinical improvement occurred in one patient but not in the other; both died within a short period. Despite the final outcome with these patients, Emerson and his associates state that: "In patients with reversible anuria this procedure might well be life-saving."

One precaution mentioned by Emerson *et al.* (1951) relates to the increased toxicity of digitalis which follows potassium withdrawal. They recommend that digitalis be discontinued during the period of administration of resin. This increased toxicity of digitalis after resin therapy has been observed by others (Hay and Wood, 1950; Feinberg and Rosenberg, 1951; Callahan *et al.*, 1952) following the oral administration of resins in other clinical states.

Exchange Resins and the Edema of Pregnancy

Edema in the obstetric patient has for some time been treated by dietary sodium restriction with the concomitant administration of agents designed to induce diuresis, e.g., hypertonic glucose or ammonium chloride. It was therefore not surprising that cation exchange resins would be tried to bring about the desired therapeutic effects, and the results of these trials have been uniformly favorable.

The dosage of resin employed has varied from 45 Gm. (Odell *et al.,* 1951; Penman, 1951, 1952) to 50 to 100 Gm. (Carey, 1953). The form has been either the hydrogen-potassium type, the ammonium-potassium type or combinations of anion and cation exchangers. From the point of view of administration, the resins have been suspended in water (Odell *et al.,* 1951), put into food, dispersed in grapefruit juice, pineapple juice, or cola beverages (Penman, 1951, 1952). Patient acceptance of resin therapy has in general been satisfactory. Odell *et al.* (1951) report that outpatients complained that the suspension "tastes not unlike suspended sand." Penman (1951, 1952) indicates that of 26 patients in his series, 7 objected. Of the 7, there were 5 who stated that they had vomited almost every dose; a sixth simply objected to the taste; the seventh gave no reason.

As stated above, therapeutic results have been uniformly favorable. Odell *et al.* (1951), using a 45-Gm. dose of potassium-hydrogen cycle resin, employed dietary regimens with 1- and 3-Gm. sodium chloride levels. Ten patients were in each series. Of the 10 on the 1-Gm. sodium chloride diet, 3 had pre-eclampsia. The average weight loss in this group was 8.0 lbs. over a 5-day period of treatment. The average weight loss figure for the group on the 3-Gm. sodium chloride dietary was 7.8 lbs. Clearly these figures indicate equal efficacy of resin therapy on a dietary involving sodium chloride ingestion varying by a factor of three. This is not in agreement with the findings of other clinicians, who have reported that the use of resins does not permit liberalization of sodium chloride intake. It is within the realm of possibility that cation exchange resin therapy may function by mechanisms other than that of sodium removal. Perhaps it is better to suggest that these resins may function in a multiple fashion, and not solely through sodium removal.

The only untoward effect observed by Odell and his associates (1951) concerned the development of a compensated acidosis. During the 5-day period of treatment, the carbon dioxide–combining power of the blood dropped on an average 7.3 volumes per cent. The period of treatment employed by these investigators is of short duration and there would be little reason to expect the development of side effects such as have been reported to occur when patients are kept for long periods of time on resin therapy.

In the studies of Penman (1951), a potassium-ammonium cycle resin form was employed in the treatment of 11 patients with fluid retention in pregnancy, all of whom were hospitalized. The resin was not employed in the treatment of pre-eclampsia or eclampsia. Three groups of patients were selected. A control group (2 patients) received a hospital diet containing 2 Gm. of sodium but no resin. Small weight losses were recorded, but at the termination of the study clinical evidence of edema persisted. The second group (7 patients) were given resin and a 2-Gm. sodium diet. All showed marked weight losses and complete mobilization of clinical edema. As an example, in one patient a weight loss of 13.5 lbs. occurred in 8 days. Removed from the resin but continued on the low sodium diet, this patient gained 1.25 lbs. in 6 days. The third group (2 patients) received resin and were on a 6- to 9-Gm. sodium intake diet. Further weight gains were prevented by this regimen, but there was no indication of weight loss. From these results, Penman concluded that the use of resins permits the daily ingestion of 2 to 3 Gm. of sodium with simultaneous elimination of edema. No untoward side effects were reported.

Subsequently, Penman (1952) investigated the efficacy of resin therapy in outpatients with fluid retention. Seventeen of the 19 patients who tolerated the resin showed rapid weight loss and reduction or complete disappearance of edema. In this group, the dietary regimen eliminated salt and salty foods but could not be regarded in any sense as a low sodium diet. Of the 2 not included in the 17, one delivered after taking about six doses; the other took the resin well but failed to derive any benefit. The fact that resin therapy does not prevent the development of pre-eclampsia is established by Penman's observation that pre-eclampsia developed in 2 of the 8 patients who experienced complete reduction of edema. In patients of the type under consideration, resin therapy is not employed over prolonged periods (not more than 7 to 20 days) and therefore no clinical evidence of side effects is reported.

Penman (1952) indicates the difficulty encountered by the physician in endeavoring to persuade the pregnant patient with edema to reduce salt intake to the point at which food becomes unpalatable, though this is essential for success in edema reduction. He feels that of the three approaches available—ammonium chloride, low sodium diets or moderate dietary restriction with resin—the last is by far the most practical for the control of edema.

The report of Carey (1953) confirms in large measure the findings of Odell *et al.* (1951) and of Penman (1951, 1952). Carey modified the regimen in that he used alternately the ammonium and the potassium cycle resins and did not give them together as the other investigators had. Laboratory studies and clinical observation in 3 cases of pre-eclampsia demonstrated reduction of total body sodium and immediate disappearance of edema. The statement is made by Carey that: "Resin therapy is in addition to low salt diets and bed rest and has its principal value in maintaining the pregnancy for a longer period than would be otherwise feasible, thus reducing complications resulting from prematurity."

Recently, Baker *et al.* (1953) have reported a series of 16 hospitalized and 32 outpatient prenatal patients, exhibiting edema and/or excessive weight gain in the last trimester of pregnancy, treated by a combination anion-cation exchanger preparation. The results were again uniformly favorable, with reduction or elimination of edema, and weight reduction in the majority of patients. Elevated blood pressures were lowered. The dietary regimen employed varied in its sodium content from 1 to 6 Gm., and it was concluded by these workers that resin therapy was most effective when the sodium intake was at one of the higher levels. The resin was given in amounts of 48 to 72 Gm. for periods of 5 to 7 days, after which the patient was removed from resin therapy or another period of resin administration was begun. With this alternating or short-period treatment, there is little danger of the development of hypokalemia, hyponatremia or acidosis; however, Baker and his associates did observe electrocardiographic changes suggestive of hypokalemia in 4 patients. Potassium supplementation with 15 mEq. of this ion in the form of the citrate, bicarbonate and acetate corrected these signs, and if such supplementation was given beforehand no manifestation of hypokalemia developed. Apparently no acidosis or hyponatremia was observed in the entire series, and this seems in keeping with the probability that no side effects of resin therapy will develop in a 5- to 7-day period. Constipation was reported as occurring and as being a factor decreasing the efficiency of resin therapy. Correction of this was usual following the concomitant administration of bulking laxatives.

These studies lead to several conclusions: (1) that cation exchange resin therapy is of definite value in edema associated with pregnancy; (2) that it is not an effective prophylactic procedure for prevention of the development of eclampsia but probably does delay the onset and reduce the severity of this unfortunate complication of pregnancy; and (3) that the short duration of the use of resin precludes the development of untoward side effects. There is much to be gained and nothing to be lost by the employment of resin therapy wherever sudden weight gains occur or in the presence of edema in the pregnant patient.

Cation Exchange Resin Therapy in Patients Receiving Cortisone or the Adrenocorticotropic Hormone

Retention of sodium and depletion of potassium frequently accompany the prolonged use of either the adrenocorticotropic hormone or of cortisone or related steroids. Logically, cation exchange resins through their capacity to retain sodium in the intestine should modify and alleviate such abnormal cation metabolism.

It was with this concept in mind that Peters *et al.* (1951) administered doses of 24 to 60 Gm. of cation exchange resins (hydrogen, ammonium, or hydrogen-potassium cycle types) to patients being treated with ACTH or cortisone. In this and a subsequent study (Greenman *et al.,* 1953*b*), the Pittsburgh group concluded that while the general effects of resin therapy were not modified by the accompanying hormone administration, the regimen did not prevent the development of complications. The resin form adopted contained 50 per cent hydrogen cycle and 50 per cent potassium cycle forms. Despite this larger proportion of potassium cycle resin, the alkalosis or hypochloremia of ACTH and cortisone therapy was not prevented, nor was the incidence of hypokalemia significantly modified. Finally, edema formation (patients on unrestricted diet) was not controlled despite the fact that the resins increased stool output of sodium.

Greenman and his associates (1953*b*) conclude that cation exchange resins do not provide "as satisfactory a method of controlling the acid-base and mineral effects of cortisone and ACTH therapy as do adequate sodium restriction plus supplementary KC1." As a generalization from their data this seems a valid conclusion, but the patient is above all else an individual, and there will doubtless be situations in which a given patient will respond as well to resin therapy as to any other regimen. The problem of patient acceptability of low sodium diets will arise and may well result in the specific indication of a resin regimen as an alternate approach.

To date, there has been but one other report relative to resins used concomitantly with ACTH or cortisone. Bonner (1952) used a sulfonic type of cation exchange resin in the ammonium cycle with potassium supplementation and reported reduction of sodium and water retention in patients receiving such hormone therapy; however, hypokalemia developed in all 3 patients studied. The latter side effect "precluded the practical use of resins for this purpose," according to Bonner.

The case for possible use of resins with ACTH or cortisone hardly seems closed. The number of patients studied has been small (a total of 8) and beneficial effects have been noted (decreased water and sodium retention). The major complication would seem to be the development of hypokalemia, a situation subject to correction either by potassium supplementation or the use of resins higher in the potassium cycle form. Another future potentiality is the development of resins with greater selectivity for sodium. Clearly, however, the presently reported investigations demonstrate the validity of the assertion that the resin forms, when used as stated, do not offer a practical solution to the problem of the toxicity of cortisone or ACTH.

Cation Exchange Resins as Clinical Indicators

An ingenious application of cation exchange resins to the field of clinical indicators has been made by Segal and his co-workers (1950a, b). Ion exchange is a reversible process governed by laws of mass action and ionic characteristics. Further, as with all such systems, the exchange reactions are dynamic, not static. There will be in any biological system a constant stream of cations going on and off the electronegative exchange groups fixed to the insoluble resin structure. In the case of the carboxylic type of cation exchanger the exchange grouping (the carboxyl radical) is a comparatively weak acid and tends to retain hydrogen ions or revert to the hydrogen ion cycle if the pH is less than a certain critical value. Segal *et al.* (1950a, b) took advantage of these facts and constructed a quininium resin compound which exchanged the quinine cation for the free hydrogen ion of the gastric juice. If no free gastric acid were present, no exchange would occur and no quinine would be liberated. The liberated quinine would be absorbed and subsequently excreted, mainly in the urine, and could be determined. Its presence would indicate some free gastric acid; its absence none. Thus they had devised a method for the determination of gastric acidity without intubation.

The preparation of the indicators is simple. The resin is converted into the hydrogen cycle form and is then allowed to react with a solution of quinine hydrochloride in water. The amount of quinine hydrochloride is so controlled as to provide 20 mg. for adsorption on 1 Gm. of the resin. Obviously, there are many other potentialities for selection of cation to function as the indicator, e.g., a whole range of cation dye molecules, and inorganic ions, either radioactive or those not normally found in biological fluids. Future developments may well indicate the abandonment of the quininium form for one more easily adaptable to determination.

The exact technic employed by Segal *et al.* (1950*b*) involves the administration to the patient at 8:30 A.M. of 50 cc. of 7 per cent alcohol (histamine or caffeine sodium benzoate may be used as stimulant to gastric juice secretion). No breakfast is permitted. At 9:00 A.M. the patient is instructed to urinate and the resin indicator compound is given in a 2-Gm. dose suspended in water. One hour later the first urine sample is taken, followed at 2 hours by the second. The amount of quinine contained in the samples is determined by the Kelsey and Geiling (1942) procedure, which involves extraction of the urine with ether in suitable separatory funnels, subsequent transfer to an aqueous sulfuric acid medium, and finally determination of the amount of quinine by ultraviolet light in a fluorophotometer or by some parallel technic. Unfortunately, the procedure is cumbersome and difficult to carry out. Furthermore, it requires special equipment. It is to be hoped that further study will result in a different approach involving simplification of the technic. Three samples of urine must be assayed for fluorescence—the control sample taken before the administration of quininium dye indicators and the 1- and 2-hour samples after. Fluorescence of the control sample must be deducted from that of the others in order to achieve a reasonably accurate result. Urine contains many substances which are highly fluorescent and may be extracted as is the quinine.

Interpretation of data by Segal *et al.* (1950*a, b*) resulted in the creation of three categories:

1. The group with free gastric hydrochloric acid showing quinine in the first- and second-hour urine samples.

2. The group with no free gastric acid secreting no quinine into the urine during the first or second hours.
3. The third group is small and constitutes those patients showing quinine in the second-hour sample but not in the first. Interpretation here depends upon the quantity of quinine excreted during the second hour.

Table 33, from Segal (1951), illustrates the accuracy of the test. Of the 223 individuals tested, all fell into the proper categories as shown by relating determinations of free gastric acid made by intubation. There were 5 patients with no free gastric acid who excreted quinine during the second hour and 6 with gastric acid who did not

TABLE 33
Time Interval Between Oral Administration of IEC-QH and Appearance of Quininium Cations in Urine of Individuals with and Without Free Gastric Hydrochloric Acid

(From Segal, H. L., *M. Clin. North America*, 35: 593, 1951)

Free HCl secretion after alcohol stimulation (intubation technic)	No. of individuals tested	No. of individuals showing quininium cations in urine		
		Control	Hour of quinine excretion	
			1st	2nd
Present	180	0	174	180
Absent	43	0	0	5

excrete quinine during the first hour but did during the second. Of the former group, the quinine excreted during the second hour was 0.012 mg. or less; for the latter group, the corresponding value was 0.023 mg. or more. Thus from the quantitative values a distinction could easily be established and the proper diagnosis made.

Segal (1951) emphasizes that the test reveals only the presence or absence of free gastric acid and does not indicate pH, nor does it give the clinical units of hydrochloric acid present. He recommends the test primarily for clinical diagnosis of gastric cancer, pernicious anemia or gastric polyps, in cases of which achlorhydria is general.

REFERENCES

AARON, R. S., and R. E. WESTON. *Arch. Int. Med.,* **90:** 182, 1952.

BAKER, J. P., J. J. LEHMAN, H. A. CLAIBORNE, and W. S. BAKER, JR. *Am. J. Obst. Gynec.,* **65:** 969, 1953.

BARKER, R. A., and J. R. MACKAY. *Lancet,* **2:** 758, 1951.

BECK, W. S. and H. C. GOODMAN. *Federation Proc.,* **10:** 11, 1951.

BERGER, E. Y., G. P. QUINN, and M. A. HOMER. *Proc. Soc. Exper. Biol. Med.,* **76:** 601, 1951.

BERGER, E. Y., and J. M. STEELE. *J. Clin. Investigation,* **31:** 451, 1952.

BEST, M. M. *Am. Pract. and Dig. Treatment,* **3:** 274, 1952*a*.

BEST, M. M. *J. Lab. Clin. Med.,* **40:** 777, 1952*b*.

BONNER, C. D. *New England J. Med.,* **247:** 158, 1952.

CALLAHAN, E. J., N. R. FRANK, H. KRAUS, and L. B. ELLIS. *Am. J. M. Sc.,* **223:** 117, 1952.

CAREY, H. M. *Obst. Gynec.,* **1:** 177, 1953.

CHAPMAN, D. W., F. C. PANNILL, JR., and R. H. SKAGGS. *Am. Pract. and Dig. Treatment,* **2,** 945, 1951.

CH'EN, J. S., and S. FREEMAN. *J. Lab. Clin. Med.,* **35:** 99, 1950.

COBBEY, T. S., JR., R. H. WILLIAMS, N. MACRAE, and B. T. TOWERY. *Federation Proc.,* **8:** 352, 1949.

CRAIG, P. E. *M. Times,* **80:** 92, 1952.

CRISMON, J. M. *Federation Proc.,* **8:** 30, 1949.

CURRENS, J. H., T. COUNIHAN, and M. ROURKE. *J. Clin. Investigation,* **29:** 807, 1950.

DANOWSKI, T. S., L. GREENMAN, F. M. MATEER, W. B. PARSONS, F. A. WEIGAND, H. MERMELSTEIN, and J. H. PETERS. *J. Clin. Investigation,* **30:** 984, 1951*a*.

DANOWSKI, T. S., L. GREENMAN, J. H. PETERS, F. M. MATEER, F. A. WEIGAND, and R. TARAIL. *Ann. Int. Med.,* **35:** 529, 1951*b*.

DOCK, W. *Tr. A. Am. Physicians,* **59:** 282, 1946.

DOCK, W., and N. R. FRANK. *Am. Heart J.,* **40:** 638, 1950.

DUNCAN, L. E. JR. *Am. J. Med.,* **14:** 425, 1953.

ELKINTON, J. R., J. K. CLARK, R. D. SQUIRES, L. W. BLUEMLE, JR., and A. P. CROSLEY, JR. *Am. J. M. Sc.,* **220:** 547, 1950.

ELKINTON, J. R., R. D. SQUIRES, and W. C. KLINGENSMITH, JR. *Circulation,* **5:** 747, 1952.

EMERSON, K., JR., S. S. KAHN, J. W. VESTER, and K. D. NELSON. *Arch. Int. Med.,* **88:** 605, 1951.

FASHENA, G. J., and T. R. HARRISON. In Harrison, T. R., *et al.* (eds.), *Principles of Internal Medicine.* Philadelphia: Blakiston, 1950.

FEINBERG, A. W., and B. ROSENBERG. *Am. Heart J.,* **42:** 698, 1951.

FLANAGAN, T. L., M. F. SAX, and A. E. HEMING. *Federation Proc.,* **10:** 295, 1951*a*.

FLANAGAN, T. L., M. F. SAX, and A. E. HEMING. *J. Pharmacol. Exper. Therap.,* **103:** 215, 1951*b*.

FRIEDMAN, I. S., S. ZUCKERMAN, and T. D. COHN. *Am. J. M. Sc.,* **221:** 672, 1951.

FRIEDMAN, I. S., S. ZUCKERMAN, and E. McCATTY. *Am. J. M. Sc.,* **225:** 399, 1953.

GABUZDA, G. J., JR., G. B. PHILLIPS, and C. S. DAVIDSON. *New England J. Med.,* **246:** 124, 1952.

GILL, R. J., and G. G. DUNCAN. *New England J. Med.,* **247:** 271, 1952.

GILL, R. J., and G. G. DUNCAN. *Am. Pract. Dig. Treatment,* **4:** 68, 1953.

GREENBLATT, J. J., and M. E. GILWOOD. Abstracts, 113th Meeting Am. Chem. Soc., 2c, April, 1948.

GREENMAN, L., J. B. SHALER, and T. S. DANOWSKI. *Am. J. Med.,* **14:** 391, 1953a.

GREENMAN, L., F. A. WEIGAND, and T. S. DANOWSKI. *Am. J. M. Sc.,* **225:** 1, 1953b.

GRIFFITH, R. S., O. M. HELMER, and K. G. KOHLSTAEDT. *Federation Proc.,* **11:** 59, 1952.

GROFF, D. N. *New York State J. Med.,* **51:** 758, 1951.

HALD, P. M., A. J. HEINSEN, and J. P. PETERS. *J. Clin. Investigation,* **26:** 983, 1947.

HAY, S. H., and J. E. WOOD, JR. *Ann. Int. Med.,* **33:** 1139, 1950.

HEGSTED, D. M., D. WILSON, G. McPHEE, and F. J. STARE. *Am. J. Physiol.,* **164:** 695, 1951.

HEMING, A. E., and T. L. FLANAGAN. *Federation Proc.,* **10:** 307, 1951.

HOLLEY, H. L. Discussion of Voyles and Orgain, *South. M. J.,* **45:** 439, 1952.

IRWIN, L., E. Y. BERGER, B. ROSENBERG, and R. JACKENTHAL. *J. Clin. Investigation,* **28:** 1403, 1949.

KAHN, S. S., and K. EMERSON, JR. *J. Clin. Investigation,* **29:** 827, 1950.

KATTUS, A. A., JR. *M. Clin. North America,* **36:** 953, 1952.

KEITH, N. M., H. B. BURCHELL, and A. H. BAGGENSTOSS. *Am. Heart J.,* **27:** 817, 1944.

KELSEY, F. E., and E. M. R. GEILING. *J. Pharmacol Exper. Therap.,* **75:** 183, 1942.

KLEIBER, E. E., and G. PICKAR. *Ann. Int. Med.,* **34:** 407, 1951.

KLINGENSMITH, W. C., JR., and J. R. ELKINTON. *Circulation,* **5:** 842, 1952.

KRAUS, H. *J. Clin. Investigation,* **29:** 829, 1950.

LEFKEN, E. B., D. K. HAWLEY, and A. IGLAUER. *Postgraduate Med.,* **12:** 537, 1952.

LIPPMAN, R. W. *Arch. Int. Med.,* **88:** 9, 1951.

McCHESNEY, E. W. *J. Lab. Clin. Med.,* **38:** 199, 1951.

McCHESNEY, E. W. *Am. J. Physiol.,* **168:** 44, 1952a.

McCHESNEY, E. W. *Federation Proc.,* **11:** 103, 1952b.

McCHESNEY, E. W. *J. Lab. Clin. Med.,* **39:** 629, 1952c.

McCHESNEY, E. W. *Proc. Soc. Exper. Biol. Med.,* **79:** 531, 1952d.

McCHESNEY, E. W., W. DOCK, and M. L. TAINTER. *Medicine,* **30:** 183, 1951.

McCHESNEY, E. W., and J. P. McAULIFF. *Am. J. Physiol.*, 160: 264, 1950.

McHARDY, G., D. C. BROWNE, R. McHARDY, and S. WARD. *New Orleans M. S. J.*, 104: 187, 1951.

McHARDY, G., D. C. BROWNE, S. WARD, and J. BECHTOLD. *South. M. J.*, 45: 636, 1952.

MARCHAND, J. F., and C. A. FINCH. *Arch. Int. Med.*, 73: 384, 1944.

MARTIN, G. J., S. ALPERT, and M. J. SULLIVAN. *Proc. Soc. Exper. Biol. Med.*, 82: 373, 1953.

MARTZ, B. L., K. G. KOHLSTAEDT, and O. M. HELMER. *J. Lab. Clin. Med.*, 36: 962, 1950.

MARTZ, B. L., K. G. KOIILSTAEDT, and O. M. HELMER. *Circulation,* 5: 524, 1952.

MATEER, F. M., L. H. ERHARD, M. PRICE, F. A. WEIGAND, J. H. PETERS, T. S. DANOWSKI, R. TARAIL, and L. GREENMAN. *J. Clin. Investigation*, 30: 1018, 1951.

MELCHOIR, N. C. Abstracts, 122nd Meeting Am. Chem. Soc., 48c, September, 1952.

MOSER, R. H., B. D. ROSENAK, R. D. PICKETT, and C. FISCH. *Gastroenterology,* 19: 336, 1951.

ODELL, L. D., G. A. JANSSEN, J. C. NOVELLI, and D. G. RALSTON. *Am. J. Obst. Gynec.*, 62: 121, 1951.

PAYNE, W. W., and R. H. WILKINSON. *Lancet*, 2: 101, 1951.

PENMAN, W. R. *Am. J. M. Sc.*, 222: 193, 1951.

PENMAN, W. R. *Am. J. M. Sc.*, 223: 657, 1952.

PETERS, J. H., T. S. DANOWSKI, L. GREENMAN, F. A. WEIGAND, C. E. CLARKE, K. GARVER, F. M. MATEER, and R. TARAIL. *J. Clin. Investigation*, 30: 1009, 1951.

ROSENAK, B. D., R. H. MOSER, R. D. PICKETT, R. K. ALLEN, and T. MALINOWSKI. *Gastroenterology*, 22: 575, 1952.

SEGAL, H. L. *M. Clin. North America*, 35: 593, 1951.

SEGAL, H. L., L. L. MILLER, and J. J. MORTON. *Proc. Soc. Exper. Biol. Med.*, 74: 218, 1950a.

SEGAL, H. L., L. L. MILLER, J. J. MORTON, and H. Y. YOUNG. *Gastroenterology*, 16: 380, 1950b.

SMITH, G. W. *Am. Dyestuff Reporter*, 23: 313, 1934.

SULLIVAN, M. J., S. ALPERT, and G. J. MARTIN. *J. Am. Pharm. A. (Scient. Ed.)*, 42: 357, 1953.

VOYLES, C., JR., and E. S. ORGAIN. *New England J. Med.*, 245: 808, 1951.

VOYLES, C. M., JR., and E. S. ORGAIN. *South. M. J.*, 45: 439, 1952.

WESTON, R. E., J. GROSSMAN, E. R. BORUN, H. A. GUERIN, H. MARK, T. D. ULLMAN, M. WOLFMAN, and L. LEITER. *Am. J. Med.*, 14: 404, 1953.

WINKLER, A. W., H. E. HOFF, and P. K. SMITH. *J. Clin. Investigation*, 20: 119, 1941.

WOOD, J. E., JR., D. H. FERGUSON, and P. LOWRENCE. *J.A.M.A.*, 148: 820, 1952.

CHAPTER 7

Medical Applications of Combinations
of Exchange Materials

EFFECT OF EXCHANGE MATERIALS ON TOXIC
CHEMICALS OF ENDOGENOUS OR EXOGENOUS
ORIGIN

MEDICAL APPLICATIONS OF COMBINATIONS OF
EXCHANGE MATERIALS

MULTIPLE ADSORBENTS AND EXCHANGERS IN THE
TREATMENT OF DIARRHEA IN PEDIATRICS

COMMENTS

EFFECT OF EXCHANGE MATERIALS ON TOXIC CHEMICALS OF ENDOGENOUS OR EXOGENOUS ORIGIN

THE human gastrointestinal tract is a major subdivision of the microcosm that is man. The enzymatic concatenation in constant activity for anabolism and catabolism is of endogenous and exogenous origin. The microorganisms present supply a multiplicity of catalytic reactions not inherent in the secretions. Knowledge of the toxic agents produced in the gut is meager. For every known toxic agent, there are doubtless dozens unknown. Similarly, our knowledge of the deleterious action of these toxic substances is largely confined to their acute effects; chronic studies are few in number and those published concern comparatively short periods of time.

Man has poured forth his technological ingenuity in an effort to control his external environment. His success is attested by air conditioning, thermostatic temperature controls, ultraviolet health lamps and thousands of other devices. Strangely, he has failed to control his internal environment, his gastrointestinal composition; and yet it is to the content of this complex tube that he is exposed during every second of his life span. It is well within reason that exposures of 40 and 50 years to extremely minute amounts of toxic chemicals will produce profound physiological alterations. Further, it is the summation of the effect of many such deleterious agents that constitutes the pathological straw breaking the back of physiological normality.

With these premises in mind, investigations were made of the capacity of various exchange and adsorption materials to remove under simulated physiological conditions toxins of known and unknown composition.

In a study conducted by Martin and Wilkinson in 1947, indole, skatole, histamine, guanidine and tyramine were used as examples of toxic chemicals endogenously produced. These studies were extended (Martin and Alpert, 1950) from the initial two exchange or adsorbing materials to thirty-five such chemicals. The results are presented in Table 34.

From this table it is to be noted that a major degree of selectivity exists. For example, the anion exchange resins are effective in removing histamine, skatole, and indole but ineffective in a comparative sense against tyramine and putrescine; the activated charcoals are effective against all of these chemicals except putrescine. This selectivity dictates the necessity for the use of multiple adsorbing and exchange material compositions for broad-spectrum toxin removal. It can be concluded from this study that no single adsorbing or exchange agent is likely to be found which will selectively remove all toxins.

A further deduction from the evidence of Table 34 is that different anion exchange resins are strikingly unlike one another in their capacity for the removal of a given toxic chemical, e.g., resin A as contrasted to resin C for mercuric chloride removal. Once again, the point is to be made that one anion exchange resin is not like another; they should never be used interchangeably. On the other hand, many more standard adsorbing agents are relatively constant in their effect, e.g., the charcoals. Martin and Alpert (1950), consequent to the paper of Mutch (1937), in which he reported kaolin as an effective histamine adsorber, obtained six different samples of kaolin and also isolated the kaolin from one marketed preparation. With these seven samples, histamine adsorption powers were determined and found to vary in their capacity from 18 to 42 per cent. The conclusion was reached that there is little variation in kaolin samples as obtained and marketed in the United States. It is noteworthy that neither kaolin nor aluminum hydroxide, two agents of most common use in the treatment of diarrhea, is an effective adsorbing agent for any of the chemicals under test.

TABLE 34

Comparative Adsorption Study

(From Martin, G. J., and S. Alpert, *Am. J. Dig. Dis.*, **17**: 151, 1950)

Adsorbent (conc., 4 Gm./100 cc. except where indicated)	Skatole, % adsorption (conc. 10 mg./100 cc., pH, 8.0–8.5)	Indole, % adsorption (conc., 50 mg./100 cc., pH, 8.0–8.5)	Tyramine hydrochloride, % adsorption (conc., 100 mg./100 cc., pH, 8.0–8.5)	Putrescine dihydrochloride, % adsorption (conc., 150 mg./100 cc., pH, 8.0–8.5)	Histamine dihydrochloride, % adsorption (conc., 250 mg./100 cc., pH, 8.0–8.5)	Mercuric chloride, % adsorption (conc., 2 Gm./100 cc., pH, 1.5)
1 Insoluble polyamine anion exchange resin A, commercial sample, 200-mesh	96.0	96.0	24.5	36.7	60.0	97.7
2 Insoluble polyamine anion exchange resin B, chloride salt, commercial sample, 200-mesh	98.0	99.2	25.5	10.0	None	100.0
3 Insoluble polyamine anion exchange resin C, commercial sample, 200-mesh	97.0	95.6	20.5	None	None	8.0
4 Insoluble polyamine anion exchange resin D, commercial sample, 200-mesh	92.0	77.5	16.5	None	28.0	73.0
5 Insoluble polyamine anion exchange resin E, commercial sample, 200-mesh	64.0	58.0	11.0	10.0	24.0	100.0
6 Insoluble polyamine anion exchange resin F, commercial sample, 200-mesh	53.6	47.0	10.0	8.0	72.0	100.0
7 Cation exchange resin A, hydrogen-activated commercial sample, 200-mesh	99.0	100.0	95.0	96.5	72.0	3.5
8 Cation exchange resin B, hydrogen-activated commercial sample, 200-mesh	98.0	100.0	99.5	96.2	98.0	13.0

No.	Sample						
9	Cation exchange resin C, hydrogen-activated commercial sample, 200-mesh	95.0	100.0	100.0	97.3	100.0	9.0
10	Cation exchange resin D, hydrogen-activated commercial sample, 200-mesh	98.5	100.0	96.5	94.7	92.0	7.5
11	Cation exchange resin E, hydrogen-activated commercial sample, 200-mesh	100.0	100.0	72.0	7.0	20.0	99.3
12	Cation exchange resin F, carboxylic acid type commercial sample, 200-mesh	98.8	72.0	98.5	97.3	100.0	15.0
13	Cation exchange resin G, carboxylic acid type commercial sample, 200-mesh	49.0	48.0	79.5	96.0	92.0	1.5
14	Cation exchange resin H, sodium-activated commercial sample, 200-mesh	85.0	72.0	100.0	98.0	100.0	11.0
15	Cation exchange resin C, sodium-activated commercial sample, 200-mesh	81.0	78.8	92.5	96.6	100.0	17.0
16	Cation exchange resin I, sodium-activated commercial sample, 200-mesh	61.0	47.0	100.0	99.0	99.0	9.0
17	Colloidal magnesium aluminum silicate gel (conc., 40 cc./100 cc.)	24.0	14.0	71.3	96.3	61.0	4.0
18	Synthetic magnesium silicate	16.0	18.0	17.0	35.0	16.0	10.0
19	Synthetic sodium aluminum silicate, 200-mesh	19.0	23.0	62.0	98.0	64.0	None
20	High-capacity synthetic sodium aluminum silicate, 200-mesh	12.0	8.0	31.5	92.7	0.5	12.4
21	Polyamine anion exchange resin A (10%), synthetic sodium aluminum silicate (10%), suspended in colloidal magnesium aluminum silicate gel (conc., 40 cc./100 cc.)	82.0	62.0	41.0	95.3	72.0	79.0
22	Activated charcoal A	100.0	100.0	100.0	10.0	90.0	100.0
23	Activated charcoal B	100.0	100.0	100.0	12.5	86.0	100.0

TABLE 34 (*Continued*)

Adsorbent (conc., 4 Gm./100 cc. except where indicated)	Skatole, % adsorption (conc. 10 mg./100 cc., pH, 8.0–8.5)	Indole, % adsorption (conc., 50 mg./100 cc., pH, 8.0–8.5)	Tyramine hydrochloride, % adsorption (conc., 100 mg./100 cc., pH, 8.0–8.5)	Putrescine dihydrochloride, % adsorption (conc., 150 mg./100 cc., pH, 8.0–8.5)	Histamine dihydrochloride, % adsorption (conc., 250 mg./100 cc., pH, 8.0–8.5)	Mercuric chloride, % adsorption (conc., 2 Gm./100 cc., pH, 1.5)
24 Activated charcoal C	100.0	100.0	100.0	27.5	84.0	84.5
25 Activated bauxite (essentially, Al_2O_3)	15.0	12.0	18.0	20.0	None	5.0
26 Fuller's earth (essentially SiO_2)	13.0	15.0	46.0	40.6	38.0	4.5
27 Diatomaceous earth	15.0	12.0	9.0	6.0	32.0	3.7
28 Kaolin	14.0	15.0	18.0	6.7	22.0	1.7
29 Talc	12.0	12.0	15.5	None	10.0	3.0
30 Bentonite	26.4	None	89.0	95.4	99.2	3.4
31 Bauxite	16.0	16.0	14.0	3.0	None	None
32 Filtrol adsorbent	20.0	16.0	70.0	91.7	64.0	11.0
33 Aluminum hydroxide gel	16.0	16.0	15.0	30.0	30.0	10.0
34 Magnesium trisilicate	14.5	20.0	77.0	97.4	44.0	5.0
35 Aluminum hydroxide powder	8.0	10.0	19.5	16.6	None	None

The question is often raised whether or not there is a correlation between *in vitro* adsorption studies and *in vivo* effects. Joachimoglu (1920) concluded from such investigations with strychnine that no correlation existed. On the other hand, Martin and Wilkinson (1947), having established the efficacy of anion exchange resins for the adsorption of indole and of sodium aluminum silicate for the adsorption of guanidine, tested these agents *in vivo*. Table 35 presents the results.

TABLE 35
Biological Results with Ion Exchange Materials and Toxic Putrefactive Chemicals

(From Martin, G. J., and J. Wilkinson, *Arch. Biochem.*, **12**: 95, 1947)

Toxic chemical*	Amount used (Gm./kg.)	Adsorbing agent	Amount used	No. of mice	Deaths (%)	Controls (%)
Indole	0.4	Amberlite IR-4	10% in diet	20	20	50
	0.5			20	30	60
	0.6			20	60	70
	0.4	Amberlite IR-4	10% in diet	20	10	50
	0.5		+5% in	20	30	60
	0.6		suspension	20	30	70
Guanidine acetate	0.4	Permutit	10% in diet	10	10	30
	0.5			10	30	50
	0.6			10	40	50
	0.4	Permutit	10% in diet	10	20	30
	0.5		+5% in	10	20	50
	0.6		suspension	10	30	50

* Indole was administered in 5% suspension and guanidine acetate in 5% solution.

The *in vitro* and *in vivo* results compare favorably and tend to establish the merit of *in vitro* screening procedures.

A general principle underlying the medical application of ion exchange and adsorption therapy is that of differential adsorption. The combination of materials used must remove toxic chemicals while permitting normal absorption of all nutrients. This point was emphasized by the work of Melnick *et al.* (1945), in which they demonstrated that fuller's earth but not kaolin markedly reduced the availability of thiamin. Studies with sodium aluminum silicate (Martin and Wilkinson,

1947) and with anion exchange resins (Martin and Wilkinson, 1946) have demonstrated that the feeding of diets containing 5 per cent of these materials does not interfere with normal nutrition.

The results of unpublished experiments on exchange materials and aging have established the nontoxicity of these agents over periods exceeding 3 years. Rats kept for such prolonged periods actually manifested complete normality in growth rate, hematology, pathology, and blood biochemistry.

Of all abnormal states primarily afflicting the gastrointestinal tract, the most common is "food poisoning." The syndrome associated is a manifestation of the toxic, poisonous elements brought into the gut via the food. Clearly, under such conditions treatment must be related to the ability of the medication to prevent the absorption of the toxins into the system and to prevent irritation of the surfaces by the toxic materials. It seemed logical to use paralytic shellfish poison as a typical example of this general category of deleterious principles, the nonbacterial "food poisons."

The paralytic poison is apparently a component of the dinoflagellate (*Gonyaulax catenella* Whedon and Kofoid), which is consumed by the shellfish (Riegel *et al.*, 1949). Its chemistry has been studied by Müller (1935), who reported that kaolin, sea sand and Lloyd's reagent adsorbed the active principle; Norite A, aluminum hydroxide and diatomaceous earth did not. Swayne and Martin (1950) studied a series of exchangers and adsorbers for their capacity to remove the paralytic poison from aqueous and alcoholic solutions (Table 36).

Kaolin, aluminum hydroxide and charcoal—three of the most commonly employed intestinal adsorbents—were completely inactive under the experimental conditions. On the other hand, magnesium trisilicate, sodium aluminum silicate, bentonite, sulfonic cation exchange resins, carboxylic cation exchange resins and polyamine anion exchangers were highly active. It seems probable that a successful intestinal adsorbent for the treatment of food poisoning should be composed of one or more of the chemicals found effective. Conservatively, it may be stated that the currently used preparations, comprised of kaolin and aluminum hydroxide, will be comparatively ineffective in such therapeutic procedures.

Another general category of "food poisoning" is bacterial in origin. For *in vitro* screening of the efficacy of exchangers and similar materials, Moss and Martin (1950) investigated the activity of these agents against the toxins of *Shigella dysenteriae, Eberthella typhosa*

TABLE 36
Adsorption of Paralytic Shellfish Poison (0.2 cc. of Solution Injected Intraperitoneally in Mice)

(From Swayne, V. R., and G. J. Martin, *Am. J. Dig. Dis.*, **17**: 39, 1950)

Adsorbent	Gm. adsorbent (ratio vol. in cc. of solution)	Type of solution		No. of mice	% Deaths	Death time
		Alcoholic	Aqueous			
Polyamine anion exchange resin A	10/20	x		6	0	
	10/40	x		3	100	5 min.
	10/20		x	3	33⅓	3 hrs.
	10/40		x	3	0	
Polyamine anion exchange resin B	10/20	x		6	100	5 min.
	10/40	x		3	100	5 min.
	10/20		x	3	0	
	10/40		x	3	33⅓	5 min.
Cation exchange resin A, carboxylic	10/20	x		3	100	5 min.
	20/20	x		3	33⅓	18 hrs.
	10/40	x		6	100	5 min.
	35/10	x		3	33⅓	
	10/20		x	3	66⅔	1 hr. 18 hrs.
	10/40		x	3	66⅔	18 hrs.
Cation exchange resin B, carboxylic	10/20		x	3	0	
	10/40		x	3	100	5 min.
Cation exchange resin A, sulfonic	10/20	x		3	0	
	10/40	x		6	100	<30 min.
	10/20		x	3	0	
	10/40		x	3	0	
Bentonite	10/20	x		3	0	
	10/40	x		3	100	10 min.
	10/20		x	3	0	
	10/40		x	3	100	20 min.
Kaolin	10/20	x		3	100	7 hrs.
	10/20		x	3	100	5 min.
	10/40		x	3	100	5 min.
Sand	35/20	x		3	100	8 min.
	10/20	x		3	100	7 min.
	10/20		x	3	100	5 min.
	10/40		x	3	100	5 min.
Silica	10/20	x		3	100	5 min.
	10/20		x	3	100	6 min.
	10/40		x	3	100	5 min.

TABLE 36 (*Continued*)

Adsorbent	Gm. of adsorbent (ratio vol. in cc. of solution)	Type of solution		No. of mice	% deaths	Death time
		Alcoholic	Aqueous			
Synthetic magnesium alumi-	10/20	x		3	100	5 min.
num silicate	10/40	x		6	100	5 min.
	10/20		x	3	100	5 min.
	10/40		x	3	100	5 min.
Sodium aluminum silicate	10/20	x		3	0	
	10/40	x		3	100	5 min.
	35/20	x		3	0	
	10/20		x	3	0	
	10/40		x	3	0	
Aluminum hydroxide	10/20	x		3	100	5 min.
	10/40	x		3	100	5 min.
	10/20		x	3	100	5 min.
	10/40		x	3	100	5 min.
Magnesium trisilicate	10/20	x		6	0	
	10/40	x		6	100	5 min.
	10/20		x	3	0	
No adsorbent		x		6	100	5 min.
			x	6	100	5 min.

and *Esch. coli.* The toxins were prepared in accordance with the procedures of Branham and Hable (1946). To these toxins, the material under study was added with thorough mixing, filtered, and the filtrate subsequently injected in mice. The results of a series of agents are presented in Table 37. Of the material under test only bentonite and the carboxylic cation exchange resins were broad-spectrum agents, removing the toxins of all three bacterial species.

There seems little reason to consider the possible removal of bacterial cells by exchangers or adsorbing agents as a procedure applicable to the gastrointestinal tract. The enormous number of cells normally comprising intestinal content dwarfs the number which would be removed in this manner. It seems possible that such agents might remove from the medium nutrients essential to the growth of the bacterial cells, but if this occurred in the gut the logical corollary would be that the body would also be deprived of the adsorbed food substances. A similar opinion has been expressed by Gunnison and Marshall (1937) following studies of intestinal flora after feeding charcoal and kaolin.

There were no changes. Selective and differential absorption or adsorption of the toxic chemicals elaborated by bacteria and other microorganisms represents the only practical applicable procedure in the retention in the gut of deleterious principles.

TABLE 37

Adsorption of Toxic Substances from Bacterial Lysates

(From Moss, J., and G. J. Martin, *Am. J. Dig. Dis.*, **17**: 18, 1950)

Adsorbent	Approximate M.L.D. per ml.		
	S. dysenteriae (Shiga)	E. typhosa	Esch. coli
Aluminum hydroxide (powdered)	50	>10	12
Bentonite	0.5-1.0	0-1	0
Vegetable charcoal	>40	0	0
Carboxylic cation exchange resin	<10	0.5-1.0	1
Kaolin	20	12	5
Hydrated sodium aluminum silicate (a synthetic zeolite) 10 mg./cc.	50	1	1-3
Hydrated sodium aluminum silicate (a synthetic zeolite) 20 mg./cc.	50	1	5
Synthetic zeolite (5%) + polyamine resin (5%)	50	0-1	10
Synthetic zeolite (10%) + polyamine resin (10%)	50	0.5	>5.0
Polyamine anion exchange resin	>50	10	5
Silica	>40	2	0
Magnesium aluminum silicate	<50	10	10
Toxin controls	40	50	10-12 10-12 24

Another feature for consideration relative to normalization of the gastrointestinal tract in the diarrheal disease states lies in the inhibition of enzymes. It has been suggested, for example, that limitation or reduction in the activity of trypsin might favorably affect the course of chronic ulcerative colitis and that the case might be similar with reference to lysozyme (Chapter 5). From the charts presented in Chapter 5, it is clear that certain anion exchange resins do not inhibit either lysozyme or trypsin. The exceptions lie in the ability of some anion exchangers to block trypsin. In the treatment of pathological states in the intestine, wherever inhibition of these enzymes was deemed indicated, the anion exchangers would have to be supplemented by use in combination with other exchange or adsorption materials. As an example of this, a combination of anion exchange resin, a sodium aluminum silicate and a magnesium aluminum silicate proved synergistic in the inhibition of lysozyme (Moss and Martin, 1948) and trypsin (Alpert and Martin, 1950).

The most attractive theory of etiology of chronic ulcerative colitis lies in a combination of ideas expressed by various groups (Meyer *et al.*, 1948; Grace *et al.*, 1949; Gray *et al.*, 1950) and supplemented by the present author. Emotional states, reactions to stress situations, psychic trauma—all stimulate nervous mechanisms resulting in localized ischemia. Altered oxygen tensions in isolated areas of the intestinal mucosa increase the activity of lysozyme, which in turn hydrolyzes the mucin and heightens thereby the susceptibility of the surface to adverse reactions, one of which is the accelerated kinetics of tryptic and other proteolytic enzymes. The chain reaction could be broken at any one of several points; this concept might account for the multiplicity of therapeutic procedures which seem to give some but not full relief. Logic therefore dictates a multiple approach to any pathological state of the gastrointestinal tract.

One feature of paramount significance in the consideration of these clinical states is the fact that irritated mucosal surfaces will increase markedly the absorption of toxic substances from the gut. The correlative is that treatment should involve a simultaneous attempt to restrict these deleterious principles to the tract, and as has been indicated this can be accomplished through the application of multiphasic adsorption and exchange compositions.

MEDICAL APPLICATIONS OF COMBINATIONS OF EXCHANGE MATERIALS

The potential applications of polyphasic exchange and adsorption therapy are legion. Restriction in scope to the diarrheal diseases would be illogical, as countless clinical states not primarily associated with the gastrointestinal tract have as a component of their etiology the abnormal gut. It seems highly probable that chronic degenerative disease in some measure develops as a result of abnormal function in the digestive tube. To establish in a positive sense the association of many clinical entities with abnormal gut physiology will be difficult, as studies must be conducted over long periods in well-controlled groups. Such research is extremely expensive and difficult to undertake, as adequate facilities are rare. It seems highly probable that in many instances the government, through federal subsidies, will necessarily underwrite such investigations.

For the present, discussion must be restricted to those disease states in which concrete proof of the efficacy of such treatment can be obtained. Prime among these are the diarrheal diseases. Diarrhea is a symptom resulting from an inflammatory reaction in or irritation to the intestinal mucosa, with consequent stimulation of nerve channels precipitating in turn increased peristalsis. It may also result from purely psychoneurotic reactions. Basically, the tendency of the past to regard diarrhea as no more than an annoying symptom is unsound, as it represents excessive water, salt and essential nutrient loss. Furthermore, in a positive sense, it will invariably be associated with altered absorption from the tract, resulting in systemic action of poisonous principles elaborated in the gut.

The magnitude of the water and salt effect is indicated by the fact that diarrhea may cause the loss of as much as 500 to 5,000 ml. of water and 2 to 45 Gm. of sodium chloride (Leake, 1949), this in contrast with the normal figures of approximately 100 ml. of water and 0.2 Gm. of sodium chloride.

A brief summary of the classification of the diarrheas will serve to indicate the importance of specific therapy and to underline the significance of adjuvant treatment designated for immediate relief of this distressing symptom. The major subdivisions of the classification are the acute and the chronic diarrheas.

The acute diarrheas are classified as being caused by food, microorganisms, systemic toxins, and psychic factors; more specifically as related in origin to bacillary dysentery, amebiasis, staphylococcal food poisoning, *Salmonella* food poisoning, allergic reactions, chemical irritants, cholera, schistosomiasis, etc. With most of these specific disease states manifesting diarrhea as a symptom, there is some abnormality of gastrointestinal flora or ingestion of foods containing toxic materials elaborated by microorganisms. In other words, the etiology can in an immediate sense be related to chemicals of greater or lesser complexity formed in the biosynthetic processes of metabolism in microorganisms. It is not beyond logic to ponder the probability that the sole deleterious action of many microorganisms commonly associated with disease states may be that of synthesis of toxic agents. This concept is not advanced as a counter to the present use of specific therapy but rather to emphasize the importance of the multiple approach.

The chronic diarrheal states are classified as due to amebiasis, ulcerative colitis, regional enteritis, cancer, tuberculosis, colitis, uremia, amyloid disease, leukemias, pancreatitis, cystic disease of the pancreas, sprue, pellagra, and similar conditions. With this chronic group, the factor of absorption into the system of toxic chemicals becomes of increasing importance. The issue is there whether or not the etiology is associated with microorganisms. As Leake (1949) has emphasized, there is a balance among the intestinal flora. Any disturbance of this relationship may so upset the economy as to cause normally nonpathogenic bacteria to produce reactions and local irritations leading to a diarrheal state. It is therefore apparent that the so-called normal flora of the tract may under certain circumstances precipitate a pathological state which would not normally be diagnosed as having its origin in bacterial metabolism.

MULTIPLE ADSORBENTS AND EXCHANGERS IN THE TREATMENT OF DIARRHEA IN PEDIATRICS

In 1950, Joslin of Baltimore reported the study of a combination of exchanger and adsorbent materials in the management of diarrhea in pediatric practice. Diseases manifesting diarrhea as a symptom were in the past responsible for as many deaths among infants as all other diseases combined. In the United States this no longer holds true, but in other areas of the world it is today the fact. Dr. Joslin had found that diarrhea in infants in Baltimore was of the proteolytic rather than the fermentative type. The composition used consisted of 10 per cent of a polyamine formaldehyde anion exchange resin, 10 per cent of a synthetic sodium aluminum silicate, and 1.25 per cent of a magnesium aluminum silicate. The dose adopted was a tablespoonful three or four times daily, or if the diarrhea was severe, a tablespoonful of the mixture was given after each bowel movement. No other medication was employed. As a tablespoon contains approximately 15 ml., it is seen that the average daily dose consisted of 4.5 Gm. each of the polyamine resin and the sodium aluminum silicate, and approximately

TABLE 38
Statistics of Pediatric Patient Group Treated by Multiple Adsorbents

(From Joslin, C. L., *Delaware State M. J.*, **22:** 35, 1950)

Average age of the 50 patients	13.8	mos.
Youngest	1	mo.
Oldest	60	mos.
Average duration of diarrhea before treatment	11.22	days
Shortest	1	day
Longest	120	days
Average no. of stools per day before treatment	5.3	
Smallest	4	
Largest	7	

TABLE 39
Results of the Treatment of Diarrhea in Pediatrics by Multiple Adsorbents

(From Joslin, C. L., *Delaware State M. J.*, **22:** 35, 1950)

No. of cases	Average age (mos.)	Average duration of diarrhea (days)	Average no. of stools per day	Diarrhea controlled (days)
19	14.70	5.9	5.3	1
12	8.58	9.5	5.3	2
6	18.70	14.0	5.2	3
3	13.60	9.7	5.3	4
5	6.80	13.3	5.3	5
6	17.00	10.0	6.0	6
2	18.00	6.5	5.2	7
1	60.00	120.0	4.0	30

0.5 Gm. of the magnesium aluminum silicate. Tables 38 and 39 illustrate the finding reported.

The tables list 6 patients treated with smaller doses (a teaspoonful three or four times daily), subsequently established to be inadequate. In all 44 patients receiving the larger doses, the diarrhea was controlled within 24 to 48 hours. Joslin recommends the continuation of treatment with the combination of exchangers for a period of several weeks as a prophylactic measure to insure against recurrence. It is most interesting to note that in the series studied there were 5 cases of infectious diarrhea, 4 with *Salmonella* and 1 with dysentery, who were first given sulfonamides and penicillin in an attempt to control the diarrhea. When this regimen had failed, they were transferred to the adsorbent and controlled within 24 to 48 hours. This raises the point made previously that all therapeutic regimens should be multiple in nature, using not only the specific but also the palliative drugs.

TABLE 40

Comparative Figures of Patients Treated with Sulfa Drugs and Resion, and Those Treated with Sulfa Drugs Alone

(From Quintos, F. N., *J. Philippine M. A.*, **26:** 155, 1950)

Type of diarrhea	Group I, sulfa drugs with Resion		Group II, sulfa drugs only	
	No. of cases	%	No. of cases	%
Severe	17		56	
Improved	11	64.7	30	53.6
Not improved	6	35.3	26	46.4
Moderately severe	30		30	
Improved	28	93.3	27	90.0
Not improved	2	6.6	3	10.0

In the Philippine Islands, infectious infantile diarrhea is the major cause of child mortality despite the use of sulfonamides and antibiotics. Quintos (1950) states that: "It caused 50% of the deaths in the Children's Ward of the Philippine General Hospital (95 deaths), although the number of cases of infantile diarrhea admitted was only 33% of the total number of admissions (694 out of 2,106)." This investigator studied some 312 patients with infantile diarrhea, divided into four general groups: (1) those treated with sulfonamides and the adsorbent combination; (2) those treated with sulfonamides alone; (3) those treated with sulfonamides plus streptomycin plus the adsorbent combination; and (4) those treated with sulfonamides plus streptomycin. In all cases, the therapeutic regimen included proper adjustments of fluid and electrolyte balances. The results of the experiment involving sulfonamides alone as compared with sulfonamides plus adsorbent combination are presented in Table 40.

The results clearly demonstrate the value of the multiple approach to the therapeutic problem, as there were roughly 50 per cent fewer failures in the series treated with sulfonamide and adsorbent combination. This is in complete agreement with theory. The specific, the sulfonamide, could do no more than cause a stasis of the growth of the

TABLE 41
Comparative Figures of Patients Treated with Streptomycin-Sulfa Drugs and Resion, and Those Treated with Streptomycin and Sulfa Drugs Alone

(From Quintos, F. N., *J. Philippine M. A.*, **26:** 155, 1950)

Type of diarrhea	Group III, streptomycin-sulfa drugs and Resion		Group IV, streptomycin-sulfa drugs alone	
	No. of cases	%	No. of cases	%
Severe	17		38	
Improved	11	64.7	23	60.5
Not improved	6	35.3	15	39.5
Moderately severe	19		14	
Improved	19	100.0	8	57.0
Not improved	0		6	43.0
Moderate	6		25	
Improved	6	100.0	25	100.0
Not improved	0		0	
Total no. of patients	42		77	
Improved	36	85.7	56	72.7
Not improved	6	14.3	21	27.2

bacteria involved. This requires time. During this period, water and electrolyte loss continue, and while this can be corrected by intravenous fluids, the continued absorption from the gut of toxic chemicals cannot be controlled by any procedure other than that of adsorption and exchange. Table 41, also from the work of Quintos, shows the findings from the experiment involving the use of streptomycin with sulfonamides as compared with the use of streptomycin plus sulfonamides and adsorbent combination.

Once again, the concept of multiple therapy is vindicated. The incidence of failures is 50 per cent lower. This series is of interest, as it offers a basis for raising the point of possible adsorption of the antibiotic by the adsorption and exchange combination. In the case of streptomycin, the results of Quintos (1950) establish synergism of antibiotic

TABLE 42

Adsorption of Antibiotics by Various Adsorbents

(Antibiotic Adsorbed per Mg.)*

(From Moss, J., *et al.*, unpublished data, 1953)

Adsorbent	Peni-cillin-G (U.)	Aureo-mycin (μg.)	Chloro-mycetin	Poly-myxin (μg.)	Neo-mycin (μg.)	Baci-tracin (U.)	Terra-mycin (μg.)	Strepto-mycin (μg.)
XE-67	900	<711	N	N	N	N	725	19.4
XE-64	N	24.7	N	66.5	N	37.5	N	12.4
XE-58	850	43.9	N	N	N	N	N	N
XE-65	N	N	N	N	100	N	N	667
Natrinil	80	N	N	79.2	469	334	N	1000
XE-88	900	711	N	93.8	815	27.7	N	1000
Veegum	N	71.3	N	995	474	N	N	800
Al(OH)$_3$	N	71.3	N	N	N	N	N	N
Charcoal	900	830	70 μg.	92.5	14.8	120	N	71.3
Bentonite	N	830	N	995	100	16.9	N	81.0
Mg trisilicate	800	830	N	93.8	81.5	N	N	64.1
Kaolin	—	N	N	N	N	16.5	N	N
Na carboxycellulose	N	N	N	N	N	N	N	N
Folin Decalso	N	N	N	81.3	N	13.9	N	71.3
Permutit	N	N	N	79.2	81.5	N	N	83.8
Resion mix†	>900	800	N	99.5	1000	400	815	N

* N = negative.
† Permutit, −10 ⎫
  Bentonite, −5 ⎪ mg./cc.
  Veegum, −5 ⎬
  Xe-58, −5 ⎭

with adsorbent; if adsorption did occur it was beneficial in the sense that it may have been responsible for retention of the antibiotic in the gut for a longer period, permitting as a result greater local chemotherapeutic efficacy. In order to clarify this problem, an entire series of antibiotics and adsorbents were studied in the following manner (Moss *et al.*, 1953).

The antibiotic being tested was dissolved in distilled water and treated with 1 mg. and 10 mg. per cubic centimeter quantities of the adsorbing agent. The antibiotic-adsorbent mixtures were shaken at room temperature for 2 hours, filtered, and the filtrate was stored in the deep freeze until the assay period. Assays were performed by employing modified agar disc methods and measuring zone of inhibition. *Staphylococcus aureus* 209 and 9144 were used for bacitracin and penicillin assays; *Esch. coli* 9661 for streptomycin, neomycin, and terramycin; *Sarcina lutea* 9341 for Chloromycetin and aureomycin; *Brucella bronchiseptica* 4617 for polymyxin.

Elution of adsorbed antibiotic was carried out by treating the adsorbent with 0.05 N hydrochloric acid or 4 per cent sodium bicarbonate. The filtrates collected after this treatment were in turn assayed and compared with suitable controls. Table 42 shows the general picture of the activity of the adsorbing agents tested. Generally, repeat tests did not vary. However, in some cases 20 per cent differences in results did occur. This is to be expected since the dilution factor required to obtain workable solutions of antibiotics is large, thereby probably increasing the experimental error.

The results in Table 43 show the amount (per cent) of adsorbed antibiotic which was eluted by acid or base treatment. In many cases it was difficult to filter materials such as magnesium aluminum silicate, Permutit and Resion mixture. The results with these materials may be arbitrary.

The duration of diarrhea following the institution of therapy is of great practical importance, as it is during this period that there will be absorbed into the blood stream toxic substances which may produce immediate manifestation or which may be the initiating factor in tissue and organ damage not to be shown for years. The findings of Quintos (1950) establish the fact that combination adsorbent therapy reduced the duration of treatment from a period averaging 2.7 to 4.2 days to one of 2.3 to 3.2 days.

From the reports of Joslin (1950) and Quintos (1950), it can be seen that *in vitro* laboratory results on toxic chemical adsorption and enzyme inhibition parallel in large measure the *in vivo* clinical studies. This summation of laboratory and clinical results is further extended by the observations of Rollins (1950), who found the combination of adsorption and exchange materials effective adjuncts in the treatment of a variety of gastrointestinal disease states, including diverticulitis, gastroenteritis, colitis and infantile diarrheas.

TABLE 43
Elution of Various Adsorbed Antibiotics

(From Moss, J., *et al.*, unpublished data, 1953)

Antibiotic	Adsorbent	Acid*	Base*
Penicillin	XE-58	N	N
	XE-67	N	40%
	XE-88	N	N
	Charcoal	N	N
Polymyxin	XE-64	100%	100%
	XE-88	27	75%
	Natrinil	100%	80%
	Veegum	N	N
	Charcoal	N	N
	Bentonite	N	N
	Mg trisilicate	30%	30%
	Decalso	100%	70%
	Permutit	80%	80%
	Resion	N	N
Neomycin	XE-65	N	100%
	Natrinil	100%	37%
	XE-88	53%	100%
	Veegum	Did not filter	
	Charcoal	55%	30%
	Bentonite	Not done	
	Mg trisilicate	27%	100%
	Permutit	N	100%
	Resion	N	N
Streptomycin	XE-67	Not done	Not done
	XE-64	Not done	Not done
	XE-65	48%	62%
	Natrinil	62%	62%
	XE-88	69%	12%
	Veegum	Not done	Not done
	Charcoal	100%	25%
	Bentonite	NN	23%
	Mg trisilicate	100%	100%
	Decalso	100%	N
	Permutit		

* N = negative.

Lichtman (1951), in a study involving 300 patients, compared the efficacy of a regimen based upon the use of exchangers and adsorbents with one based upon the use of bismuth and kaolin. The experimental group of 200 patients received a tablespoonful of a combination of 10 per cent anion exchange resin, 10 per cent sodium aluminum silicate and 1.25 per cent magnesium aluminum silicate every hour for four doses, and then a tablespoonful every 3 hours, while awake, for 48 hours. The severe cases were also given retention enemas consisting of 2 tablespoonfuls of the combination suspended in 1 pint of tepid water. The control group of 100 patients received 1 Gm. of bismuth subcarbonate and 8 Gm. of kaolin every hour for 4 hours, and then at 3-hour intervals while awake until the symptoms subsided.

The results demonstrated the superiority of the exchanger combination, as in the experimental group diarrhea, vomiting, nausea and cramps were relieved by two doses in a period of 2 hours for the milder cases and by four doses in a period of 4 hours for the more severe cases. In contrast, the control group receiving bismuth and kaolin continued to manifest symptoms for 24 to 48 hours and in the more severe cases up to 5 days.

There is therefore a striking correlation between the *in vitro* laboratory testing of exchangers for their capacity to absorb or adsorb toxic chemicals and their *in vivo* clinical effect. Kaolin failed to adsorb significantly any of the toxic chemicals produced endogenously (Martin and Alpert, 1950), to remove bacterial toxins (Moss and Martin, 1950), to adsorb paralytic shellfish poison (Swayne and Martin, 1950) or to inhibit lysozyme (Moss and Martin, 1948). In view of these negative findings *in vitro,* it is not surprising that those agents effective in the above systems would prove more efficacious in the clinic. The observations of Lichtman (1951) are exceptionally valuable, as this direct comparison of kaolin plus bismuth and of a polyamine anion exchange resin with silicate is made. Better controls could not have been designed. It is important to note that with this study correlation of *in vitro* and *in vivo* results is found to be not only qualitatively but also quantitatively comparable.

Three lines of evidence and thinking led Fitzpatrick *et al.* (1951) to attempt the control of nausea and vomiting of pregnancy through the use of multiphasic adsorbent and exchange materials. The first was the observation that histamine and similar agents induce vomiting when applied directly to the vomiting center (Best and Taylor, 1943); the second was the concept that histamine is an important etiological factor in nausea and vomiting of pregnancy (Hofbauer, 1926; Kapeller-Adler and Adler, 1943); and the third was the possibility that toxic substances of the histamine type, but not necessarily histamine, might be formed by bacterial action in the gut and absorbed, causing the distressing clinical syndrome. In their series of 94 ambulatory patients, the routine treatment with frequent small dry feedings and nutrient supplements was effective in 66. The remaining 28 patients were tried on pyridoxine and then on an antihistaminic preparation. Twenty-five patients did not respond to any of these procedures and were given a multiphasic intestinal exchange and adsorbent combination. Eighteen of these refractory patients responded; the 7 who did not respond were felt to be those with a heavy psychiatric overlay.

The implication contained in these results is that toxic chemicals other than histamine were involved, as the antihistaminic did not prove effective, while the intestinal exchangers and adsorbents did give relief. It is not improbable that the impression gained from this work will in fact apply not only to the nausea and vomiting of pregnancy but to an entire host of clinical syndromes not generally regarded as having any part of their etiology based upon the gastrointestinal tract.

COMMENTS

With reasonable certainty it can be stated that no currently existing product represents the ultimate potential to be achieved via the intestinal adsorbent and exchanger. To date, in fact, there is but one such item (containing a resinous exchanger) available. Perhaps by attempting to define the ideal product of this sort, some idea can be obtained of current limitations and of the magnitude of the problem. The ideal intestinal adsorbent and exchanger will possess the following qualifications:

1. Maximum capacity for the removal of toxic amines, such as tyramine, histamine, putrescine, and cadaverine.
2. Maximum capacity for the removal of toxic bacterial metabolites, such as indole and skatole.
3. Maximum capacity for the removal of toxic substances of bacterial origin but of unknown composition.
4. Maximum capacity for the removal of agents comparable to paralytic shellfish poison (probably responsible for "food poisoning").

5. Maximum capacity for the removal of all irritant chemicals whether toxic or nontoxic.
6. Maximum capacity for the inhibition of lysozyme.
7. Absence of any tendency to remove essential food factors such as minerals, vitamins, or amino acids.
8. Nontoxicity, generally through total insolubility.
9. Patient acceptability.

Virtually the entire list consists of factors reflecting the concept of differential exchange and adsorption. There is no direct correlation between molecular structure and adsorption on a given material; there is a direct correlation between the strength of an acid or base, its valence and similar factors and ion exchange materials; however, it seems probable that all ion exchange materials also possess the physical characteristics of adsorbers. Mixed-bed principles add to the complexity of the problem in that an exchange material, and probably also an adsorbent, will not necessarily behave in combination as each will as a separate entity. The fact remains that extensive investigations must be conducted in a purely empirical manner before a material can be designated as possessing in maximum degree the capacity to remove a given toxic chemical under specified hydrogen ion concentrations.

Selective adsorption and exchange phenomena do occur, and this fact, combined with the lack of broad-spectrum materials, renders essential the use of multiple adsorption and exchange agents. It seems highly probable that no single material will ever be found possessing in maximum degree a capacity for the removal of the host of toxic chemicals biosynthesized in the gut. Further, it is not necessarily true that the toxic chemicals are identical with those responsible for irritation of the mucosal surfaces. Specifically, there is no knowledge today of the identity of those chemicals resulting from bacterial metabolism which are primarily responsible for the irritation produced by lysed bacterial cultures introduced into the gastrointestinal tract. This line of approach should prove most fruitful.

Lysozyme doubtless plays some role in the normalization of the gut. Its function being that of destruction of mucin, one might assume that the correlative was true, namely that the presence of mucin is essential to the control of normal permeability and normal resistance to irritating chemicals on the part of the mucosa; this is to be doubted, as the mere fact of mucin presence would be without significance unless its location were known. In other words, mucin at the surface of the mucosal cells is one thing; mucin not adherent and simply present in the intestinal content is quite another. Limitation of the activity of lysozyme seems logical for the protection of the mucosal surface of the tract. Whether or not the same situation may hold for other enzymes in the intestine remains an unknown feature. It is not improbable that the interplay of biologically antagonistic forces underlies the etiology of ulcerative colitis and that re-establishment of the proper balance in such patients can come only through inhibition of a series of enzymes rather than with any one. The proteolytic enzymes, trypsin and erepsin, may play some role in ulcerative disease of the lower tract just as pepsin does in peptic ulceration. Enzyme inhibitors directed against the proteolytic team may prove beneficial in intestinal disease.

The point for greatest emphasis lies in the certainty that the microorganisms of the tract produce a host of highly toxic agents and that these agents, even if absorbed in minute quantities, will in the long run precipitate pathological states. Increased production of such toxic elements may result from a qualitative modification in the flora, from imbalance in normal flora, and from alteration in the medium supplied to the microorganisms by virtue of the dietary habits of the host. Suspicion naturally leads to the proteolytic bacteria and to diet high in protein. Certainly one would expect a diet high in protein combined with a flora high in proteolytic bacteria to produce more toxic chemicals associated with protein breakdown such as histamine, putrescine, cadaverine, tyramine and similar amino acid decarboxylation products.

REFERENCES

ALPERT, S., and G. J. MARTIN. *Rev. Gastroenterol.*, **17**: 251, 1950.

BEST, C. H., and N. B. TAYLOR. *The Physiological Basis of Medical Practice* (3rd ed.). Baltimore: Williams and Wilkins, 1943.

BRANHAM, S. E., and K. HABEL. *J. Immunol.*, **54**: 305, 1946.

FITZPATRICK, V. deP., R. E. HUNTER, and C. E. BRAMBEL. *Am. J. Dig. Dis.*, **18**: 340, 1951.

GRACE, W. J., P. H. SETON, S. WOLF, and H. G. WOLFF. *Am. J. M. Sc.*, **217**: 241, 1949.

GRAY, S. J., R. W. REIFENSTEIN, J. C. G. YOUNG, H. M. SPIRO, and E. P. CONNOLLY. *J. Clin. Investigation*, **29**: 1595, 1950.

GUNNISON, J. B., and M. S. MARSHALL. *J. Bacteriol.*, **33**: 401, 1937.

HOFBAUER, J. *Am. J. Obst. Gynec.*, **12**: 159, 1926.

JOACHIMOGLU, G. *Chem. Ztg.*, **44**: 780, 1920.

JOSLIN, C. L. *Delaware State M. J.*, **22**: 35, 1950.

KAPELLER-ADLER, R., and E. ADLER. *J. Obst. Gynaec. Brit. Emp.*, **50:** 177, 1943.

LEAKE, C. D. *Postgrad. Med.*, **6:** 1, 1949.

LICHTMAN, A. L. *Exper. Med. Surg.*, **9:** 90, 1951.

MARTIN, G. J., and S. ALPERT. *Am. J. Dig. Dis.*, **17:** 151, 1950.

MARTIN, G. J., and J. WILKINSON. *Gastroenterology*, **6:** 315, 1946.

MARTIN, G. J., and J. WILKINSON. *Arch. Biochem.*, **12:** 95, 1947.

MELNICK, D., M. HOCHBERG, and B. L. OSER. *J. Nutrition*, **30:** 233, 1945.

MEYER, K., A. GELLHORN, J. F. PRUDDEN, W. L. LEHMAN, and A. STEINBERG. *Am. J. Med.*, **5:** 496, 1948.

MOSS, J., and G. J. MARTIN. *Am. J. Dig. Dis.*, **15:** 412, 1948.

MOSS, J., and G. J. MARTIN. *Am. J. Dig. Dis.*, **17:** 18, 1950.

MOSS, J., N. MOORE, J. M. BEILER, and G. J. MARTIN. Unpublished data, 1953.

MÜLLER, H. *J. Pharmacol Exper. Therap.*, **53:** 67, 1935.

MUTCH, N. *Brit. M. J.*, **1:** 595, 1937.

QUINTOS, F. N. *J. Philippine M. A.*, **26:** 155, 1950.

RIEGEL, B., D. W. STANGER, D. M. WIKHOLM, J. D. MOLD, and H. SOMMER. *J. Biol. Chem.*, **177:** 7, 1949.

ROLLINS, C. T. Personal communication, 1950.

SWAYNE, V. R., and G. J. MARTIN. *Am. J. Dig. Dis.*, **17:** 39, 1950.

CHAPTER 8

Chemistry and Medical Applications of Nonresinous Ion Exchange and Adsorption Materials

---

CHARCOAL

KAOLIN

MAGNESIUM TRISILICATE

ALUMINUM HYDROXIDE

BISMUTH COMPOUNDS

BARIUM SULFATE

BENTONITE

SODIUM ALUMINUM SILICATE

ALGINIC ACID

CELLULOSE DERIVATIVES

CONCLUSIONS

ION exchange materials possess adsorptive capacities distinct from those associated with exchange. It is equally true that agents generally considered to be adsorptive are also in some measure capable of ion exchange. In view of this, it seems logical to review briefly some of these materials which have found or probably will find application in the world of medicine. A large number of such agents are known, but unfortunately comparatively few have been investigated with any degree of thoroughness. As the rational approach to gastrointestinal adsorption and exchange therapy lies in complete knowledge of the behavior of all such materials, with subsequent use of those with the greatest selectivity, it is to be hoped that research will be directed toward this goal.

228

CHARCOAL

The therapeutic use of charcoal goes back to ancient times; it was used in the treatment of anthrax, epilepsy, vertigo, and many other conditions. One of the first applications was in the adsorption of poisons.

Voronina (1945) studied the relative adsorption capacities of granular carbons compared to finely powdered charcoals. The adsorption capacity was much lower in the granular forms. In a study designed to determine the most applicable type of charcoal, Laqueur and Sluyters (1925) had compared the adsorptive capacity of various types for oxalic acid, potassium oxalate, mercuric chloride, strychnine nitrate, morphine sulfate, methylene blue and iodine. Supra Norite was reported as being markedly superior. Sjogren and Wallden (1935) warn against any attempt to assume that the *in vitro* testing of adsorptive agents reflects their *in vivo* capacity to reduce the lethal dose of any given toxic agent. They had attempted to correlate the capacity of some twenty different medicinal charcoals for adsorption of methylene blue with their capacity to protect the animal against mercuric chloride poisoning.

The probability that charcoal will actually remove a toxic chemical from the gut wall was established by Dingemanse and Laqueur (1926), who found that 47 per cent of the mercuric chloride was adsorbed from the gut wall by charcoal.

Yoshida (1939), in a thorough study of lead poisoning and charcoal, found that he was able to double and even triple the excretion of lead following the intravenous injection of lead acetate into rabbits if he fed an activated charcoal. The adsorption of lead ions by the charcoal prevented their reabsorption in the digestive tract. The point of lack of correlation of *in vitro* adsorptive power with protective action *in vivo* had been emphasized by Joachimoglu (1920), who determined the adsorptive power of charcoals for iodine and then checked their capacity to prevent strychnine poisoning. There was no correlation whatever. Leibenson (1928) makes the point clear that charcoal can even be used to decrease the toxicity of agents given subcutaneously. Thus, morphine is excreted through the gastrointestinal tract and can be effectively removed, preventing readsorption.

Andersen (1944) has recently determined the capacity of charcoal to adsorb a series of drugs including strychnine, morphine, atropine sulfate, nicotine, mercuric chloride, diethylbarbituric acid and sulfanilamide. The studies were carried out *in vitro* and *in vivo*. In 1946, he added studies of Medinal, Alurate, Dial, Evipal, Phanodorn, salicyclic acid, phenol, alcohol and potassium cyanide. The importance of pH and concentration for maximum adsorption by a charcoal is emphasized by Andersen (1947). He concludes that the maximum adsorption of nicotine, which is a weak base, occurs from dilute solutions at an alkaline pH. Weak acids (such as phenols and barbiturates) are best adsorbed at an acid pH and ampholytes such as sulfanilamide at the isoelectric point. As one would expect, the adsorption of ethyl alcohol is unaffected by pH.

The chemical toxin, solanine, found in fresh potato sprouts, is effectively removed by charcoal (Smerha, 1948). Diets containing sprouting potato tubers caused a decrease in the weight of rats by 19 per cent. With 4 per cent animal charcoal added to the diet, detoxication was almost complete. Solanine is typical of those chemicals associated with "food poisoning"; another such agent is that elaborated by the dinoflagellate *Gon. catenella* Whedon and Kofoid. By contrast with solanine, the toxic chemical of paralytic shellfish poison is not adsorbed on charcoal (Riegel *et al.,* 1949; Swayne and Martin, 1950).

Of extreme importance in the consideration of adsorption agents for their medicinal value is their capacity for the adsorption of toxic chemicals produced endogenously. In this connection, charcoals were found effective in the removal of skatole, indole, tyramine, mercuric chloride and histamine but ineffective against putrescine (Martin and Alpert, 1950).

Whether or not adsorbing agents actually adsorb bacteria remains an open question. Gunnison and Marshall (1937) found that the apparent adsorption of *Esch. coli, Cl. welchii* and *L. acidophilus* by particulate kaolin, Lloyd's reagent, calcium carbonate, aluminum hydroxide and barium sulfate was not marked *in vitro*. Charcoal did effectively remove *L. acidophilus* but did not significantly remove *Esch. coli* and *Cl. welchii*. It was effective against staphylococci. The general impression received from the work of these authors is that alterations in intestinal flora produced by administration of inert particulate agents are not due to adsorption of bacterial cells. It is clear that adsorbing agents possess two distinct mechanisms of action on bacteria—a physical adsorption of cells and removal of nutrient materials from the medium, thereby preventing or inhibiting growth.

Charcoal definitely adsorbs toxins and antitoxins, including those of diphtheria and tetanus. It is also able to adsorb viruses such as those of sheep pox and hoof and mouth disease. Kraus and Barbará (1915*a*) established the ability of charcoal to adsorb diphtheria, tetanus and dysentery toxins. Further studies (Kraus and Barbará, 1915*b*) demonstrated that rabbits which had received intravenous injections of dysentery toxin were saved by the administration of animal charcoal per os. Following this approach, Lemétayer and Uhry (1937) attempted to reduce the toxicity of tetanus toxin by the intravenous injection of charcoal and found it ineffective.

In addition to toxins, antitoxins and a miscellaneous group of chemicals, charcoals have been reported to adsorb hormones, vitamins, enzymes and drugs. Extensive work has been done on the adsorption of enzymes, and there is no need to review it beyond considering the action of these agents on the enzymes of the gastrointestinal tract. Strauss (1916) reported the adsorption of both hydrochloric acid and pepsin from gastric juice. Most recently, Alpert and Martin (1949) noted the power of activated charcoal for the inhibition of pepsin *in vitro*. Fifteen milligrams of charcoal per 5 ml. completely inhibited the activity of 1.5 mg. of 1:3,000 N.F. pepsin per each 5 ml. In a similar study, Moss and Martin (1948) found that lysozyme was specifically inhibited by an activated carbon; certain hydrated aluminum silicates, however, were more active.

The effectiveness of charcoals in adsorbing hormones is well illustrated by the work of Sklow (1943), who tested animal and plant charcoals, kaolin, kieselguhr, fuller's earth, calcium carbonate, benzoic acid and Lloyd's reagent and found that of these only the charcoals prolonged the action of estrogenic hormones following the implantation of adsorbates. Somewhat similar efforts have been made to use charcoal adsorbates for the administration of various pharmacological agents. Goiffon (1930) adsorbed eserine on charcoal and used it effectively in the treatment of atonia of the intestine. Through this technic he avoided secondary reactions. Similarly, this investigator used an adsorbate of hydroxyaminophenylarsonic acid against amebic, parasitic and certain bacterial infections of the gut. Atropine is adsorbed by charcoal and is subsequently released in the gastrointestinal tract, providing thereby a depotlike action and reducing the incidence of side effects (Lefevre, 1930). In general, this is a sound approach and has been neglected in the field of medicine. Atropine is generally conceded to be an exceptionally good antispasmodic, limited in application by the unfortunate incidence of side effects, e.g., drying of the mouth and blurring of vision. Although millions have been spent in research aimed at antispasmodics retaining the efficiency of atropine but without the side effects, it is questionable whether this goal has yet been achieved. Strangely, charcoal or other adsorbates of antispasmodic molecules such as atropine may resolve the issue. With such adsorbates there are no peaks and troughs in the curve of absorption of the drug from the gut; the result is a prolonged and more constant level of drug action. It is to be assumed that the peaks in the absorption curve of a drug like atropine give the points of incidence of side effects and that the troughs in this same curve are the points of lowered efficacy. Preventing this waving curve, leveling it out, will automatically bring efficiency and absence of side effects. Further, sterilization of the intestinal tract remains a problem. One approach to the resolution of this problem is via the pathway of adsorbates of antibiotics or other similar antibacterial agents. Such adsorbates would release their cargo of chemotherapeutic drug slowly and steadily, providing constant and continued antiseptic action.

The constipating effect of charcoal has been demonstrated by Bauer (1928). Using rats, he observed a doubling of the period for material to pass through the intestinal canal. Charcoal, in his experiments, possessed the power to inhibit increased peristalsis induced by castor oil. Further evidence of the capacity of activated charcoals to modify gastrointestinal physiology and biochemistry has been presented by Kuribayashi (1934), who observed that this agent delayed the increase in residual nitrogen of the blood following a meal in a manner paralleling the effects of astringents.

It is well known that charcoals are effective adsorbents for vitamins, e.g., pantothenic acid (Williams *et al.*, 1938), and therefore it is not surprising that reports have been made on the development of deficiency states induced by the feeding of these agents.

For example, Almquist and Zander (1940) observed that a chick diet adequate for normal growth and health was rendered deficient in vitamins A and K, pantothenic acid and the gizzard factor by the addition of charcoal. Again, Cailleau and Adrian (1948) noted the unfavorable growth effect of charcoal fed at 4 per cent of the diet. The decrease observed was almost 50 per cent and was attributed to the adsorbing power of the charcoal for thiamin and riboflavin. Similarly, Cailleau and Chevillard (1949) demonstrated interference by these adsorbing agents in thiamin and riboflavin absorption through urinary excretion studies of these vitamins. Nicotinic acid as well was reduced in urinary concentration as a result of the charcoal, but, strangely, pantothenic acid was not significantly affected. This effect of charcoal may be on fat-soluble as well as water-soluble factors, as evidenced by the work of Matet and Matet (1945), who reported the precipitation of an avitaminosis A through the inclusion of 2 per cent charcoal in the diet of rats. These findings are another signpost indicating the necessity for investigation of the effects of all adsorbing and exchange agents on nutritional status prior to the general introduction of such materials into the medical world.

Koenig (1928) listed the applications of charcoal in medicine as follows:

1. Acute poisoning with metal salts, such as mercuric chloride, arsenic, phosphorus, lead compounds; poisoning with organic compounds like strychnine, morphine, cocaine, nicotine and in general food poisoning.
2. Infectious diseases; cholera, dysentery, intestinal catarrh.
3. Autointoxication.
4. Hyperacidity of the stomach.
5. Peptic ulcer.
6. Intestinal complaints owing to excessive formation of gas and occurrence of large quantities of bacteria.

Of this list, items 1, 2 and 3 remain a part of modern therapeutics, but the other indications have fallen into disrepute. Whether or not this is deserved remains an open question.

While charcoal is recommended today in therapeutics in severe diarrheal conditions, such as cholera, dysentery or ulcerative colitis (dose, 1 to 5 Gm. three or four times daily), Bastedo (1947) states that in his experience charcoal has little or no value in these conditions; however, its use in the treatment of the milder forms of diarrhea is well established. Again, the use of this adsorbent in the treatment of poisoning due to strychnine and similar agents is accepted, but efficacy in food poisoning of bacterial origin is not regarded as established (Werch, 1948). In flatulence, there seems little doubt that charcoal is an ineffective agent (Calvert, 1922), as once moistened it will not adsorb gases of any kind.

Some rather bizarre applications of charcoal have been made, including those of its use intravenously for the treatment of various infections such as erysipelas (Gonzalez and Schteingart, 1936) and its use as a substitute for Antabuse in the treatment of chronic alcoholism (Moench, 1950). Topically, charcoals have been used on surface wounds, particularly those with bad odors (Peyer, 1940), and for decreasing malodor from colostomies and ileostomies (Anonymous, 1947).

Considering the historical role of charcoal in therapeutics, it is surprising that there is so little sound data on its use in medicine. Activated charcoals adsorb toxins, hormones, enzymes, drugs, vitamins and a host of other chemicals. They are valuable in preventing absorption of many toxic chemicals and in the treatment of diarrhea. Other potential applications are not established, and such questions as the possible interference of charcoal with nutrition are open and unresolved. It seems that much of the work reported must be repeated and that the dozens of potential clinical uses for these agents should be rechecked. Unfortunately, the sphere of activity is old and few investigators consider it a promising one. Progress will therefore be slow until some group or groups become interested.

KAOLIN

Kaolin is a native hydrated aluminum silicate, called variously China clay, porcelain clay, bolus alba, terra alba, white bole or argilla. It is a grayish-yellow, fine, inert powder commonly used in ceramics, as a filler for paper and textiles, and for pencils. Samples of kaolin have been found to differ markedly (Mukherjee and Gupta, 1946) in their content of silicon dioxide, ferric oxide, calcium oxide, magnesium oxide and aluminum. Mukherjee and Das Gupta (1946) and Rae (1928) emphasize these differences and state that capacity for adsorption is not ensured by knowledge of the chemical composition, particle size, exchangeable base content, etc. In the author's laboratory, eight different samples of kaolin obtained from the United States and elsewhere were checked for their ability to adsorb histamine. In these experiments, a solution of histamine hydrochloric acid was prepared containing 250 mg. per 100 cc. Twenty-five cubic centimeter portions of this solution were shaken with 1 Gm. of different samples of kaolin after adjusting the pH to 8.0 to 8.5. The mixtures were then centrifuged and the supernatant liquid assayed for histamine concentration. The results were as indicated in Table 44. From these figures, it is apparent that there was no significant difference among the various samples of kaolin with respect to their capacity to adsorb histamine. It is doubtful that marked differences do exist among such materials with respect to their adsorptive capacity. The data cited certainly do not prove the point, but the evidence to the contrary is not on a firm basis.

Kaolin is one of the oldest remedies used in medicine. The Greeks and Persians used it, and for centuries the Chinese physicians have regarded it as a specific in the treatment of diarrheas. Modern science has sought a rationale for the use of this adsorptive agent in its effects on enzymes, toxic chemicals and nutritional status.

Direct studies of the toxicity of kaolin early demonstrated its essentially inert character. Thus Goldfeder (1929) observed that kaolin given in levels of 80 per cent of the diet for a short period had no effect

TABLE 44

Adsorption of Histamine by Various Samples of Kaolin

Sample	Supplier	Histamine adsorbed (%)
Kaolin-English (Electros Brand)	C. B. Crystal Co.	22
Kaolin Colloidal N.F.	Whitaker, Clark and Daniels	18
Kaolin N.F.	C. B. Crystal Co.	28
Kaolin No. 347 (same as colloidal kaolin, English Kaolin)	Whitaker, Clark and Daniels	34
Kaolin No. 372 (English Kaolin)	Whitaker, Clark and Daniels	30
Kaolin No. 34 (English Kaolin)	Whitaker, Clark and Daniels	42
Kaolin from marked intestinal adsorbent		33

on the mouse. Such studies do not answer the question of the possible interference of kaolin with nutrition, but this had been studied by Messerli (1922), who demonstrated that rats and pigeons fed a diet of decorticated rice developed an avitaminosis more rapidly and severely if either charcoal or kaolin was added to the diet. Melnick *et al.* (1945), in studies with human subjects, demonstrated that while fuller's earth did reduce markedly the availability of thiamin, kaolin did not interfere with the utilization of this factor. These investigators emphasized that the continuous use of large doses of adsorbing agents is accompanied by the danger of production of some nutritional abnormality. With kaolin as with all aluminum preparations, there is a danger of interference with other factors, specifically the phosphates. In this relation, Deobald and Elvehjem (1935) found that rickets developed in a greater degree in chicks given oral doses of kaolin and related compounds. They noted a definite drop in the blood phosphorus as early as the fifth day.

Another possible complication of the use of kaolin is indicated in the work of Long *et al.* (1935), who noted polyposis in the rat intestine produced by the incorporation of kaolin into the diet. They felt, however, that polyposis would be unlikely to occur in man when kaolin was used in the amounts ordinarily prescribed. It is interesting to note that there has been a report of an instance in which kaolin granuloma of the stomach was demonstrated (Cohn *et al.*, 1941). The patient had been ingesting kaolin for a long period of time, and microscopic studies proved the lesion to be a granuloma with the type of foreign body giant cells present in lesions of silicosis. Mineralogical studies established the presence of silica in the gastric tissues. Subsequently, these investigators were able to produce lesions in rabbits similar to that they had found in the human case. The potentiality that granulomas develop following the long-continued use of kaolin is remote but must be considered as possible.

Attempts have been made to place the use of kaolin in food poisoning on a fundamental basis. Muller (1935), working with mussel poison, reported that German kaolin would not remove more than 50 per cent of the toxic substances from an aqueous solution. Emphasizing differences in kaolins, Mutch (1937a) reported that an English sample of kaolin adsorbed mussel poison, mushroom poison (muscarine), and the potato poison known as solanine. Using a kaolin designated as No. 4, he found that per gram it adsorbed 94 M.L.D. of mussel toxin, 3.8 mg. of muscarine, 5 mg. of solanine, and 5 mg. of histamine phosphate. These data permit comparison with other adsorption agents under somewhat similar experimental conditions. For example, 1 Gm. of an activated synthetic zeolite adsorbed approximately 30 mg. of histamine (Martin and Wilkinson, 1947). In an attempt to determine the most efficient agent for the adsorption of paralytic shellfish poison (mussel poison), Swayne and Martin (1950) were led to the conclusion that of the three most commonly used intestinal adsorbents—kaolin, aluminum hydroxide and charcoal—not one possessed any degree of efficacy for the removal of this highly toxic agent. The inefficiency of kaolin against mussel poison is a reflection of its lack of capacity to adsorb such endogenously produced toxic chemicals as skatole, indole, tyramine, putrescine and histamine (Martin and Alpert, 1950).

With reference to enzymes, kaolin has been reported to inhibit the activity of digestive enzymes (Strauss, 1916; Petersen, W. F., 1917; Petersen, S. R., 1932). In the studies conducted by Martin and Alpert (1949), kaolin did not inactivate pepsin in a ratio of 0.2 to 0.3 Gm. of pepsin 1:3,000 N.F. This study was carried out at the pH of gastric juice. With reference to trypsin, however, the result was quite different. One-tenth gram of kaolin removed 73 per cent from a solution of 8 mg. of the enzyme dissolved in 100 cc. Repetition of the pepsin studies with larger amounts of kaolin also revealed that kaolin was a moderately effective inhibitor of this enzyme. Kaolin did not inhibit the action of lysozyme in any concentration up to the maximum tested, which was 10 mg. per milliliter in the presence of 10 to 200 units of lysozyme (Moss and Martin, 1948). It is probable that kaolin at the optimum pH would remove and inactivate most enzymes, but under physiological conditions and as commonly employed in medicine the chances are good that no enzyme other than trypsin would be inhibited to any significant degree.

In 1915, Hektoen and Rappaport used kaolin in cases of diphtheria and found it useful. They proposed that its action was physical and that through this effect it removed pathogenic bacteria from the pharynx. In 1921, Walker offered a rationale for the use of kaolin, concluding that its action was both mechanical and adsorptive. It formed an adherent coating on the wall of the gut and enclosed and carried with it a large number of bacteria. Further support of this concept came with the work of Eisler (1924), who reported that kaolin combined with cholera vibrions but not with typhus bacilli.

A much more detailed report by Braafladt (1923) demonstrated the neutralizing effect that kaolin had on toxins and toxic products of pathogenic intestinal microorganisms. His technic involved treating cultures, centrifuging and then injecting the supernatant fluid into animals. Adsorption was offered as explanation of the successful use of kaolin in Asiatic cholera, bacillary dysentery, acute enteritis, typhoid, meat poisoning and botulism. Kaolin combined with the toxins and toxic products of *V. cholerae, B. dysenteriae* (Shiga), *B. enteritidis, B. diphtheriae, B. botulinus, B. typhosus* and *B. paratyphosus B,* and seemed to combine with toxic products of putrefactive and proteolytic bacteria. Kaolin changed the bacterial flora of the gut from a predominantly proteolytic type to an aciduric one.

The problem of adsorption of bacteria by kaolin was studied in some detail by Gunnison and Marshall (1937). The adsorptive agent had little capacity to remove bacteria such as *Esch. coli, Cl. welchii* and *L. acidophilus.* It did remove *Staph. aureus, S. lutea* and *B. subtilis.* These investigators concluded that alteration in intestinal flora could not be due to the physical adsorption and subsequent removal of bacteria by the kaolin.

Moss and Martin (1950) studied the adsorption of bacterial toxins from lysates of bacteria and found that kaolin was ineffective in removing the toxic substances produced by *E. typhosa* and only weakly active against those of *S. dysenteriae* or *Esch. coli.* Similarly, Eyre and Durch (1925) found kaolin to possess only slight ability to adsorb diphtheria toxin.

There have been many medical applications of kaolin, and in general no specific effects have been claimed; rather, the material is used, and properly so, as adjuvant to more specific therapy. One of the first papers to appear recommending the use of kaolin was that of Meunier (1913). He used the material in the form of a thick paste for hyperacidity and stomachic hypersecretion, an application which has largely fallen into disuse. Shortly thereafter Stumpf (1914) and Stoerck (1915) indicated the successful use of kaolin in chronic dysentery. Also in 1915, Aaron recommended kaolin in any condition manifesting an inflamed or ulcerated intestinal mucosa. Specifically, he found it highly effective in enteritis when used in doses of 60 to 100 Gm.

As with dysentery, cholera offered a potential application for adsorption therapy, and in the work of Kuhne (1918) this potentiality was made practice. He reduced the mortality rate in this disease from 50 per cent to around 3 per cent. Later, Walker (1921) included ulcerative colitis, cholera, diphtheria, ptomaine poisoning and bacillary dysentery among the list of indications for kaolin therapy. Extension of the use of kaolin to rheumatism, neuritis and asthma was proposed by Jordan (1923), who also recommended its use in bronchitis, pharyngitis and infantile diarrhea. Furthermore, in his hands, measles, whooping cough and other children's diseases responded well to this therapeutic measure. Finally, he observed benefit and even complete alleviation of morning sickness of pregnancy by kaolin.

Many of the above-mentioned indications for kaolin therapy rest on sketchy clinical material, but there can be no question of the value of kaolin in food poisoning. The first record of successful application of kaolin in the treatment of toxemia resulting from unsuitable food is that of Jordan (1925). Fundamentally, his work lacked scope, and it remained for others to really establish this use of kaolin. McRobert (1934) referred to an outbreak of bacterial food poisoning in Burma in 1932. The outbreak occurred within 3 hours of the evening meal and involved a number of elderly men and women. Before McRobert reached the spot kaolin therapy had been instituted and he reported that nothing more was required. The work of Schwartz (1946) places this usage on a firm basis. He observed 110 patients suffering from acute gastroenteritis following a staphylococcal food poisoning in which kaolin and mild sedation were the only measures used, with marked success.

A most interesting use of kaolin is its topical application in the therapy of excoriations around external gastrointestinal fistulas (CoTui, 1933). CoTui treated 162 such patients with kaolin powder, with results that were uniformly good. He considered the treatment a specific in that it removed the enzyme trypsin. The therapeutic regimen consisted of the application of the powder over the osteum of the fistula and all around it. The material was changed every 2 or 3 hours in patients with duodenal fistulas and every 4 to 8 hours in those with ileostomies.

One of the basic premises advanced in this volume rests on the fact that no single adsorption agent can be as effective for general application as combinations. While this concept did not underlie the thinking of those investigators using kaolin combinations, it is interesting to consider the large number of such combinations employed. For example, Jordan (1923) used kaolin with paraffin or mineral oil for intestinal stasis not only for its adsorptive properties but also for its bulking action. Similarly, Bargen (1931) found a mixture of kaolin, bismuth and tribasic calcium phosphate of value in the treatment of uncomplicated chronic ulcerative colitis. Further examples of this combined therapy include kaolin with bismuth subnitrate in the treatment of general gastrointestinal disturbances (Hayem, 1931), kaolin with calcium gluconate in the treatment of bacillary dysentery (Greene and Block, 1938), kaolin with calcium lactate or gluconate in diarrheas (Tumen, 1942), and a kaolin, thiamin and lactose combination for the treatment of avitaminosis and secondary anemia associated with diseased conditions of the gastrointestinal system (Stein and Kotin, 1937). Of all such combinations the one most widely studied is that of kaolin and aluminum hydroxide.

The first report on this mixture was presented in 1934 by Swalm, who treated a series of some 65 cases of various gastrointestinal disorders and observed that 86 per cent were definitely improved. He stressed its local action in the lumen of the stomach and intestine by virtue of its mildly astringent and adsorptive properties. The combination was recommended in hypermotile states in doses of 1 tablespoonful containing 20 per cent kaolin and 2.5 per cent aluminum hydroxide. This was to be repeated three times a day.

In 1937, several reports appeared advocating combinations of kaolin and aluminum hydroxide. Smith, W. (1937), found the dual product more effective in adsorbing bacteria from fecal samples. His results indicated that if enough of the kaolin-alumina mixture was present, almost complete adsorption of the bacteria of fecal samples occurred, with 100 per cent removal of *Esch. coli*. The mixture as used contained 20 per cent kaolin and 2.5 per cent aluminum hydroxide gel. On the clinical side, Eyerly and Breuhaus (1937) obtained beneficial results in ulcerative colitis using retention enemas of kaolin and aluminum hydroxide. These investigators state that they believe the use of the combination to be rational because the adsorption of bacteria and their metabolic products reduces irritation and decreases the absorption of toxins. The astringent action was also claimed to be beneficial. The potential danger of fecal impaction resulting from the use of kaolin alone was emphasized, and it was claimed that this would not occur with the use of the mixture. The point made by these workers relative to the dangers of kaolin alone had been emphasized by Bungart (1917), who noted accumulations of the adsorbent in the intestines; however, he felt that serious complications such as impaction were most unlikely. Also in 1937, Fradkin published his results in using the mixture with patients having ulcerative colitis. The results were satisfactory except that the frequency of administration of large doses interfered with patients' digestion and had to be discontinued. Fradkin then resorted to the use per rectum of a mixture of 20 per cent kaolin, 10 per cent mineral oil, and 70 per cent aluminum hydroxide gel. The results of the treatment were reported to be strikingly beneficial. The therapy was recommended only in the convalescent patient whose stools continued to be streaked with blood.

It is not intended to cover the literature on kaolin but rather to indicate the manner in which this agent and mixtures containing it fit into the general pattern of therapeutic application of ion exchange and adsorption agents. For this reason only a few additional aspects will be considered. In support of the use of kaolin-alumina mixtures are the findings of Spiesman (1943), who obtained good results in the treatment of chronic cases such as those of functional diarrhea, spastic colon and chronic ulcerative colitis. He recommended the use of the combination in the management of tropical dysenteries, diarrheas and functional colonic conditions. One complication of the use of preparations containing aluminum hydroxide is the development of constipation. Neuwelt and Steigmann (1942) maintain that this does not happen with combinations of these agents, due to the maintenance of a fine state of dispersion. It seems probable that any aluminum-containing preparations will in some measure be constipating. The formation of aluminum ions will occur and these ions possess an astringent effect; this may in many instances, however, be beneficial rather than harmful. In general, combinations of the aluminum hydroxide and kaolin type are used in states associated with excessive intestinal motility, and in these conditions astringence with reduction of motility is indicated. In peptic ulcer the problem is different and it is difficult to justify the use of the mixture.

Another interesting application of such combinations was made by Shelanski *et al.* (1942) in the treatment of conditions characterized by intestinal parasitism. Using three 1-oz. doses of a combined kaolin–aluminum hydroxide preparation, he reported the elimination of infections of *Trichuris trichiura, Oxyuris vermicularis, Ascaris lumbricoides, Strongyloides stercoralis, Hymenolepsis nana, Endamoeba coli, Endolimax nana, Iodamoeba bütschlii, Dientamoeba fragilis, Retortomonas hominis, Chilomastix mesnili, Giardia lamblia* and *Trichomonas intestinalis*. The treatment was continued for a period of 3 or 4 weeks, with elimination of all parasites except *T. trichiura*.

In summary, from the laboratory standpoint kaolin is far from the ideal agent. In fact, in comparison with a number of other agents, it is not effective in its capacity to adsorb toxic chemicals, enzymes or bacteria. Clinically, it is effective in the treatment of those diarrheal states caused by an agent capable of being adsorbed, including those due to food poisoning and bacterial or parasitic infestations of the intestinal tract. The doses are very high; approximately 50 to 100 Gm. must be given every 3 or 4 hours until the desired effect is obtained. The literature would seem to substantiate the logic of the use of kaolin as an adjuvant in the treatment of chronic ulcerative colitis. Certainly it is not a specific in any instance and must always be considered as an adjuvant. Combinations of kaolin with other agents, particularly aluminum hydroxide, would seem to offer advantages in the sense of reduction of potential impaction. Adequate studies have not been made establishing clearly the merit of such combinations, but it is to be assumed that multiple adsorption therapy is in every instance superior to the use of a single agent. If kaolin is to be used alone it should be with the thought that impaction can occur, although the potentiality is quite remote. In general, as an absorbent, kaolin offers little, if anything, not possessed in greater measure by other agents capable of being employed in medical practice.

MAGNESIUM TRISILICATE

Magnesium trisilicate, a tasteless white powder insoluble in water, was first introduced into medical practice by Mutch (1936a), who stated that its adsorptive affinities covered acid and basic dyes, alkaloids, bacterial toxins, putrefactive amines and food poisons. The silicate selectively removed tetanus toxin and paralytic shellfish poison but failed to adsorb the toxin of *Amanita phalloides*. In the second paper of his initial series Mutch (1936b) reported that magnesium trisilicate was nontoxic and did not disturb the normal action of the bowel. He indicated that it possessed a prolonged action in acid neutralization and that pepsin was adsorbed. As it neutralized, the chemical was decomposed, freeing hydrated silica, which in turn possessed marked adsorptive powers. In the recommended doses, magnesium trisilicate produced no side effects; appetite, digestion and bowel action were all normal. Reported in this same paper were his studies of toxicity in rats, mice and men; all indications were for complete nontoxicity at almost any levels compatible with experimental technic. The third paper published by Mutch (1936c) on magnesium trisilicate pointed out the fact that pepsin adsorbed on the agent did not entirely lose its proteolytic properties, and this quality was regarded by him as advantageous in that digestion was not halted by the chemical. Similarly, he felt that the inability of magnesium trisilicate to reduce gastric pH to the alkaline side was a merit of considerable import, as no alkalosis could ensue from its use. The specific regimen recommended by Mutch (1937b) involved the ingestion of approximately 0.5 Gm. of magnesium trisilicate five or six times at spaced intervals during the day. In 1949, Mutch elaborated upon the action of magnesium trisilicate relative to pepsin, pointing out that the pepsin–magnesium trisilicate complex was insoluble and devoid of proteolytic properties but that the silica gel liberated by the acid from the silicate formed a complex which still carried out digestive functions on protein substrates. In general, therefore, it would be expected that this adsorptive agent would reduce but not eliminate peptic activity.

In our laboratories, we have found magnesium trisilicate to be among the more effective inhibitors of pepsin (Alpert and Martin, 1949), and of trypsin (Alpert and Martin, 1950). It was not effective in the adsorption of toxic substances from the lysates of *S. dysenteriae*, *E. typhosa* or *Esch. coli* (Moss and Martin, 1950), nor was it active against paralytic shellfish poison (Swayne and Martin, 1950). Another criterion of the efficacy of intestinal adsorbents employed in this laboratory has been that of removal of endogenously produced toxic chemicals. In this system of study, magnesium trisilicate adsorbed tyramine and putrescine with some degree of specificity but failed against skatole, indole, and histamine (Martin and Alpert, 1950).

Many papers have appeared on the antacid qualities of magnesium trisilicate and on its use in the treatment of peptic ulcer (Hurst, 1936; Hardy, 1937; Hunt, 1937; Levin, 1937; Mann, 1937; Kraemer, 1938, 1941; Tidmarsh and Baxter, 1938; Goldstein, 1939; Kurtz, 1939; Page and Thomas, 1939; Reid, 1939; Kirsner and Palmer, 1940; Kraemer and Aaron, 1940; Breuhaus and Eyerly, 1941; Silverman and Katz, 1941; Rossett and Flexner, 1943). In general, they have supported the contention of Mutch to the effect that it is an effective agent, the neutralizing power being less prompt but the duration of action somewhat longer than with other antacids available for study at that time. For example, Wyllie (1940), in a series of seventy-eight tests involving half-hourly analysis of gastric contents throughout 12 hours on each of 24 patients, found that magnesium trisilicate and aluminum hydroxide were superior, in duration of antacid effects and absence of undesirable side effects, to milk, modified Sippy powders, and tribasic magnesium phosphate. He was able to control free gastric acid satisfactorily by giving milk feedings of 6 oz. every 2 hours, and 1 dr. (6.8 Gm.) of magnesium trisilicate half an hour after the feeding. Similarly, Page and Thomas (1939) strongly recommended magnesium trisilicate for its antacid, antienzyme and adsorbent qualities. They employed doses of 1 Gm. every 1 or 2 hours for the control of nonspecific food poisoning, in fact for all nonspecific diarrheas. In the opinion of these workers, the sustained antacid power of the trisilicate was a cardinal attribute. The degree of absorption of silica which follows use of magnesium trisilicate has been indicated by the excretion of an average of 17.6 mg. of silicon dioxide daily prior to treatment

(Page *et al.,* 1941) and an elevation of silica excretion to 444 mg. daily following ingestion of 20 Gm. of the silicate. Page and his co-workers (1941) assumed that silica absorption from the gastrointestinal tract would be a function of the alkalinity of intestinal content and that such absorption would exert no deleterious effect.

Critical views of the merit of magnesium trisilicate have come from various laboratories. Among the first such reports was that of Schiffrin and Komarov (1941), in which they stated that magnesium trisilcate failed to inactivate pepsin at pH values of 1.0 to 2.0, indicating that the trisilicate functioned to modify peptic activity only through shift in pH. In other words, the trisilicate did not in itself inactivate pepsin but rather, by causing a shift in pH beyond the range of optimal activity of the enzyme, brought about decreased activity. In 1947, this same group of investigators (Shay *et al.*) reported a series of studies designed to determine the greatest protection afforded by single agents against gastric ulceration produced experimentally in rats. In the group treated with magnesium trisilicate, 62 per cent showed ulcers; with the use of sodium aluminum silicate the corresponding figure was 35 per cent, but neither of these agents was any match for aluminum hydroxide or sodium lauryl sulfate. Experimentally, therefore, the stature of magnesium trisilicate was materially reduced.

There have also been several clinical reports critical of the trisilicate. West and Pennoyer (1945) found markedly depressed serum calcium levels and elevated serum magnesium levels following the administration of 6 Gm. daily of the trisilicate. The magnesium blood levels were so high as to cause drowsiness. On an average they found that 6.5 per cent of the magnesium content of the trisilicate ingested was absorbed and excreted in the urine. Another complication reported was that of interference with protein digestion and amino acid assimilation. Another negative report was made in 1947 by Batterman and Ehrenfeld, who stated that magnesium trisilicate in peptic ulcer therapy was relatively ineffective for symptomatic relief and provided little improvement. Twenty-one per cent of the patients became worse, 14 per cent showed no change and 64 per cent showed some degree of improvement. When the dose was raised (1 to 5 Gm. every 4 hours) to give adequate therapeutic effect, gastrointestinal irritation occurred, and as a result any observable beneficial effects were overshadowed by borborygmi, abdominal colic and laxation. They concluded that the use of magnesium trisilicate was not justified in the treatment of peptic ulcer.

The irritative capacities of the magnesium ion have been recorded by many investigators (Mutch, 1937*a*; Tidmarsh and Baxter, 1938; Page and Thomas, 1939; Silverman and Katz, 1941), resulting in the general conclusion that the dose required for therapeutic response causes marked laxation. This has led investigators to attempt to combine the laxation-inducing magnesium trisilicate with the constipating aluminum hydroxide in the hope that the two unpleasant side effects would cancel out. In some measure this concept has found justification in actual practice. Combinations of aluminum hydroxide and magnesium trisilicate have been reported to be effective in the treatment of gastric hyperacidity, peptic ulcer, gastroenteritis, food poisoning and in the vomiting of pregnancy (Cushing, 1942; Hammarlund and Rising, 1949). Extension of this general line of reasoning has led to the use of combinations of magnesium trisilicate and aluminum hydroxide with kaolin (Goldstein, 1938) and with gastric mucin (Hardt and Brodt, 1947; Hardt and Steigmann, 1950). At present, the reported observations are not sufficiently extensive to permit conclusions concerning the merits of further additions such as mucin or kaolin to the basic combination of magnesium trisilicate and aluminum hydroxide.

The logic associated with use of agents in combination as adsorbents is clearly established; however, certain questions remain to be answered relative to the aluminum hydroxide–magnesium trisilicate family. The combined agents would not reduce the absorption of magnesium systemically and therefore would not eliminate the sedative effects of the absorbed magnesium ions. Another question remaining unanswered concerns the nature of the counteracting effects of the two agents. It is not improbable that elimination of the constipating effect of the aluminum ion is directly associated with elimination of many of its therapeutic effects.

Summarizing the literature leads to the conclusion that magnesium trisilicate used alone is inadequate. Its use with aluminum hydroxide is an unquestioned advance, but such combinations remain to be established. To date no basic comparison has been made with other currently available exchange and adsorption combinations.

ALUMINUM HYDROXIDE

Aluminum hydroxide has become the most generally used of all intestinal adsorbents. It is not the author's intention to review the literature on aluminum hydroxide in its entirety but rather to present an attempted analysis of those points permitting the medical research worker to study the situation to his own satisfaction. In 1929, Crohn made the first report on the value of aluminum hydroxide in the treatment of peptic ulcer. The literature today is replete with papers (Rutherford and Emery, 1939; Jones, 1940; McIntosh and Sutherland, 1940; Spangenberg *et al.,* 1941; Winkelstein *et al.,* 1942; Rossett and Flexner, 1943; Miller, T. G., 1944; Collins, 1945) on this subject. It was the first nonsystemic antacid (Einsel and Rowland, 1932) and there are few today who debate the dangers of alkalinizing the body with soluble antacids (Schiffrin and Warren, 1942; Rossett and Flexner, 1943). A second point favoring aluminum hydroxide is its reported capacity to inactivate pepsin. The importance of pepsin in the production of peptic ulcers has been repeatedly demonstrated. The entire emphasis of the concept of etiological factors in gastric and duodenal ulcers has shifted from hydrochloric acid to a recognition of the dominant role of pepsin.

Schiffrin and Warren (1942), using cats, perfused isolated loops of the small intestine with hydrochloric acid plus pepsin and produced typical ulcers. Hydrochloric acid alone was not as productive of ulcers. In the absence of biliary and pancreatic secretions the duodenum was more susceptible to the action of acid alone than was either the jejunum or ileum. Similar results have been reported by Driver *et al.* (1945) and by Matzner *et al.* (1936). More recently, LeVeen (1947) observed the induction of ulcers in the small bowel of dogs by irrigation with acid pepsin solutions. He offered evidence showing that this effect of acid is dependent upon its enhancement of pepsin activity rather than upon injury by the acid itself. Commenting editorially in the same issue of *Gastroenterology,* Grossman (1947) stated that: "There is little question that pepsin enormously increases the injurious effect of acid." From such statements and publications it has come to be generally felt that a highly effective therapeutic agent in peptic ulcer must not only alter acid concentrations but must primarily reduce pepsin activity. Complete elimination of peptic activity would not be fatal to protein digestion because the intestinal enzymes are quite capable of carrying on this function (Bockus, 1944).

A given agent may eliminate the action of pepsin and thus bring about a therapeutic effect either directly or indirectly. Indirectly, the action is by way of altered pH, with reduced peptic activity due to that alteration. Directly, it may prevent the action of the enzyme without changing the pH. If the agent reduces peptic activity there will be a therapeutic effect even if no change in hydrogen ion concentration occurs. It is even probable that excessive reduction of gastric acidity is illogical (Miller, T. G., 1944) as the antibacterial action of the highly acid gastric content would be eliminated, thus permitting living bacteria to pass through to the intestine. This is a decidedly unphysiological state. Since the time of Spallanzani and Beaumont, who first observed the antiseptic action of gastric juice, a fund of knowledge has developed showing that persons having a copious and acid gastric juice are less liable to infection by typhoid and cholera than those with less acid gastric juice. The acid juice provides protection against parasites of all kinds—bacteria, molds, protozoa, etc. Of particular importance is the power of this acidity in checking fermentation. In general, any reduction of gastric acid is apt to be followed by a bacterial or yeast fermentation in the stomach, with resultant production of irritating organic acids and gas.

With the foregoing facts in mind, the importance of reports that aluminum compounds precipitate pepsin at low pH is clear (Komarov and Komarov, 1940; Schiffrin and Komarov, 1941; Komarov, 1942; Schiffrin and Warren, 1942; Rossett and Flexner, 1943). The basis of the action is the precipitation of pepsin by aluminum ions, forming an aluminum proteinate. It must be kept in mind that it is extremely probable that this same formation of aluminum ions, with consequent reaction, is the basis of the constipating effects of such preparations. Further, a parallel etiology undoubtedly underlies the production of intestinal obstruction which so frequently follows the continued use of aluminum preparations. Both Havens (1939) and Kraemer (1938) have reported on the severity of constipation and the occurrence of fecal impaction following the use of aluminum hydroxide. The case reported by Havens was one with a bleeding duodenal ulcer. Aluminum hydroxide was used for its astringent effect, an action doubtless due to the presence of aluminum ions. He felt that there was danger in the use of aluminum preparations in older or very ill patients whose energy is depleted and whose intestinal tract may lack normal tonus.

Schiffrin and Komarov (1941) found aluminum phosphate to be markedly inferior to aluminum hydroxide in relative capacity for pepsin inactivation. The phosphate is also less constipating than is the hydroxide (Winkelstein *et al.*, 1942). These findings would tend to indicate that aluminum ion formation is the feature common to all actions of these preparations, whether of value therapeutically or classed as side effects. In the author's laboratory, aluminum hydroxide has been found to markedly inhibit pepsin (Alpert and Martin, 1949) at pH 1.5 and trypsin at pH 8.5 to 8.8 (Alpert and Martin, 1950). In fact, the suggestion was made (Alpert and Martin, 1950) that any agent such as aluminum hydroxide inhibiting both pepsin and trypsin should be regarded as nonselective and associated with the potentiality for interference with protein digestion. Generally, the literature is in agreement with the concept of pepsin inhibition at pH 1.5 by aluminum ions in solution; however, in the interests of coverage it should be pointed out that there are those who feel that a direct correlation of pH changes and peptic activity reduction exists (Shoch and Fogelson, 1942).

Many other possibilities for favorable therapeutic action by aluminum hydroxide are apparent. The colloid would probably adsorb toxins generally because it is known to adsorb diphtheria antitoxin (Hansen, 1938) and the corresponding toxin (Schmidt, 1935). It does not, however, remove toxic materials present in the lysates of cultures of *S. dysenteriae, E. typhosa* or *Esch. coli* (Moss and Martin, 1950) nor does it adsorb paralytic shellfish poison (Swayne and Martin, 1950). Further, at the pH of the intestinal tract, aluminum hydroxide does not effectively adsorb skatole, indole, tyramine, putrescine or histamine (Martin and Alpert, 1950). Polyphasic adsorption principles would strongly indicate that this aluminum preparation is not in itself a particularly effective agent for intestinal efficacy. This contention is supported by the work of Wallbach (1935), who found that no single adsorbent was effective against all diarrhea-producing agents; thus, aluminum silicate was most active against podophyllin, bolus alba against castor oil, and so on. He decided upon and used a mixture of equal parts of animal charcoal, talcum and aluminum hydroxide in his adsorptive combinations. Similarly, it is known that neither aluminum hydroxide nor kaolin is as effective singly as in combinations when tested for removal of fecal matter (Smith, W., 1937).

It is necessary that constant vigilance be maintained for differential adsorption, i.e., the differences between the capacity of any given adsorption agent to remove harmful elements and to remove dietary ingredients vital to life. Beazell *et al.* (1938) first undertook an investigation of this type. In dogs, they reported that aluminum hydroxide did not alter nitrogen or fat content of the feces. This was interpreted to indicate no major interference with digestion. Similar findings were reported by Grondahl and West (1945), who found in human subjects no interference with carbohydrate, fat or protein utilization. On the other hand, interference by alumina gels with both vitamin A nutrition and phosphate metabolism had been reported (Hoffman and Dyniewicz, 1946). Aluminum phosphate gels did not interfere with vitamin A tolerance curves, indicating no interference with this phase of nutrition. Some disturbances of amino acid, ascorbic acid and glucose metabolism were noted; by contrast, fat metabolism seemed normal. Aluminum hydroxide reduced the available phosphate to such a degree as to potentially interfere with phosphorylation. This phase of phosphate metabolism and its modification by aluminum hydroxide had been previously investigated by Fauley *et al.* (1939, 1941), who found that the most unfavorable effect occurred in the absence of adequate pancreatic secretion. This group found aluminum phosphate completely satisfactory in this respect.

Inasmuch as aluminum ions doubtless bring about a therapeutic effect through the precipitation of pepsin and also cause such side effects as constipation by a similar protein precipitation mechanism, it is interesting to note the appearance of so-called nonreactive aluminum hydroxide gels. Smith (1947) failed to find any difference from the standpoint of therapeutic efficacy between reactive and nonreactive gels. The advantages of the nonreactive form noted in the course of this investigation were "lack of any taste and the decreased incidence of nausea and constipation in patients receiving this medication." Nonreactive aluminum hydroxide is produced by precipitation of the gel from aluminum chloride and a great excess of ammonium hydroxide. The aluminum hydroxide thus formed is in a nonreactive state and will not dissolve in 0.1 N hydrochloric acid. Theoretically and at the laboratory level such nonreactive forms can be achieved, but it is highly improbable that similar gels can be produced commercially. The nonreactive aluminum hydroxide gel remains a laboratory curiosity. This is not meant to indicate that commercial preparations may not have had small amounts of nonreactive forms, but that they consisted wholly of this form is not within the realm of possibility. The fact remains that the less reactive the aluminum hydroxide, the fewer aluminum ions will be formed and the less will be the constipation produced. There is a product now marketed containing an aluminum hydroxide gel which is probably less reactive than the standard variety in combination with magnesium trisilicate, and this combination has received favorable clinical recognition (Miller, T. G., 1944; Collins, 1945; Seley, 1946).

Aluminum phosphate possesses less pepsin-inactivating capacity, is less apt to produce phosphate loss, and is not as constipating as aluminum hydroxide, due to a decreased formation of aluminum ions. If aluminum ions are primarily responsible for the therapeutic efficacy, one would expect that the phosphate would be less valuable than the hydroxide. It is difficult to find a direct comparison, but there are many favorable reports on the clinical effect of the phosphate. Lichstein *et al.* (1945) noted favorable therapeutic activity with lowered incidence of constipation and no changes in mineral metabolism. Similar results are recorded by Fauley and his associates (1941). Emphasis on adequate dosage was the cardinal feature of the work of Upham and Chaikin (1943). They found doses of 3 tablespoonfuls every 2 hours and 6 tablespoonfuls at night essential for therapeutic efficacy, and when such doses were employed the incidence of constipation was comparable to that seen with aluminum hydroxide. This work would therefore tend to support the contention that the therapeutic effect of aluminum preparations and their side effects are due to one and the same thing, the aluminum ion.

Thus, it seems that the major problem in the clinical application of the aluminum preparations is constipation. In support of this statement is the work of Batterman and Ehrenfeld (1947), who found 16 to 33 per cent incidence of constipation in patients treated with reactive aluminum hydroxide gels; 30 to 35 per cent with so-called nonreactive aluminum hydroxide gels; 22 per cent with aluminum phosphate; 14 to 15 per cent with magnesium trisilicate; 20 per cent with sodium aluminum silicate; 29.2 per cent with a mixture of calcium caseinate and calcium carbonate; and 9.7 per cent with a mixture of magnesium trisilicate, magnesium oxide and calcium carbonate. Of the antacid preparations studied, a combination of aluminum hydroxide and magnesium trisilicate gave the best ratio of effectiveness to incidence of constipation; however, the incidence of constipation was approximately 12 per cent.

In summary, aluminum hydroxide possesses limited capacity for adsorption of toxic agents *in vitro* and seems to exert its therapeutic effect in peptic ulcer treatment via the formation of aluminum ions, which also produce undesirable side effects, namely constipation and even fecal impaction. Combinations of aluminum hydroxide with magnesium trisilicate are superior to either agent used singly, but the question of magnesium ion absorption remains unanswered. The logic of the correction of constipation induced by aluminum ions through the use of laxation-inducing magnesium ions is also questionable. In any event, there can be no doubt that aluminum hydroxide preparations are the most popular of the antacids available today. This would seem to be a tribute to their immediate effects rather than to any fundamental research structure.

BISMUTH COMPOUNDS

Bismuth subgallate and subsalicylate were once, in general, used as intestinal protectives and mild antiseptics. These salts have been largely replaced by bismuth subnitrate and subcarbonate, which when administered orally give mechanical protection to inflamed and irritated mucous membranes of the gastrointestinal tract. The bismuth goes into solution to some degree and the result is astringence. In the colon, bismuth salts are converted into the black sulfide form and also by reduction to metallic bismuth. Cases of nitrite poisoning have been reported from the use of bismuth subnitrate.

While in general the bismuth salts can be said to possess no therapeutic merit as adsorption agents, it is of interest to document in some degree the story of these materials, as they indicate by their fate in the intestinal tract the multiplicity of forces operating at that site. The initial introduction of bismuth salts was for the treatment of amoebic dysentery, but actually the bismuth salts have very low amoebicidal powers. They were in some measure effective, as they controlled the diarrhea. In 1909, Beck first reported evidence on the toxicity of these agents. The subnitrate was found to be reduced by certain bacteria in the intestines of children, with resultant nitrite formation and the production of methemoglobinemia. Deaths were observed. In his studies, Beck found children and adults with intestinal putrefaction to be the most susceptible to nitrite poisoning resulting from the administration of bismuth subnitrate. Confirmation of these findings has been made by Constantinescu and Jonescu (1920). An attempt was made by Stieglitz (1930) to utilize this bacterial reduction of nitrate to nitrite for the treatment of hypertension. *Esch. coli* was found to be the microorganism causing the reduction (Stieglitz and Palmer, 1936). The nitrite production varied in accordance with the number of bacteria, the pH, the amount of nitrate available and with other factors. The inherent variability of the reaction probably accounts for the failure of Ayman (1932) to obtain any favorable effect in a series of well-controlled hypertensive patients who were treated with bismuth subnitrate. In any event, this application has not found a place in the medical armamentarium.

Another use of bismuth salts was in the treatment of ulcerative colitis, but this use has in recent times been largely replaced by other more effective measures. Further, it seems that bismuth in large doses becomes detrimental by covering the intestinal mucosa with concretions. Another complication is the development of methemoglobinemia, which has been reported to occur in patients with ulcerative colitis undergoing treatment with bismuth subnitrate (Miller, R. C., 1944).

In summary, the bismuth salts seem to possess no merit when compared to other inactive, inert adsorbing agents with the same or greater adsorptive capacity.

BARIUM SULFATE

Barium sulfate is extensively used in roentgenology but has never found application as an intestinal adsorbent. It is probable that fear of barium poisoning limits its general application, although doses of 300 to 400 Gm. are commonly given in the form of a suspension prior to radiology. The only report known to the present author referring to the use of barium sulfate is that of Spadolini (1927), who recommended this chemical in the treatment of intestinal toxemias, especially those in association with parathyroid insufficiency.

In summary, there has been essentially no attempt to study this adsorbent either *in vitro* or *in vivo,* and its potential value remains unknown.

BENTONITE

Bentonite is a colloidal, hydrated aluminum silicate. When added to water the dry powder swells to approximately twelve times its volume and forms a gel which has great adsorptive capacity. It is widely used as a suspending agent in pharmaceutical preparations. In veterinary medicine, bentonite-nicotine combinations are employed as anthelmintics (Harwood and Stunz, 1945).

Bentonite should receive increasing attention in the future, as it has been demonstrated to inhibit lysozyme (Moss and Martin, 1948), pepsin (Alpert and Martin, 1949) and trypsin (Alpert and Martin,

1950), to remove toxic substances from bacterial lysates (Moss and Martin, 1950), to adsorb paralytic shellfish poison (Swayne and Martin, 1950), and to adsorb effectively toxic chemicals of endogenous origin such as histamine, tyramine and indole (Martin and Alpert, 1950).

SODIUM ALUMINUM SILICATE

Sodium aluminum silicate is variously designated as Zeolite, Decalso or Permutit. As is the case with bentonite, sodium aluminum silicate has a greater role in the future than it has played in the past. Laboratory studies have established its remarkable capacity for the adsorption of paralytic shellfish poison (Sommer *et al.*, 1948; Swayne and Martin, 1950). In this capacity, such commonly employed intestinal adsorbents as kaolin, aluminum hydroxide and charcoal possess no power whatever. When tested as adsorbents against toxic material in bacterial lysates, the sodium aluminum silicates were highly effective against lysates of *E. typhosa* and *Esch. coli* but ineffective against that of *S. dysenteriae* (Moss and Martin, 1950). Another *in vitro* criterion, that of the adsorption of endogenously produced toxic chemicals, showed sodium aluminum silicate to be active against tyramine, putrescine and histamine but generally ineffective against skatole and indole (Martin and Alpert, 1950).

For enzyme inactivation the synthetic sodium aluminum silicates have been found to be exceptionally effective against lysozyme (Moss and Martin, 1948), moderately active against pepsin (Alpert and Martin, 1949) and highly efficient for trypsin (Alpert and Martin, 1950).

Recently sodium aluminum silicate in combination with a polyamine anion exchange resin and magnesium aluminum silicate has found application as an intestinal adsorbent. This combination is discussed in detail in Chapter 7.

ALGINIC ACID

Sodium alginate is a gelatinous material obtained from seaweed. It is made up of D-mannuronic acid units and its gel-forming characteristics have made it of value in the manufacture of cosmetics and pharmaceuticals.

In medical practice, this naturally occurring cation exchange material has found application in the form of alginate dressing for the aural surgeon (Passe and Blaine, 1948). Such dressing can be left *in situ* for 3 or 4 weeks and tends to prevent the formation of excessive granulation tissue. Similarly, Blaine (1944) has used calcium action to promote healing in scleral wounds. An additional action of alginic acid on wounds is that of hemostasis (Smith, 1946; Frantz, 1948; Eberl and George, 1950). Smith (1946) offers in explanation of this hemostatic effect the power of alginic acid to combine with calcium at the bleeding point, thus forming a coagulum and sealing the wound. He used topical alginic acid in 100 cases of extractions and minor oral surgery, with complete absence of untoward reaction, and prompt healing. The results of Frantz (1948) would not support those of Smith, as the former concluded that toxic reaction occurred following the use of alginates. It seems highly probable that the degree of purity of such natural materials might well explain discrepancies in results.

Parenteral administration of sodium alginate produces toxic effects characterized by an accelerated sedimentation rate and the appearance of a precipitate of calcium alginate (Solandt, 1941). Further studies of the toxic action of alginates by Chenoweth (1948) revealed the formation of large intracardiac clots and injury to the brain, kidneys and liver. The results of Meunier *et al.* (1950) offer additional material in explanation of the toxic action of parenteral sodium alginate. The sodium form shortened the coagulation time of plasma. These investigators also esterified the alginic acid molecule, forming the sulfated complex, and found that this molecular species prolonged coagulation time, as do most sulfonated polyhydroxylated macromolecular agents.

The oral administration of sodium alginate to adult human beings did not modify the calcium balance in an experiment in which 8 Gm. of the chemical were ingested each day for 7 days (Millis and Reed, 1947). Similar results were obtained with experimental animals fed alginic acid products at levels ten times higher than those which might be used in food or pharmaceuticals (Nilson and Wagner, 1951).

From such evidence of the nontoxicity of alginic acid on oral administration, combined with *in vitro* studies establishing the cation exchange capacity of this agent as 4.2 mEq. per gram (Ludwig *et al.*, 1952), Feldman and his associates (1952) studied its efficacy clinically. While the acid was well tolerated when ingested at levels of 45 Gm. daily, it had only approximately one-fifth to one-sixth of the capacity of the commonly used resins for sodium removal via the intestine. Confirmation of these findings has been presented by Gill and Duncan (1952).

The story of sodium alginate has been reviewed in detail in order to emphasize the number of potential adsorption and exchange agents known in some degree but almost totally unknown in relation to their capacity for the selective removal of toxic agents formed in the gastrointestinal tract or brought into the tract from without. A large amount of work remains to be done before any clear idea can be achieved concerning the relative power and selectivity of an entire host of such agents. While this research effort will be long and arduous, there is every chance that it will be most rewarding.

CELLULOSE DERIVATIVES

In recent years, two cellulose derivatives have come into general use; they are sodium carboxymethylcellulose and methyl cellulose. These materials are of such molecular magnitude as to preclude absorption from the intestinal tract. In general, such macromolecular agents are toxic when given intravenously (Hueper, 1942, 1945; Katzenstein *et al.*, 1943; Cugurra, 1947) and totally without toxicity when given orally (Deichmann and Witherup, 1943; Machle *et al.*, 1944; Shelanski and Clark, 1948; Hodge *et al.*, 1950; Bauer and Lehman, 1951; Ellingson and Massengale, 1952). One specific point of danger with methyl cellulose would lie in the potentiality for metabolic rupture of the ether linkage, with consequent formation of methanol. Machle *et al.* (1944) clearly demonstrated that if such rupture does occur it is of slight degree and does not create any toxicity. Chronic toxicity studies in rats extending over three generations gave no sign of deleterious effect on growth, reproduction or any tissue as evidenced by histopathological examinations (Bauer and Lehman, 1951). Even when rats are kept on low vitamin intakes, specifically with reference to thiamin and vitamin A, the simultaneous administration of methyl cellulose does not significantly alter the growth curves, establishing the absence of interference by this cellulose ester with nutrition (Ellingson and Massengale, 1952). Another cellulose derivative of low toxicity is sodium cellulose sulfate (Morrow *et al.*, 1952). The latter compound is mentioned here as an example of still another macromolecular agent the potentialities of which for intestinal adsorption are unknown.

In 1943, Tainter introduced methyl cellulose as a colloidal laxative, reporting that each gram of methyl cellulose ingested increased the stools by approximately 10 Gm. Since that time many papers have appeared recommending the use of either methyl cellulose or sodium carboxymethylcellulose as a laxative (Blake, 1948; Fittipoldi and Davis, 1948; Schweig, 1948; Bargen, 1949; Blythe *et al.*, 1949; Marks, 1949; Newey and Goetzl, 1949; Schultz, 1949; Keeler and Rusk, 1952).

Blythe and his associates (1949) selected sodium carboxymethylcellulose from an entire series of natural gums and synthetic cellulose compounds as the most promising because it did not dissolve in simulated gastric juice and yet possessed great hydrophilic capacity, forming a viscous, homogeneous solution under conditions similar to those in the intestine. In general, the cellulose derivatives have found a place for themselves in the therapy of constipation. They are not without defects, however, and have in recent times come to be used primarily in combination with a mild-acting irritant laxative (Marks, 1949).

Another application of sodium carboxymethylcellulose has been in the antacid field, where, it is claimed, success equal to that with other antacids has been achieved (Brick, 1949). This cellulose derivative avoids, as do other antacids, the constipating effects seen with the more commonly employed aluminum hydroxide–containing preparations. More recently, carboxymethylcellulose has been used in combination with magnesium oxide, which adds materially to its antacid power (Bralow *et al.*, 1951; Necheles *et al.*, 1951).

Evidence that cellulose derivatives do, in fact, possess adsorptive capacities comes from several lines of research. The first of these is the use of such compounds in the control of diarrhea (Bargen, 1949). It is true that such action may be due to the coating effect of the macromolecular agent, but the probability remains that adsorption of toxic or irritant materials may also play a role. Another line of evidence suggesting a specific role as adsorbent is the use of these chemicals with terramycin as a mechanism of controlling nausea and vomiting, which often accompanies the use of this antibiotic (Parsons and Wellman, 1951). Yet another support for the contention of adsorptive capacity of carboxymethylcellulose is the report by Feinblatt *et al.* (1950) on the use of this agent with digitoxin for the elimination of peaks of acute activity of the drug. It would seem that the cellulose derivatives adsorbed the digitoxin and then slowly released it for absorption.

CONCLUSIONS

We have endeavored in this chapter to review a few of the many adsorption agents, some of which are in use, the majority remaining unknown quantities. Such agents need not be inorganic but can with equal certainty be complex macromolecular organic units. Among the materials not yet studied are included: many permutations and modifications of the customary anion or cation exchange resins, fuller's earth, diatomaceous earth, talc, bauxite, filtrol, bentonite, barium sulfate, graphite powder, large molecular dye molecules, a large number of natural gums, various cellulosic derivatives, sulfonated carbohydrates, natural and synthetic polymers, etc. If this discussion has given some idea of the marked limitations manifested by research in this field, the goal has been achieved. Even those agents most commonly employed as intestinal adsorbents have not been studied to the degree merited by the importance of the field. This is a strange situation, as it reflects our desire to bring about a result in a few days, whereas we are well aware of the fact that the human body reacts after years to repeated stresses against it. Pathology as seen in medical practice is today far more the result of long-continued insults against the bodily economy than it is an immediate and precipitate result of an invasive agent. Sulfonamides, antibiotics and similar drugs have met the challenge of the acute, and now we turn in the medical crusade toward those states most generally characterized as the chronic degenerative diseases. Of these, the most important is aging. It is not a state predestined to be the fate of man; it is rather a reflection of the failure of man to provide protection against those minor and infinitely repeated blows leading directly to pathology of major impact. We have sought, and with reward, for the immediate, the spectacular, the wonder drug; now we must seek those agents designed to cushion the shock of time. There will be no spectacular result, no one jumping out of bed to rush through the hospital corridors; only the reward of the golden period of age without the attributes of that state which are accepted at present. We speak of the potential life span as being 150 years or more but give little thought to the fact that 75 of those years spent in senility are better denied. The path of progress in this sphere may be a relay of geriatric scientists handing a program from generation to generation to form the underlying principles of the true medicine of the world to come.

REFERENCES

AARON, C. D. *Diseases of Digestive Organs.* Philadelphia: Lea and Febiger, 1915.

ALMQUIST, H. J., and D. ZANDER. *Proc. Soc. Exper. Biol. Med.,* **45**: 303, 1940.

ALPERT, S., and G. J. MARTIN. *Am. J. Dig. Dis.,* **16**: 10, 1949.

ALPERT, S., and G. J. MARTIN. *Rev. Gastroenterol.,* **17**: 251, 1950.

ANDERSEN, A. H. *Dansk. Tids. Farm.,* **18**: 21, 1944.

ANDERSEN, A. H. *Acta pharmacol. toxicol.,* **2**: 69, 1946.

ANDERSEN, A. H. *Acta pharmacol. toxicol.,* **3**: 199, 1947.

Anonymous. Queries and Minor Notes. *J.A.M.A.,* **135**: 132, 1947.

AYMAN, D. *J.A.M.A.,* **90**: 545, 1932.

BARGEN, J. A. *Northwest Med.,* **30**: 205, 1931.

BARGEN, J. A. *Gastroenterology,* **13**: 275, 1949.

BASTEDO, W. A. *Pharmacology.* Philadelphia: Saunders, 1947.

BATTERMAN, R. C., and I. EHRENFELD. *Gastroenterology,* **9**: 141, 1947.

BAUER, H. *Arch. exper. Path. Pharmakol.,* **134**: 185, 1928.

BAUER, R. O., and A. J. LEHMAN. *J. Am. Pharm. A. (Scient. Ed.),* **40**: 257, 1951.

BEAZELL, J. M., C. R. SCHMIDT, and A. C. IVY. *Am. J. Dig. Dis.,* **5**: 164, 1938.

BECK, E. G. *J.A.M.A.,* **52**: 14, 1909.

BLAINE, G. *Tr. Ophth. Soc. U. Kingdom,* **64**: 187, 1944.

BLAKE, A. D., JR. *Am. J. Dig. Dis.,* **15**: 336, 1948.

BLYTHE, R. H., J. J. GULESICH, and H. L. TUTHILL. *J. Am. Pharm. A. (Scient. Ed.),* **38**: 59, 1949.

BOCKUS, H. L. *Gastroenterology.* Philadelphia: Saunders, 1944, Vol. 2.

BRAAFLADT, L. H. *J. Infect. Dis.,* **33**: 434, 1923.

BRALOW, S. P., M. SPELLBERG, H. KROLL, and H. NECHELES. *Am. J. Dig. Dis.,* **18**: 7, 1951.

BREUHAUS, H. C., and J. B. EYERLY. *Ann. Int. Med.,* **14**: 2285, 1941.

BRICK, I. B. *Am. J. Dig. Dis.,* **16**: 315, 1949.

BUNGART, E., 1917. Reference in Sollman, T., *A Manual of Pharmacology.* Philadelphia: Saunders, 1942.

CAILLEAU, R., and J. ADRIAN. *Bull. Soc. scient. hyg. aliment.,* **36**: 114, 1948.

CAILLEAU, R., and L. CHEVILLARD. *Ann. pharm. franç.,* **7**: 132, 1949.

CALVERT, R. L. *J. Am. Pharm. A.,* **11**: 798, 1922.

CHENOWETH, M. B. *Ann. Surg.,* **127**: 1173, 1948.

COHN, A. L., A. S. WHITE, and H. B. WEYRAUCH. *J.A.M.A.,* **117**: 2225, 1941.

COLLINS, E. N. *J.A.M.A.,* **127**: 899, 1945.

CONSTANTINESCU, C. D., and A. JONESCU. *Presse méd.,* **28**: 155, 1920.

COTUI, F. W. *Ann. Surg.,* **98**: 242, 1933.

CROHN, B. B. *J. Lab. Clin. Med.,* **14**: 610, 1929.

CUGURRA, F. *Farm. sci. tec.* (*Pavia*), **2:** 307, 1947.

CUSHING, R. G. *M. Times,* **70:** 200, 1942.

DEICHMANN, W., and S. WITHERUP. *J. Lab. Clin. Med.,* **28:** 1725, 1943.

DEOBALD, H. J., and C. A. ELVEHJEM. *Am. J. Physiol.,* **111:** 118, 1935.

DINGEMANSE, E., and E. LAQUEUR. *Biochem. Ztschr.,* **169:** 235, 1926.

DRIVER, R. L., R. H. CHAPPEL, and E. B. CARMICHAEL. *Am. J. Dig. Dis.,* **12:** 166, 1945.

EBERL, J. J., and W. L. GEORGE. U.S. Patent 2,512,616, June 27, 1950.

EINSEL, I. H., and V. C. ROWLAND. *Ohio State M. J.,* **28:** 173, 1932.

EISLER, M. *Biochem. Ztschr.,* **150:** 350, 1924.

ELLINGSON, R. C., and O. N. MASSENGALE. *Proc. Soc. Exper. Biol. Med.,* **79:** 92, 1952.

EYERLY, J. B., and H. C. BREUHAUS. *J.A.M.A.,* **109:** 191, 1937.

EYRE, J. W. H., and M. S. DURCH. *Lancet,* **1:** 1124, 1925.

FAULEY, G. B., S. FREEMAN, A. C. IVY, A. J. ATKINSON, and H. S. WIGODSKY. *Arch. Int. Med.,* **67:** 563, 1941.

FAULEY, G. B., A. C. IVY, L. TERRY, and W. B. BRADLEY. *Am. J. Dig. Dis.,* **5:** 792, 1939.

FEINBLATT, H. M., T. M. FEINBLATT, and E. A. FERGUSON. *New York State J. Med.,* **50:** 2461, 1950.

FELDMAN, H. S., K. URBACH, C. F. NAEGELE, F. D. REGAN, and A. A. DOERNER. *Proc. Soc. Exper. Biol. Med.,* **79:** 439, 1952.

FITTIPOLDI, J., and P. L. DAVIS. *Gastroenterology,* **10:** 667, 1948.

FRADKIN, W. Z. *J. Lab. Clin. Med.,* **22:** 896, 1937.

FRANTZ, V. K. *Ann. Surg.,* **127:** 1165, 1948.

GILL, R. J., and G. G. DUNCAN. *Am. J. M. Sc.,* **224:** 569, 1952.

GOIFFON, R. *Semana méd.,* **37:** 1133, 1930.

GOLDFEDER, A. *Biochem. Ztschr.,* **209:** 154, 1929.

GOLDSTEIN, H. I. *Med. Rec.,* **148:** 417, 1938.

GOLDSTEIN, H. I. *J. Internat. Coll. Surgeons,* **2:** 379, 1939.

GONZALEZ, H. D., and M. SCHTEINGART. *Prensa méd. argent.,* **23:** 371, 1936.

GREENE, B. L., and L. H. BLOCK. *Am. J. Dig. Dis.,* **5:** 684, 1938.

GRONDAHL, R. D., and E. S. WEST. *Am. J. Dig. Dis.,* **12:** 197, 1945.

GROSSMAN, M. I. *Gastroenterology,* **8:** 678, 1947.

GUNNISON, J. B., and M. S. MARSHALL. *J. Bact.,* **33:** 401, 1937.

HAMMARLUND, E. R., and L. WAIT RISING. *J. Am. Pharm. A.* (*Scient. Ed.*), **38:** 586, 1949.

HANSEN, A. *Compt. rend. Soc. biol.,* **129:** 216, 1938.

HARDT, L. L., and L. P. BRODT. *Arch. Surg.,* **55:** 584, 1947.

HARDT, L. L., and F. STEIGMANN. *Am. J. Dig. Dis.,* **17:** 195, 1950.

HARDY, T. L. *Practitioner,* **138:** 434, 1937.

HARWOOD, P. D., and D. I. STUNZ. *Proc. Helminthol. Soc. Washington, D.C.,* **12:** 1, 1945.

HAVENS, W. P. *J.A.M.A.,* **113:** 1564, 1939.

HAYEM, G. *Bull. Acad. Med., Paris,* **106:** 224, 1931.

HEKTOEN, L., and B. RAPPAPORT. *J.A.M.A.,* **64:** 1985, 1915.

HODGE, H. C., E. A. MAYNARD, W. G. WILT, JR., H. J. BLANCHET, and R. E. HYATT. *J. Pharmacol. Exper. Therap.*, 99: 112, 1950.

HOFFMAN, W. S., and H. A. DYNIEWICZ. *J. Lab. Clin. Med.*, 31: 497, 1946.

HUEPER, W. C. *Arch. Path.*, 33: 1, 1942.

HUEPER, W. C. *Am. J. Path.*, 21: 1021, 1945.

HUNT, T. *Practitioner*, 138: 139, 1937.

HURST, A. F. *Practitioner*, 137: 409, 1936.

JOACHIMOGLU, G. *Chem. Ztg.*, 44: 780, 1920.

JONES, C. R., JR. *Pennsylvania M. J.*, 43: 468, 1940.

JORDAN, A. C. *Lancet*, 1: 432, 1923.

JORDAN, A. C. *Lancet*, 1: 1274, 1925.

KATZENSTEIN, R., W. C. WINTERNITZ, and J. MENEELY. *Yale J. Biol. Med.*, 16: 571, 1943.

KEELER, K. C., and H. A. RUSK. *New York State J. Med.*, 52: 75, 1952.

KIRSNER, J. B., and W. L. PALMER. *Am. J. Dig. Dis.*, 7: 85, 1940.

KOENIG, F. *Pharm. Ztg.*, 73: 1602, 1928.

KOMAROV, S. A. *Rev. Gastroenterol.*, 9: 165, 1942.

KOMAROV, S. A., and O. KOMAROV. *Am. J. Dig. Dis.*, 7: 166, 1940.

KRAEMER, M. *Am. J. Dig. Dis.*, 5: 422, 1938.

KRAEMER, M. *Am. J. Dig. Dis.*, 8: 56, 1941.

KRAEMER, M., and B. AARON. *Am. J. Dig. Dis. Nutrition*, 7: 57, 1940.

KRAUS, R. and B. BARBARÁ. *Deutsche med. Wchnschr.*, 41: 393, 1915a.

KRAUS, R., and B. BARBARÁ. *Wien. klin. Wchnschr.*, 28: 524, 1915b.

KUHNE, V. *Rev. méd. Suisse Rom.*, 38: 555, 1918.

KURIBAYASHI, H. Proc. 8th Meeting Japanese Pharmacol. Soc., in Japan. *J. M. Sc. (Pharmacol.)*, 8: 60, 1934.

KURTZ, P. *J. Lab. Clin. Med.*, 24: 1015, 1939.

LAQUEUR, E., and A. SLUYTERS. *Biochem. Ztschr.*, 156: 303, 1925.

LEFEVRE. *Semana méd., Buenos Aires*, 37: 133, 1930.

LEIBENSON, E. A. *Zhur. eksp. Biol. Med.*: 10, 58, 1928.

LEMÉTAYER, E., and P. UHRY. *Compt. rend. Soc. biol.*, 125: 823, 1937.

LEVEEN, H. H. *Gastroenterology*, 8: 648, 1947.

LEVIN, M. B. *Am. J. Dig. Dis.*, 4: 574, 1937.

LICHSTEIN, J., S. SIMKINS, and M. BERNSTEIN. *Am. J. Dig. Dis.*, 12: 65, 1945.

LONG, C. F., J. A. KOLMER, and W. A. SWALM. *J. Lab. Clin. Med.*, 20: 475, 1935.

LUDWIG, B. J., W. T. HOLFELD, and F. M. BERGER. *Proc. Soc. Exper. Med.*, 79: 176, 1952.

MACHLE, W., F. F. HEYROTH, and S. WITHERUP. *J. Biol. Chem.*, 153: 551, 1944.

McINTOSH, J. F., and C. G. SUTHERLAND. *Canad. M. A. J.*, 42: 140, 1940.

McROBERT, G. R. *Brit. M. J.*, 2: 304, 1934.

MANN, W. N. *Guy's Hosp. Rep.*, 87: 151, 1937.

MARKS, M. M. *Am. J. Dig. Dis.*, 16: 215, 1949.

MARTIN, G. J., and S. ALPERT. *Am. J. Dig. Dis.,* 16: 10, 1949.

MARTIN, G. J., and S. ALPERT. *Am. J. Dig. Dis.,* 17: 151, 1950.

MARTIN, G. J., and J. WILKINSON. *Arch. Biochem.* 12: 95, 1947.

MATET, A., and J. MATET. *Bull. Soc. chim. biol.,* 27: 513, 1945.

MATZNER, J. J., C. WINDWER, A. E. SOBEL, and S. H. POLAYES. *Proc. Soc. Exper. Biol. Med.,* 34: 243, 1936.

MELNICK, D., M. HOCHBERG, and B. L. OSER. *J. Nutrition,* 30: 233, 1945.

MESSERLI, N. *Arch. internat. physiol.,* 19: 103, 1922.

MEUNIER, L. *Bull. sci. pharmacol.,* 20: 641, 1913.

MEUNIER, P., D. MOLHO, J. MORAUX, and J. COTTE. *Compt. rend. Soc. biol.,* 144: 141, 1950.

MILLER, R. C. *Proc. Staff Meet., Mayo Clin.,* 19: 308, 1944.

MILLER, T. G. *M. Clin. North America,* 28: 403, 1944.

MILLIS, J., and F. B. REED. *Biochem. J.,* 41: 273, 1947.

MOENCH, G. L. *New York State.J. Med.,* 50: 308, 1950.

MORROW, P. E., H. C. HODGE, W. F. NEUMAN, E. A. MAYNARD, H. J. BLANCHET, JR., D. W. FASSETT, R. E. BIRK, and S. MANRODT. *J. Pharmacol Exper. Therap.,* 105: 273, 1952.

MOSS, J. N., and G. J. MARTIN. *Am. J. Dig. Dis.,* 15: 412, 1948.

MOSS, J., and G. J. MARTIN. *Am. J. Dig. Dis.,* 17: 18, 1950.

MUKHERJEE, S., and K. K. DAS GUPTA. *Quart. J. Pharm. Pharmacol.,* 19: 21, 1946.

MULLER, H. *J. Pharmacol. Exper. Therap.,* 53: 67, 1935.

MUTCH, N. *Brit. M. J.,* 1: 143, 1936a.

MUTCH, N. *Brit. M. J.,* 1: 205, 1936b.

MUTCH, N. *Brit. M. J.,* 1: 254, 1936c.

MUTCH, N. *Brit. M. J.,* 1: 595, 1937a.

MUTCH, N. *Brit. M. J.,* 2: 735, 1937b.

MUTCH, N. *Lancet,* 1: 859, 1949.

NECHELES, H., H. KROLL, S. P. BRALOW, and M. A. SPELLBERG. *Am. J. Dig. Dis.,* 18: 1, 1951.

NEUWELT, F., and F. STEIGMANN. *Illinois M. J.,* 82: 450, 1942.

NEWEY, J. A., and F. R. GOETZL. *Permanente Found. M. Bull.,* 7: 67, 1949.

NILSON, H. W., and J. A. WAGNER. *Proc. Soc. Exper. Biol. Med.,* 76: 630, 1951.

PAGE, R. C., R. R. HEFFNER, and A. FREY. *Am. J. Dig. Dis.,* 8: 13, 1941.

PAGE, R. C., and E. G. THOMAS. *Mil. Surgeon,* 85: 307, 1939.

PARSONS, W. B., and W. E. WELLMAN. *Proc. Staff Meet., Mayo Clin.,* 26: 260, 1951.

PASSE, E. R. G., and G. BLAINE. *Lancet,* 2: 651, 1948.

PETERSEN, S. R. *Mikrochemie,* 12: 215, 1932.

PETERSEN, W. F. *J.A.M.A.,* 68: 1234, 1917.

PEYER, W. *Pharm. Zentralhalle,* 81: 1, 1940.

RAE, J. *Pharm. J.,* 121: 150, 1928.

REID, C. G. *Am. J. Dig. Dis.,* 6: 267, 1939.

RIEGEL, B., D. W. STANGER, D. M. WIKHOLM, J. D. MOLE, and H. SOMMER. *J. Biol. Chem.*, **177:** 7, 1949.

ROSSETT, N. E., and J. FLEXNER. *Ann. Int. Med.*, **18:** 193, 1943.

RUTHERFORD, R. B., and E. S. EMERY, JR. *New England J. Med.*, **220:** 407, 1939.

SCHIFFRIN, M. J., and S. A. KOMAROV. *Am. J. Dig. Dis.*, **8:** 215, 1941.

SCHIFFRIN, M. J., and A. A. WARREN. *Am. J. Dig. Dis.*, **9:** 205, 1942.

SCHMIDT, S. *Biochem. Ztschr.*, **278:** 257, 1935.

SCHULTZ, J. *Am. J. Dig. Dis.*, **16:** 319, 1949.

SCHWARTZ, I. R. *Gastroenterology*, **6:** 105, 1946.

SCHWEIG, K. *New York State J. Med.*, **48:** 1822, 1948.

SELEY, S. A. *Am. J. Dig. Dis.*, **13:** 238, 1946.

SHAY, H., S. KOMAROV, H. SIPLET, and M. GRUENSTEIN. *Am. J. Dig. Dis.*, **14:** 99, 1947.

SHELANSKI, H. A., and A. M. CLARK. *Food Research*, **13:** 29, 1948.

SHELANSKI, H. A., W. L. PIOUS, and J. H. FRANK. *J. Parasitol.*, **28:** (Suppl.): 10, 1942.

SHOCH, D., and S. J. FOGELSON. *Proc. Soc. Exper. Biol. Med.*, **50:** 304, 1942.

SILVERMAN, D. N., and R. A. KATZ. *Southern M. J.*, **34:** 638, 1941.

SJOGREN, B., and E. WALLDEN. *Svensk. Farm. Tids.*, **39:** 617, 1935.

SKLOW, J. *Endocrinology*, **32:** 109, 1943.

SMERHA, J. *Sbornick Ceskoslov. Akad. Zemedelcke*, **20:** 177, 1948.

SMITH, C. A. H. *Science*, **103:** 634, 1946.

SMITH, F. H. *Gastroenterology*, **8:** 494, 1947.

SMITH, W. *Lancet*, **1:** 438, 1937.

SOLANDT, O. M. *Quart. J. Exper. Physiol.*, **31:** 25, 1941.

SOMMER, H., R. P. MONNIER, B. RIEGEL, D. W. STANGER, J. D. MOLD, D. M. WIKHOLM, and E. S. KIRALIS. *J. Am. Chem. Soc.*, **70:** 1015, 1948.

SPADOLINI, I. *Boll. soc. ital. biol. sper.*, **2:** 597, 1927.

SPANGENBERG, J. J., L. MUNIST, and L. M. GARCIA. *Dia méd.*, **13:** 898, 1941.

SPIESMAN, M. F. *Rev. Gastroenterol.*, **10:** 191, 1943.

STEIN, D., and E. H. KOTIN. *Clin. Med. Surg.*, **44:** 115, 1937.

STIEGLITZ, E. J. *J.A.M.A.*, **95:** 842, 1930.

STIEGLITZ, E. J., and A. E. PALMER. *J. Pharmacol. Exper. Therap.*, **56:** 216, 1936.

STOERCK, E., 1915. Reference in Sollman, T., *A Manual of Pharmacology*. Philadelphia: Saunders, 1936.

STRAUSS, H. *Deutsche med Wchnschr.*, **42:** 36, 1916.

STUMPF, J. *Münch. med. Wchnschr.*, **61:** 2050, 1914.

SWALM, W. A. *M. Rec.*, **140:** 26, 1934.

SWAYNE, V. R., and G. J. MARTIN. *Am. J. Dig. Dis.*, **17:** 39, 1950.

TAINTER, M. L. *Proc. Soc. Exper. Biol. Med.*, **54:** 77, 1943.

TIDMARSH, C. J., and R. G. BAXTER. *Canad. M. A. J.*, **39:** 358, 1938.

TUMEN, H. J. *Northwest Med.*, **41:** 42, 1942.

UPHAM, R., and N. W. CHAIKIN. *Rev. Gastroenterol.,* 10: 287, 1943.

VORONINA, L. G. *Farmakol. Toksikol.,* 8 No. 2: 43, 1945.

WALKER, R. R. *Lancet,* 2: 273, 1921.

WALLBACH, G. *Arch. internat. pharmacodyn. thérap.,* 50: 143, 1935.

WERCH, S. C. *Bull. U.S. Army M. Dept.,* 8: 199, 1948.

WEST, E. S., and C. PENNOYER. *Am. J. Dig. Dis.,* 12: 199, 1945.

WILLIAMS, R. J., J. H. TRUESDAIL, H. H. WEINSTOCK, JR., E. ROHRIMANN, C. M. LYMAN, and C. H. MCBURNEY. *J. Am. Chem. Soc.,* 60: 2719, 1938.

WINKELSTEIN, A., A. CORNELL, and F. HOLLANDER. *J.A.M.A.,* 120: 743, 1942.

WYLLIE, D. *Edinburgh M. J.,* 47: 336, 1940.

YOSHIDA, S. *Oriental J. Dis. Infants,* 26: 9, 1939.

CHAPTER 9

Chemistry and Medical Applications of Chelating Agents

CHEMISTRY, CHELATING AGENTS

CHELATION, APPLICATIONS TO CHEMOTHERAPY

CHELATION AGENTS, APPLICATION AS
ANTICOAGULANTS

CHELATING agents will with the passage of time take their rightful place in the armamentarium of the physician. The phenomenon of chelation is of fundamental biophysical significance and may even offer an explanation of the creation of life. If this seems a strong statement it will offer some idea of the importance attached by the author to these unique agents and to this field. Though the study of chelation as a chemical phenomenon is not new, the application of chelation agents to the world of medicine is current. In view of premise and fact, it seems feasible to review briefly these newcomers to the family of agents designed to modify ionic milieu.

CHEMISTRY, CHELATING AGENTS

Trace elements have long been under consideration in biochemistry and in medicine, but only with the development of the concept of chelation has there arisen a theory of the mechanism of action of these elements which in such small amounts modify the biological system. The originators of the concept (Morgan and Drew, 1920) coined the term "chelate" from the Greek word *chele,* meaning the great claw of the lobster, and applied it to those molecular structures in which rings are formed by primary and secondary valence forces. The metal ion is held in the ring of atoms as a cake of ice is held in tongs. When locked in the ring structure, the ionic characteristic of the metal disappear.

It will be recalled that primary valence forces are those in which electrons are actually transferred, thus forming the so-called hetero-polar bond, or are shared to form the covalent bond, the homopolar bond. The electrovalence system, resulting as it does from electron transfer, is typical of ionic substances, e.g., sodium chloride. The covalent bond, on the other hand, characterizes the carbon-to-carbon linkage of the organic molecule. This bond is stable and does not per-mit ionization. Whether a given system will interact in accordance with electrovalent or covalent forces depends upon the tendency of atoms to lose or gain electrons and by so doing simulate the arrange-ment of electrons in the rare gases.

In 1920, Werner introduced the concept of secondary or co-ordinate covalence, defined as the residual attraction when the primary valence is saturated. In reference to primary valence, a number is assigned representing the electrons shared or transferred. In the system of sec-ondary valence, the co-ordination number indicates the number of groups or ions held by the positive ion. Four and six are the most prevalent co-ordination numbers.

As examples of typical chelating agents, three chemicals will be discussed, each offering a different type of chelation complex. The first of these is the tetrasodium salt of ethylenediamine tetra-acetic acid (EDTA) (Figure 22).

The calcium chelate with ethylenediamine tetra-acetic acid serves as an excellent model for the discussion of the characteristics of such complex units. It is composed of two major parts, the first being the chelating structure. This is in turn subdivided into the chain of four atoms, each of which is bound by primary, covalent forces, and the chelated metallic ion. The terminal atoms in any chelating structure must form at one end an acid, and at the other a base. The metal ion is then held in the structure as one member of a ring. In the case of the metal ion calcium, as held in EDTA, all of the primary valences of the calcium are used, with the result that the ion completely loses its characteristics. The strength of this binding is indicated by the fact that metallic precipitates of calcium are dissolved by this chelating com-pound.

$$Ca_3(PO_4)_2 + 3Na_4\ EDTA \rightarrow 3Na_2(Ca\ EDTA) + 2Na_3PO_4$$
calcium
phosphate

$$CaC_2O_4 + Na_4\ EDTA \rightarrow Na_2(Ca\ EDTA) + Na_2C_2O_4$$
calcium
oxalate

If all of the primary valence forces of the chelated metallic ion are used, the characteristics of the molecule formed are primarily those of the chelating structure. In the case of the calcium chelate formed with EDTA, there are enough polar groups attached to the ring to render

FIGURE 22
Ethylenediamine Tetra-acetate

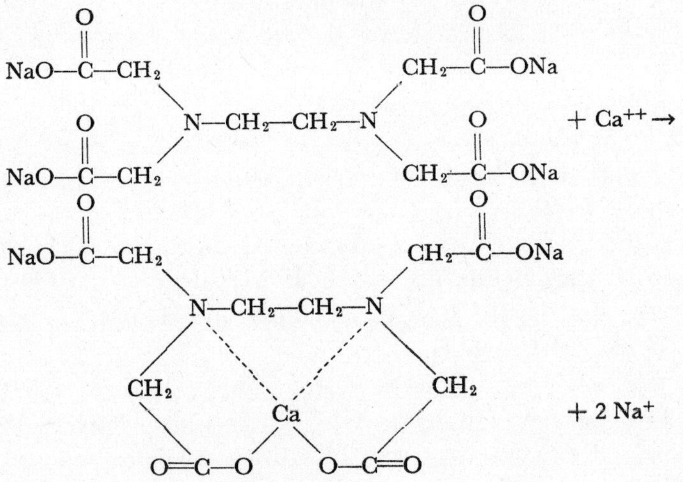

Solid lines = primary valence
Broken lines = secondary valence

the entire complex water-soluble. On the other hand, complexes may be formed in which the groups attached to the chelate ring are non-polar and the result will be solubility in organic solvents and insolubility in water. An example of this is the chelate formed between metal and thioglycolic-β-aminonaphthalide.

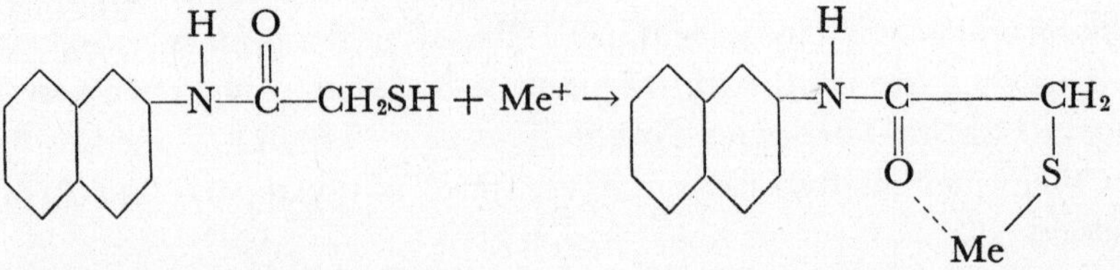

If all of the primary valence forces are not used, the entire chelate complex functions in relationship to the residual primary valence. This is seen in the case of the mordant dyes, where the chelate molecule is fixed to the fiber by the residual valences of the metallic ion. The

Turkey red color of certain cotton fabrics is the result of the interaction of the fiber, aluminum hydroxide, and alizarin. The potentialities for biochemical application of chelate complexes with residual valence forces are extremely interesting. It seems probable that such units would not behave like the free metallic ion or the chelating molecule. Fixation of antibacterial agents to certain tissues might be possible through the chelation complex structures.

The great potential for the synthesis of chelating agents is indicated by the multiplicity of organic groups which may unite with metals. Diehl (1937) lists these various groups in two subdivisions. The first includes those which unite with metals by primary valence forces: carboxyl, sulfonic, enolic hydroxyl, oxime, primary amino and secondary amino. The second list is of the group which combine with metals by secondary valence forces, and these include: primary amino, secondary amino, tertiary amino, cyclic tertiary amino, oxime, alcoholic hydroxyl, carbonyl and thioether.

In order to offer some idea of the multiplicity of chemicals now available possessing in some degree the power of chelating, Table 45 lists a series studied in the Eastman Kodak Laboratories.

The significance of chelation in biological systems is immediately recognized as paramount when it is recalled that chlorophyll is a chelate of magnesium and that hemoglobin contains hemin, which is a chelate of iron. Figure 23 gives the structural formulas for hemin and for chlorophyll and is presented as illustrative of the chelating power of the cyclic tertiary amino grouping in the four pyrrole rings present in each structure. Hemin is the chloride of heme, which is the prosthetic group of hemoglobin.

Comparatively recently, vitamin B_{12} has been designated a co-ordination complex with cobalt at its heart. The co-ordination group is the cyano grouping, which in this complex exerts none of the characteristics of the cyanide ion. Thus, cyanocobalamin is another addition to the list of vital chelate complex units functioning at the core of the life process.

Many naturally occurring organic molecules have been studied for their chelating power. Borsook and Thimann (1932) worked with the copper complexes of glycine and alanine. One most interesting chelate complex is that formed by cobaltous ions and histidine (Burk *et al.*, 1946), possessing as it does the power of combining reversibly with molecular oxygen. More recently, Albert (1947, 1950*a, b, c*) and Albert and Gledhill (1947) have studied the avidity of pterins, ribo-

TABLE 45

Calcium-Sequestering Power of Various Addends in a
Sulfite-Borate Photographic Developer

(From Henn, R. W., *Organic Chem. Bull.*, **23**: 3, 1951)

		Sequestering ($mM.$ *calcium chloride*)	
No.	*Compound*	*Per mole*	*Per acid group*
	Amino carboxylic acids		
1	Ethylenediamine tetra-acetic acid $(HOOCCH_2)_2NCH_2CH_2N—$ $(CH_2COOH)_2$	1000	250
2	Triglycine (nitrolo triacetic acid) $N(CH_2COOH)_3$	700	240
3	Methylamino diacetic acid $CH_3N(CH_2COOH)_2$	180	90
4	Aspartic acid $HOOCCH_2CH(NH_2)COOH$	35	18
5	Glycine H_2NCH_2COOH	4	4
	Oxycarboxylic acids		
6	Tartronic acid $(HOOC)_2CHOH$	200	100
7	Diglycolic acid $(HOOCCH_2)_2O$	170	85
8	Ethylene bisglycolic acid $HOOCCH_2OCH_2CH_2—$ OCH_2COOH	130	65
9	Pyruvic acid $CH_3COCOOH$	60	60
10	Gluconic acid $HOOC(CHOH)_5H$	90	90
11	Quinone tetracarboxylic acid $C_6O_2(COOH)_4$	100	25
12	Malic acid $HOOCCHOHCH_2COOH$	35	18
13	Gallic acid $3,4,5-(HO)_3C_6H_2COOH$	40	40
14	Glycolic acid $HOCH_2COOH$	6	6
15	Lactic acid $HOCH(CH_3)COOH$	6	6
16	Mandelic acid $HOCH(C_6H_5)COOH$	10	10
17	Levulinic acid $CH_3COCH_2CH_2COOH$	5	5

TABLE 45 (*Continued*)

No.	Compound	Sequestering (mM. calcium chloride)	
		Per mole	Per acid group
	Heterocyclics		
18	Imidazole-4,5-dicarboxylic acid	170	85
	HOOCC═C(COOH)N═CHNH		
19	Alloxan	75	—
	NHCONHCOCOCO		
20	Dehydromucic acid	14	7
	HOOCCOC(COOH)CH═CH		
21	Furoic acid	2	—
	HC═CHCH═C(COOH)O		
	Nitro and nitroso		
22	Nitrosoresorcinol	320	320
	$1\text{-}NOC_6H_3\text{-}2,4\text{-}(OH)_2$		
23	Picric acid	80	27
	$2,4,6\text{-}(NO_2)_3C_6H_2OH$		
	Diazo		
24	Diazomalonic acid	140	70
	HOOCCH(N═N)COOH		
	Unsaturates		
25	Maleic acid	20	10
	HOOCCH═CHCOOH		
26	Acetylene dicarboxylic acid	20	10
	HOOCC≡CCOOH		
	Mercaptocarboxylic		
27	Quinone tetrathioglycolic acid	140	35
	$C_6O_2(SCH_2COOH)_4$		
28	Thioglycolic acid	0.5	0.5
	$HSCH_2COOH$		
29	Thiodiglycolic acid	3	1.5
	$S(CH_2COOH)_2$		
	Lack sequestering action		
30	Pyromelitic acid		
	$C_6H_2\text{-}1,2,3,4\text{-}(COOH)_4$		
31	Ethylenediamine tetraglycol		
	$(HOCH_2CH_2)_2NCH_2CH_2N\text{-}$		
	$(CH_2CH_2OH)_2$		
32	Diacetyl		
	$CH_3COCOCH_3$		

FIGURE 23
Structural Formulas of Chlorophyll and of Hemin

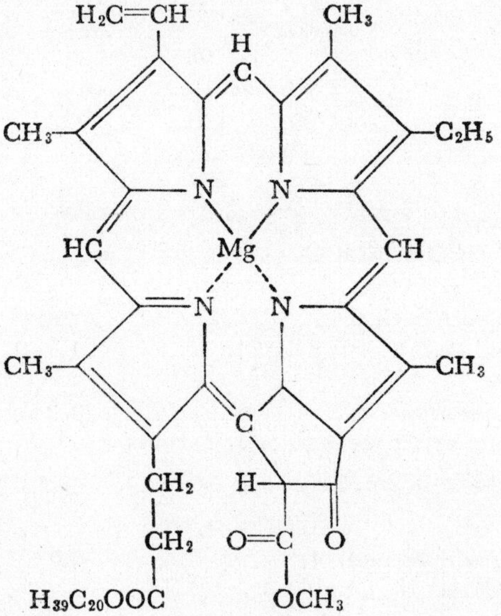

Chlorophyll-a

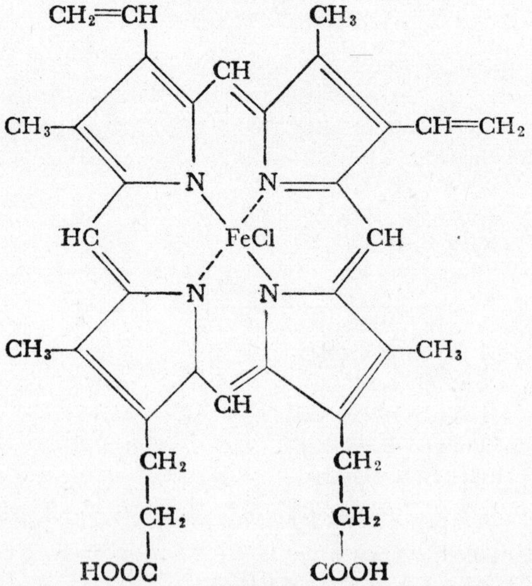

Hemin

flavin, various purines and amino acids for metallic ions. They established the following order for the stability constants of all amino acids for metallic ions:

$$Cu^{++} > Ni^{++} > Zn^{++} > Co^{++} > Cd^{++} > Fe^{++} > Mn^{++} > Mg^{++}$$

Albert emphasizes the need for data not only on the stability constant of a given naturally occurring chemical for the various metallic ions but also on the stability constants of a series of naturally occurring chemicals for a single metallic ion. The competing forces determining the ultimate fate of metallic ions in a biological system will be represented by these stability constants.

Hydrogen ion concentrations profoundly affect the efficacy with which chelating agents operate. In the case of ethylenediamine tetraacetic acid, the capacity to form complexes is greater in the more alkaline solutions. As the pH is lowered, there is no marked effect until the physiological pH is passed. If the pH drops below 7.5, magnesium, calcium and the other alkaline earth elements are complexed with slightly less efficiency than at higher pH values. With a given chelating agent, the loss of efficiency varies from metal to metal. The reverse is also true; namely, that the effect of pH on chelating power for a given metal will vary with the pK_a values of the chelating agent—the chelating species is the anion, and therefore the more of the chelator present as an anion, the greater will be its chelation potential. At the physiological pH value, 7.3, the point of dissociation of the chelate compound will be of equal importance with the avidity of the chelate compound for a given metallic ion. Albert (1950c) emphasizes this by stating: "It is already evident that the function $\bar{n}$, which represents the fraction (of the theoretically formable amount of complex) actually formed at a given pH, can be of greater interest to biochemists than the stability constant which is derived from it."

CHELATION, APPLICATIONS TO CHEMOTHERAPY

Zentmyer (1944) first reported a study which represents the direct application of chelation to the world of chemotherapy. Basing his work upon the established requirements of microorganisms for trace elements, he used complex organic molecules capable of forming chelate inner-complex salts with these elements. A good fungistatic agent, 8-hydroxyquinoline, was known to chelate with copper, manganese, iron and zinc. At those pH values at which complex formation could not occur with 8-hydroxyquinoline, Zentmyer observed an absence of fungistatic action. Next, having established the nutritional requirements of the test fungi for zinc, he added zinc in excess to the system and found that the action of the quinoline compound was nullified. Increasing amounts of the fungicide required higher quantities of zinc for reversal of action. This is doubtless an instance of the withdrawal by the chelation agent of a metal essential to the formation of a metalloprotein enzyme. In the extension of his studies, Zentmyer found ammonium nitrosophenylhydroxylamine (Cupferron) to be a good fungistatic agent.

In 1947, Albert and his associates became interested in trace metals and their relationship to chemotherapy. Of a series of papers on the subject, the first (Albert and Gledhill, 1947) reviewed the available chelating agents and considered those capable of functioning under physiological conditions. The agents were tested for their chelating power with calcium, magnesium, manganese, zinc, iron, cadmium, cobalt, lead and copper. In the second paper (Albert and Magrath, 1947), a series of derivatives of 8-hydroxyquinoline was reported. It was found that this compound alone of the seven isomeric hydroxyquinolines possessed chelating ability. The antibacterial activity of the chelating compounds formed the material for the third publication of Albert *et al.* (1947). The basis of chelation of 8-hydroxyquinoline was found to be due to the formation of a ring with the metal linked simultaneously with a phenolic oxygen via a primary valence and with nitrogen through a secondary valence (by co-ordination).

In general, the power of a compound to chelate showed a positive correlation with its ability to act as an antibacterial agent. The architectural structure, however, was a major factor, as indicated by the failure of many chelating agents to function as antibacterials. This relation of structure to antibacterial power led to the conclusion that chelation occurred with the metal on the bacterial surface and not in the medium. At least, the chelation responsible for the antibacterial power was that occurring at the surface of the bacterium. Albert *et al.* (1947) offer a conjectural location for a divalent metal in an enzyme and indicate their conception of the probable mode of attack of the quinoline (Figure 24).

In this same paper, Albert *et al.* (1947) indicate the identity of the chelated metal as being cobalt with Gram-positive bacteria and zinc or copper with the Gram-negative bacteria. In each case, the proper

FIGURE 24
Chelate Formation

(From Albert, A., *et al.*, *Brit. J. Exper. Path.*, **28**: 69, 1947)

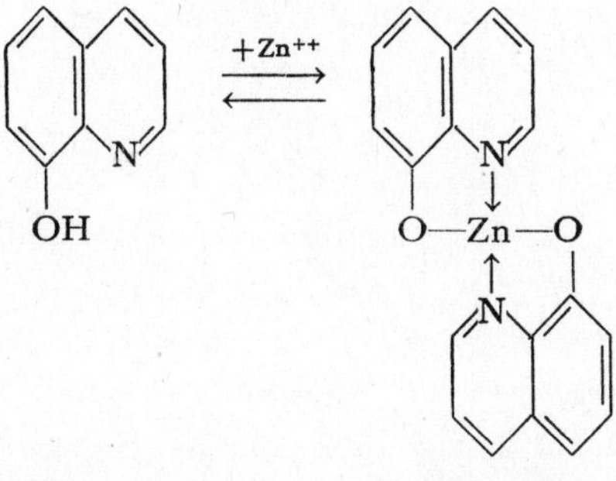

8-Hydroxyquinoline   Zinc Complex of
                              8-Hydroxy-
                              quinoline

Oxine-Metal Chelate Complex Formation

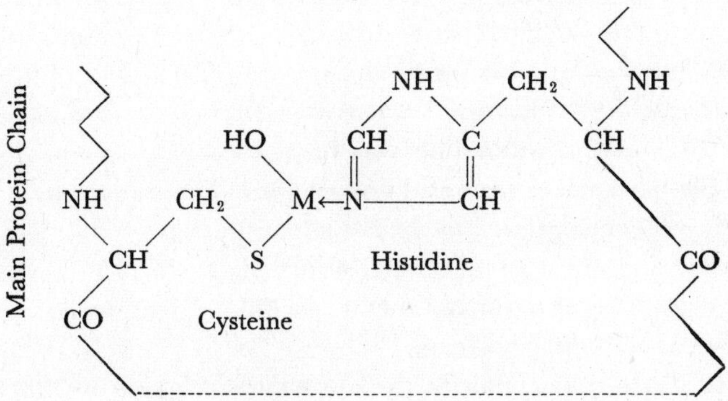

Divalent Ion, M, in Enzyme

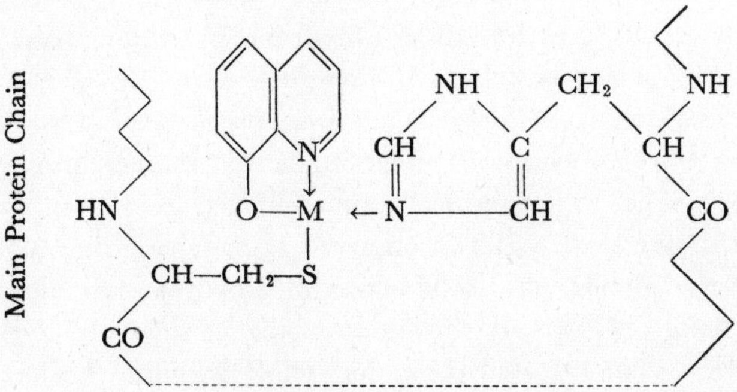

Conjectural Metal Enzyme Chelate

metal reversed the action of the 8-hydroxyquinoline. The cobalt aspect once again suggests the possibility that these agents may act to prevent the formation of vitamin B_{12}.

The tremendously important part played by trace elements in the nutrition of bacteria is indicated by the findings of Burk (1934), who calculated that *Azotobacter* required 10,000 atoms of molybdenum per cell but that *Micrococcus candicans* needed only three atoms of iron per cell. The function of cobalt in bacteria has been suggested by Albert (1947) to be that of protection of essential sulfhydryl radicals from the toxic effect of iron and copper. He offers this in explanation of the fact that concentrated solutions of 8-hydroxyquinoline do not exert their antibacterial action as rapidly as more dilute solutions. With the higher concentrations of the quinoline derivatives, all metals would be removed simultaneously and no toxic action on the sulfhydryl radicals would ensue.

In their extension of this work, Rubbo *et al.* (1950) confirmed their conclusion that cobalt is unique as an antagonist of 8-hydroxyquinoline in its action against Gram-positive bacteria and the *Neisseria.* On the other hand, the list of metal ions bearing a similar relationship to the Gram-negative bacteria was extended by the addition of iron. Their study of *Staph. aureus* in these systems was detailed and led to the conclusion that 8-hydroxyquinoline was toxic to *Staph. aureus* only because of the presence of iron and copper ions. The initial phase of the reaction involves chelation, but the actual antibacterial action is exerted by the poisoning effect of the metal either in the form of a chelation complex or by liberation of the metal ion following transport across a cell wall in the complexed form.

The relationship of cobalt to the antibacterial action of 8-hydroxy-quinoline has been reported by several other groups of investigators (Schuler and Meier, 1950; Feeney, 1951). Feeney (1951) studied inhibition of bacterial growth both by 8-hydroxyquinoline and by conalbumin (an egg white protein), finding reversal of the antibacterial actions of these agents by cobalt and iron respectively. One unique phase of this work concerns the observation that the conalbumin and 8-hydroxyquinoline were mutually antagonistic. Using an acid-fast bacterium, Sorkin *et al.* (1951) observed that copper increased and cobalt decreased the bacteriostatic action of 8-hydroxyquinoline. Vitamin B_{12} alone did not modify the action of this complexing agent.

Gale (1949) demonstrated the reduction of the internal concentration of glutamic acid coincident with the antibacterial action of

8-hydroxyquinoline (oxine). He compares this effect with that of penicillin but points out that penicillin does not inhibit uptake of glutamic acid, while oxine does. Manganese, cobalt, iron and magnesium reversed the glutamic acid assimilation defect induced by oxine. The conclusion reached by Gale placed manganese at the hub of the reaction system in that deficiency of this element, whether through chelation with oxine or by deficient media, modified glutamic acid assimilation in an identical manner.

Chelation is known to be the mechanism of action of one of the acridines, 1-hydroxyacridine, which has the same relative structure of hydroxyl to nitrogen as does 8-hydroxyquinoline (Albert *et al.*, 1945). Similarly, Freeman and Spoerri (1951) report the chelating power of 5-quinoxalinol and correlate this action with its antibacterial effect. As an antibacterial agent 5-quinoxalinol was less powerful than 8-hydroxyquinoline, and also a weaker chelating agent.

Indication that no general correlation can be found between the chelating power of various chemicals and their antibacterial action comes with the work of Schraufstätter (1950), who studied a large series of compounds for their action against *Mycobacterium tuberculosis, Trichophyton gypseum, Torulopsis minor, Staph. aureus,* and *Salmonella paratyphi* and for their chelating power with copper, cobalt and zinc. While the conclusion reached was that no direct correlation did exist, it is to be noted that a number of physicochemical factors were not controlled in these experiments and may when properly analyzed indicate a complete correlation.

Evidence exists indicating the power of chelators to inhibit enzyme activity. For example, laccase, which is a copper proteinate, is inactivated by sodium diethyldithiocarbamate, an excellent chelating agent for copper (Keilin and Mann, 1939). Phenylthiocarbamate is an inhibitor of tyrosinase and also a chelator for the copper contained in this copper proteinate (Bernheim and Bernheim, 1942). Again, Rockwood (1919) reported that fluorides decrease the activity of amylase. The probable basis for this action, and beyond question the explanation of the inhibition of enolase by fluorides, lies in the formation (in the presence of phosphates) of magnesium-fluorophosphates, which effectively remove magnesium ion from the enzyme (Warburg and Christian, 1942). Finally, the action of 2,2'-bipyridyl, a known chelator of ferrous iron, has been found effective in the inactivation of iron in the fermentation of corn mash by *Cl. acetobutyricum.* The result is an increased riboflavin production (Hickey, 1945).

CHELATION AGENTS, APPLICATION
AS ANTICOAGULANTS

The use of chelation agents in the field of chemotherapy has been reviewed in some detail in order to provide orientation in the even more complex applications of these chemicals to body fluids or to *in vivo* systems. Insoluble cation exchange resins have been used for the removal of calcium from blood with the purpose of preventing coagulation, but the more practical approach to this problem is through the use of the chelation agents as originally proposed by Dyckerhoff and his associates (1942, 1944). This group studied a series of synthetic anticoagulant substances including the sodium salt of ethylenediamine tetra-actetic acid, the potassium and sodium salts of etherified saccharic acid, the sodium salt of diglycolic acid, etherified sorbitol, saccharic acid, and tartaric acid. *In vitro,* these chemicals were found effective in the deionization of blood (calcium removal), but none of them possessed any action on intravenous injection. Quantitatively, they reported 0.5 mg. of the disodium salt of ethylenediamine tetra-acetic acid to be effective in preventing the coagulation of 1 ml. of blood (ten times more powerful than sodium citrate). This same group of German scientists observed that ethylenediamine tetra-acetic acid was able to stabilize blood *in vitro.*

The ability of ethylenediamine tetra-acetic acid to prevent blood coagulation was confirmed in 1949 by Martin *et al.* Reporting before the American Chemical Society, they stated that 0.8 to 1.0 mg. of EDTA was necessary to stop 1 ml. of blood from coagulating. The prothrombin time of the rat was not modified by 125 mg. per kilogram of the acid. At levels of 50 to 2,000 mg. per kilogram orally, the sequestering agent reduced coagulation time from a normal of 2 minutes and 40 seconds to 1 minute and 30 seconds. Given intravenously to dogs at 10 mg. per kilogram, the clotting time was reduced within 10 minutes to 1 minute and 20 seconds from an average normal of 2 minutes and 50 seconds. Proescher (1951) conducted an extensive investigation of the use of EDTA as an anticoagulant in transfusion. Blood treated with this chelator and kept at 5° C. showed no change in red cell or leucocyte counts for 3 to 5 days. The platelets were unchanged for 24 hours and then showed a drop of 6 per cent, after which there was no further change for 4 days. If sodium citrate is used in this period of time the platelets drop to 50 per cent. Hemoglobin, bilirubin, sedimentation rates, and the stainability of the cellular elements remained normal for from 3 to 7 or more days. When used for preserving human blood, disodium EDTA was used in a concentration of 1.5 Gm. dissolved in 100 ml. of 5 per cent dextrose for each 400 to 500 ml. of blood. Twenty transfusions were carried out using this material, with no ill effects. No tetany and no changes in coagulation time occurred.

It is difficult to extend consideration of the anticoagulant characteristics of this sequestering agent into the *in vivo* sphere without consideration of the toxicity of the chemical. Dyckerhoff *et al.* (1942) had observed that rabbits tolerated doses of 80 mg. per kilogram but developed tetany at the 100 mg. level. Calcium reversed the toxicological manifestations. In dogs, 50 mg. per kilogram were lethal (Martin *et al.*, 1949) unless given with calcium gluconate. Under the latter conditions, 100 mg. per kilogram given with a similar amount of calcium gluconate were well tolerated.

Proescher (1951) found that rats given the disodium salt of EDTA showed no toxic symptoms. While he gives no quantitative data, he refers to "massive doses" and indicates that some 96 per cent of the chemical was not absorbed and was found in the feces unchanged. In the experience of the present author, 150 to 800 mg. of disodium EDTA can be given intraperitoneally to rats, with no evidence of the development of tetany or any exaggerated excitability. Given 500 mg. or more (up to 800 mg.) per kilogram by this route, the animals were markedly depressed and unable to stand. Some deaths occurred at this level.

The aspect of speed of mobilization of calcium has seemed to be the decisive factor in the toxicity of EDTA in the rabbit (Popovici *et al.*, 1950). If an intravenous injection of the chelator was made in 20 seconds, the lethal dose was 100 mg. per kilogram. Hypocalcemic tetany was the immediate cause of death. By slow intravenous drip (over a 2-hour period) 2,000 mg per kilogram could be administered prior to the precipitation of a fatal serum calcium fall. In these studies, the interrelationship between toxicity and dosage is directly a function of the serum calcium levels. Administration of calcium salts at any time completely nullified the toxic action. By controlling the rate of administration and the dosage, it was possible to lower the available calcium in the serum and maintain this level. Application of EDTA in a 5 per cent water-soluble ointment to 2 human subjects resulted in a gradual fall of serum calcium levels to 8 mg. per cent, a fact proving the absorption of the sequestering agent through the skin. The ability of magnesium ions to counteract the toxicity of EDTA was noted by this group (Popovici *et al.*, 1950).

The present author conducted studies in mice of acute toxicity with EDTA (see Table 46). Table 47 indicates comparative data on toxicities from various laboratories.

A feature of importance in the interpretation of these results is that with the large doses the mice died in a short time (a few minutes), while with smaller doses the time interval was extended to 24 hours.

TABLE 46
Acute Toxicity of Ethylenediamine Tetra-acetic Acid
Disodium Salt

Group No.	No. of mice	No. dead	Mg./Kg.	L.D.	Time
Orally—acute toxicity					
1	5	0	500	0	24 hrs.
2	5	0	1000	0	24 hrs.
3	10	6	2000	60	24 hrs.
4	5	4	2200	80	24 hrs.
5	5	5	3000	100	30 min.
Intraperitoneally—acute toxicity					
1	1	1	2000	100	2 min.
2	1	1	1000	100	2 min.
3	2	2	500	100	3 min.
4	5	5	300	100	20 min.
5	10	5	250	50	24 hrs.
6	10	2	200	20	24 hrs.

This would indicate two different lethal actions. It seems probable that those killed in the shorter time intervals died of an acute ion deficiency and that those surviving for 24 hours died as a result of some other toxic effect of the drug. Gehres and Raymond (1951) obtained similar results on rapid injection, finding a M.L.D. of 150 to 250 mg. per kilogram. When this same amount of EDTA was administered over a period of 2½ hours, there was no evidence of toxicity.

Comparison of the toxicity of EDTA and o-diaminocyclohexane tetra-acetic acid (supplied by the Alrose Chemical Company through the courtesy of Dr. H. W. Zussman) shows an identical oral toxicity

level, namely a L.D.-50 of 2.0 Gm. per kilogram (Martin, 1954);
however, the ability of the diaminocyclohexane compound to prevent
clotting was only about 50 per cent of that of EDTA (1.0 mg. of
o-diaminocyclohexane tetra-acetic acid per milliliter of blood was required). This finding is mentioned to emphasize the fact that there are

TABLE 47
Toxicological Data on Ethylenediamine Tetra-acetic Acid
and Its Sodium Salts

Species	Dose (mg./ Kg.)	Result	Comment	Reference
Rabbits	80	Well tolerated	I.P.	Dyckerhoff, *et al.*, 1942
	100	Tetany	I.P.	Dyckerhoff, *et al.*, 1942
	1000	No effect	Oral	Martin, unpublished, 1949
	100	Tetany, death	I.V. (20 sec.)	Popovici *et al.*, 1950
	2000	Tetany, death	I.V. (2 hrs.)	Popovici *et al.*, 1950
Dogs	50	Lethal	I.V.	Martin *et al.*, 1949
Rats	150–800	No tetany	I.P.	Martin, unpublished, 1949
	500	Depression and some deaths	I.P.	Martin, unpublished, 1949
Mice	2000	L.D.-50	Oral	Martin, unpublished, 1949
	250	L.D.-50	I.P.	Martin, unpublished, 1949
	150–250	M.L.D.	I.P. (rapid)	Gehres and Raymond, 1951
	150–250	No effect	I.P. (given over $2\frac{1}{2}$ hrs.)	Gehres and Raymond, 1951

literally hundreds of chelating agents and that the merit of any single
molecular unit can be determined only by direct experimentation. The
organic chemist has it within his power to custom-make a host of
specific sequestering agents; the future will see the development of
molecules with greater and greater specificity for different metallic
ion units.

Chronic toxicity studies with EDTA have demonstrated it to be essentially nontoxic. Feeding tests with 100 rats kept on a diet containing 12 per cent minerals and either 0.5 per cent or 2.0 per cent EDTA for a period of 4 years showed that there was no effect on the general health, longevity or reproductive capacity (*Alrose,* 1952). Gross and microscopic tissue examinations revealed no abnormalities. The teeth were normal and the calcium content of the tibiae was within the normal range. Coagulation times were unaffected. The last observation differs from that of Martin *et al.* (1949), who reported reduction in

TABLE 48
Anticoagulant Effects of Various Salts of Ethylenediamine Tetra-acetic Acid

Salt*	Anticoagulant effect
Disodium	No coagulation
Dipotassium	No coagulation
Monomagnesium	None
Dimagnesium	Slight
Tetrasodium	Slight
Ferrous	None
Monocalcium	None
Neodymium	None
Copper	None
Cobalt	None

* Each compound tested at concentration of 0.5 mg. per milliliter of blood.

clotting time, but it is to be noted that one study was of acute toxicity and the other of chronic. The readjustment of balance would be a feature of chronic studies, and not a factor in acute findings.

The key to the internal use of chelating agents and specifically of EDTA lies in a multiplicity of factors, of which two are reasonably clear. The first of these concerns the relative toxicity of the chelated complex forms of various metals. The second is the factor of relative stability of various complexes under physiological conditions. This implies not only the stability of the complexes formed by a single sequestering agent with various metallic ions of physiological importance, but also the relative stability of complexes formed between a single metallic ion and the various sequestering and chelating molecules present in the biological system, whether native or foreign. Clearly, other factors will exist, modifying in some manner the physiological action of various sequestering agents and of the various metallic salts of these agents. The two listed have just begun to be studied, and emphasis must be placed on the magnitude of the problem. It will be a difficult path but a rewarding one.

The factor of the comparative toxicity of chelation complexes formed between metallic ions and a given sequestering agent, EDTA, was studied by Bauer *et al.* (1952) for the calcium and lead chelates. Comparative values were presented for the L.D.-50 of the lead and

TABLE 49

Toxicities of Various Chelate Salts of
Ethylenediamine Tetra-acetic Acid

Salt	*L.D.-50 (mg./Kg.)*
Disodium	400
Monomagnesium	500
Tetrasodium	350
Ferrous	350
Dimagnesium	450
Dipotassium	450
Monocalcium	500
Neodymium	1000
Copper	600
Cobalt	1000

calcium chelates when both were given as the disodium salts intra-peritoneally to rabbits; these were respectively 350 mg. per kilogram and 1000 mg. per kilogram. This would indicate that the lead chelate was roughly three times as toxic as the calcium. The corresponding values for the intravenous route were 1.0 Gm. per kilogram for the lead and an excess of 4 Gm. per kilogram for the calcium sequestrants. The relative solubilities of these forms of EDTA must be considered in evaluating such findings. Brendel *et al.* (1953) compared the anti-coagulant and toxicity power of a series of chelates of EDTA. Tables 48 and 49 show the results.

From these tables, it can be seen that only the disodium and dipotassium salts had a powerful anticoagulant effect. Since this action was due to chelation, the interpretation was that only these two salts were capable of exchanging ions with the calcium of blood. This was in accord with the report of Martell and Bersworth (1948) that the ionization of heavy-metal salts of EDTA is almost completely suppressed, indicating that any heavy-metal ions chelated in the EDTA complex would remain so and would not become available to the body. The toxicology shows little difference among the various chelates tested. In the few cases where the L.D.-50 is appreciably higher, it seems probable that poor solubility and slow absorption are involved. In all cases the toxicity symptoms were the same as those found for the disodium salts; convulsions were produced and death resulted from asphyxia. The conclusion is that from the standpoint of acute toxicity, the manifestations are not the result of chelation but rather of some inherent characteristics of the ethylenediamine tetra-acetic acid moiety.

The factor of relative stability of various complexes, native and foreign, within the body has been studied by Rubin *et al.* (1952). These values are reflected directly in the comparative toxicity data obtained with a metallic ion administered in a nonchelate form and that of the same ion in the chelate form. In this study comparison was made between ion in some simple salt form and chelated ion in the EDTA complex. In the case of mercury the ratio of toxicity for nonchelate and chelate was 3 to 1; for nickel the corresponding value was 40 to 1. In any instance in which the ratio is favorable to the chelated form, the probability is that the administration of EDTA would decrease the toxicity of the ion under study.

If the *in vitro* findings that 0.5 mg. per milliliter of EDTA is required to prevent coagulation are carried over to *in vivo* studies, a dose of 60 mg. per kilogram should prevent coagulation. This does not happen; rats can be given doses around 500 mg. per kilogram by the intraperitoneal route with no increase in the coagulation time.

One practical application of complex formation has been employed by Schubert and Wallace (1950) and by Schubert and White (1950*a, b*) for the removal of toxic elements from the body of rats. Beryllium forms a soluble, easily diffusible compound with citrate, with the result that greater excretion of the toxic element occurs. Similarly, citrate complex formation results in a threefold increase in the urinary excretion of thorium and strontium.

In 1951, White *et al.* described the protection afforded by aurin tricarboxylic acid against beryllium poisoning. Aurin tricarboxylic acid, the structural formula of which is shown following, has for some years been used as an analytical reagent for aluminum and beryllium.

HO—⟨ ⟩—C—⟨ ⟩=O
       ‖
COOH   COOH
HOOC—⟨ ⟩
       OH

The beryllium was given as the sulfate in doses of 0.7 mg. of beryllium per kilogram, and the aurin tricarboxylic acid dose was 1 to 4 mg. per mouse. In their examination of the mechanism of action of aurin tricarboxylic acid (ATA), Schubert and his group (1952) found that the agent chelated by a combination between beryllium and the ortho-carboxyl, -hydroxyl groupings in the molecule, with resultant conversion to a nondiffusible colloidal aggregate, a lake. Specifically by chelate formation, the ATA reversed the inhibition of plasma alkaline phosphatase by beryllium (Lindenbaum *et al.*, 1952). This occurred both *in vitro* and *in vivo*.

Ethylenediamine tetra-acetic acid has been used to inhibit the hematopoietic action of cobalt (Child, 1951; Child and Leonard, 1951) and to reduce the toxicity of mercury, copper and lead. This effect could be attributed either to decreased absorption of the metallic ions from the gastrointestinal tract, to inactivation of such ions through chelation in the blood stream, or to increased excretion rate induced as a result of the formation of a more soluble chelation complex. It is known that the disodium salt of EDTA does not decrease the absorption of strontium from the gastrointestinal tract (MacDonald *et al.*, 1952). Of importance to the general problem of toxic ion removal is their observation that carboxylic cation exchange resins do prevent the absorption of strontium.

Rubin and his co-workers (1952) have studied the effect of EDTA on the storage and excretion of lead in rabbits. Lead as the acetate was excreted to the extent of 1 per cent in 2 days, as contrasted to some 70 per cent excretion when the lead was in the form of the EDTA complex. Further, EDTA could bring about a mobilization and increased excretion of lead given in the form of the acetate. The prime point of mobilization of lead by EDTA was from the soft tissues. Successful clinical application of this general principle was made by Bessman and Rubin (1952) when they used the disodium calcium EDTA in the treatment of a case of lead poisoning.

Potentialities for the application of sequestering agents to the medical problem of reduction of abnormal pathological calcification sites have come from studies of the use of EDTA in the demineralization of hard tissues *in vitro* (Sreebny and Nikiforuk, 1951) and from investigations of the dissolution of urinary calculi by the same agent. Raymond and Gehres (1950) and Kissin and Natelson (1950) found EDTA an effective solvent *in vitro* for urinary calculi of the oxalate, phosphate and carbonate types. Kissin and Natelson (1950) found a 3 per cent solution of EDTA (pH 7.0) to be fairly irritating to the bladder when used for irrigation purposes. Both Gehres and Raymond (1951) and Abeshouse and Weinberg (1951) noted no irritation at levels of 3 per cent but did observe inflammation of the urinary tract with concentrations above this level. Successful solution of kidney stones other than those of urate composition was noted. It seems extremely probable that this application alone or in combination with other technics will find a permanent place in the practice of urology.

The greatest potential application of chelators of the type of EDTA would seem to lie in the mobilization of heavy-metal cations and their transfer in the chelated form across semipermeable membrane boundaries. There will be indications for the use of these agents in the removal of toxic cations from the body and doubtless indications for the use of such chemicals for gaining transfer of cations into cells. Sequestrants will serve as mechanisms of transportation for otherwise difficultly transferrable units from one site to another. Chelation is doubtless the key to those chemical forces which caused the bending, twisting and turning of protein molecules, creating as a result complex moieties endowed with the characteristics of life. Ion antagonism as a subdivision of the general field of biological antagonism will be involved; there is no more basic approach to the general field of medical practice.

REFERENCES

ABESHOUSE, B., and T. WEINBERG. *J. Urol.*, 65: 316, 1951.
ALBERT, A. *Pharm. J.*, 158: 275, 1947.
ALBERT, A. *Biochem. J.*, 46: xxxix, 1950a.
ALBERT, A. *Biochem. J.*, 47: ix, 1950b.
ALBERT, A. *Biochem. J.*, 47: 531, 1950c.
ALBERT, A., and D. J. BROWN. *Abstracts, 1st Internat. Congr. Biochem.* Cambridge, Eng.: 1949, p. 241.
ALBERT, A., and W. S. GLEDHILL. *Biochem. J.*, 41: 529, 1947.
ALBERT, A., and D. MAGRATH. *Biochem. J.*, 41: 534, 1947.

ALBERT, A., S. D. RUBBO, R. J. GOLDACRE, and B. G. BALFOUR. *Brit. J. Exper. Path.*, 28: 69, 1947.

ALBERT, A., S. D. RUBBO, R. J. GOLDACRE, M. E. DAVEY, and J. D. STONE. *Brit. J. Exper. Path.*, 26: 160, 1945.

Alrose Technical Bulletin, Sequestrene, 1952.

BAUER, R. O., F. R. RULLO, C. SPOONER, and E. WOODMAN. *Federation Proc.*, 11: 321, 1952.

BERNHEIM, F., and M. L. C. BERNHEIM. *J. Biol. Chem.*, 145: 213, 1942.

BESSMAN, S. P., and M. RUBIN. *Chem. Eng. News*, 30: 338, 1952.

BORSOOK, H., and K. V. THIMANN. *J. Biol. Chem.*, 98: 671, 1932.

BRENDEL, R., V. SWAYNE, R. PRESTON, J. M. BEILER, and G. J. MARTIN. *J. Am. Pharm. A. (Scient. Ed.)*, 42: 123, 1953.

BURK, D. *Ergebn. Enzymforsch.*, 3: 23, 1934.

BURK, D., J. HEARON, L. CAROLINE, and A. L. SCHADE. *J. Biol. Chem.*, 165: 723, 1946.

CHILD, G. P. *Science*, 114: 466, 1951.

CHILD, G. P., and P. LEONARD. *Federation Proc.*, 10: 286, 1951.

DIEHL, H. *Chem. Rev.*, 21: 39, 1937.

DYCKERHOFF, H., R. MARX, and H. BOYERLE. *Ztschr. ges. exper. Med.* 113: 291, 1944.

DYCKERHOFF, H., R. MARX, and B. LUDWIG, *Ztschr. ges. exper. Med.*, 110: 412, 1942.

FEENEY, R. E. *Arch. Biochem. Biophys.*, 34: 196, 1951.

FREEMAN, S. K., and P. E. SPOERRI. *J. Org. Chem.*, 16: 438, 1951.

GALE, E. F. *J. Gen. Microbiol.*, 3: 369, 1949.

GEHRES, R. F., and S. RAYMOND. *J. Urol.*, 65: 474, 1951.

HENN, R. W., *Organic Chem. Bull.*, 23: 3, 1951.

HICKEY, R. J. *Arch. Biochem.*, 8: 439, 1945.

KEILIN, D., and T. MANN. *Nature*, 143: 23, 1939.

KISSIN, B., and S. NATELSON. *Science*, 112: 367, 1950.

LINDENBAUM, A., M. R. WHITE, and J. SCHUBERT. *J. Biol. Chem.*, 196: 273, 1952.

MacDONALD, N. S., R. E. NUSBAUM, F. EZMIRLIAN, R. C. BARBERA, G. V. ALEXANDER, P. SPAIN, and D. E. ROUNDS. *J. Pharmacol. Exper. Therap.*, 104: 348, 1952.

MARTELL, A. E., and F. C. BERSWORTH. *Proc. Sc. Sect. Toilet Goods A.*, 10: 26, 1948.

MARTIN, G. J. Unpublished data, 1949.

MARTIN, G. J. Unpublished data, 1954.

MARTIN, G. J., V. SWAYNE, and R. BRENDEL. Abstracts, 117th Meeting Am. Chem. Soc., 16C, 1949.

MORGAN, G. T., and H. D. K. DREW. *J. Chem. Soc.*, 117: 1456, 1920.

POPOVICI, A., C. F. GESCHIKTER, A. REINOVSKY, and M. RUBIN. *Proc. Soc. Exper. Biol. Med.*, 74: 415, 1950.

PROESCHER, F. *Proc. Soc. Exper. Biol. Med.*, 76: 619, 1951.

RAYMOND, S., and R. F. GEHRES. *Proc. Soc. Exper. Biol. Med.*, 74: 715, 1950.

ROCKWOOD, E. W. *J. Am. Chem. Soc.*, 41: 228, 1919.

RUBBO, S. D., A. ALBERT, and M. I. GIBSON. *Brit. J. Exper. Path.*, 31: 425, 1950.

RUBIN, M. S. GIGNAC, and A. POPOVICI. *Abstracts, 121st Meeting Am. Chem. Soc.*, 3J, 1952.

SCHRAUFSTÄTTER, E. *Ztschr. Naturforsch.*, 5b: 190, 1950.

SCHUBERT, J., and H. WALLACE, JR. *J. Biol. Chem.*, 183: 157, 1950.

SCHUBERT, J., and M. R. WHITE. *J. Biol. Chem.*, 184: 191, 1950a.

SCHUBERT, J. and M. R. WHITE. *J. Lab. Clin. Med.*, 35: 854, 1950b.

SCHUBERT, J., M. R. WHITE, and A. LINDENBAUM. *J. Biol. Chem.*, 196: 279, 1952.

SCHULER, W., and R. MEIER. *Schweiz. Ztschr. Path. Bakt.*, 13: 463, 1950.

SORKIN, E., W. ROTH, V. KOCHER, and H. ERLENMEYER. *Experientia*, 7: 257, 1951.

SREEBNY, L. M., and G. NIKIFORUK. *Science*, 113: 560, 1951.

WARBURG, O., and W. CHRISTIAN. *Biochem. Ztschr.*, 310: 384, 1942.

WERNER, A. In Kadrer, P., *Die Wissenschaft* (4th ed.), Vol. 8. Braunschweig: Vieweg, 1920.

WHITE, M. R., A. J. FINKEL, and J. SCHUBERT. *J. Pharm. Exper. Therap.*, 102: 88, 1951.

ZENTMYER, G. A. *Science*, 100: 294, 1944.

CHAPTER 10

The Concept of Intestinal Bionomics

GENERAL

VITAMIN AND AMINO ACID SYNTHESIS IN THE
GASTROINTESTINAL TRACT
    Thiamin
    Riboflavin
    Nicotinic Acid
    Folic Acid
    Vitamin B_{12}, Cyanocobalamin
    Vitamin K and Other Fat-soluble Factors
    Amino Acids

ANTIBIOTICS

DIETARY FACTORS INFLUENCING INTESTINAL FLORA

DESTRUCTION OF NUTRIENTS BY INTESTINAL
BACTERIA

FORMATION OF TOXIC CHEMICALS BY INTESTINAL
BACTERIA

GENERAL

THE gastrointestinal tract is a manufacturing plant of such complexity as to dwarf any of modern man's industrial operations. Thousands of synthetic processes are constantly in motion; thousands of destructive metabolic mechanisms are functioning. The bacteria, forming as they do the basis of these ceaseless chemical reactions, never rest. The products of their metabolism may be beneficial to the host or they may be detrimental. As vitamins are synthesized in the gut, so are the toxic chemicals: histamine, tyramine, putrescine, cadaverine, skatole, indole and a host of others. The body is exposed during every second of its existence to the metabolic products of bacterial life. In this closing chapter it is our purpose to review in brief the complex concatenation of chemical events associated with the gastrointestinal tract and to spotlight these reactions as forming a portion of the etiological basis of the degenerative and other diseases.

The present scientific age seems unduly dedicated to the concept of the immediate. Therapeutics, not prophylactics, are the order of the day. This is doubtless in accordance with Zipf's principle of least effort as it applies to the problem of health. As long as it carries with it the necessity for self-restraint, abstinence and often the denial of the pleasure principle, prophylaxis will remain unpopular. However, the goal must be prophylaxis, and if converts are to be won to its cause, it must be made pleasant and easy.

The major premise of our discourse relates the fact that the medical history of any given individual is but the record of those irrevocable changes precipitated in the bodily economy in accordance with the second law of thermodynamics. Blum (1951) has designated this law as time's arrow and has related events in evolution with this universal determinant. The present author wishes to extend this concept and apply the same reasoning and the same law to the world of medicine and health. When through the sequence of events or through the simultaneous occurrence in time of several reactions a condition is created causing an irreversible reaction to occur, it is one of a number of such reactions bringing life to its termination. The process designated as death is but a summation of countless such irreversible reactions. Each of the physiological and biochemical manifestations of aging is no more than the summation of numberless blows dealt to the bodily economy in accordance with the second law of thermodynamics. It is our fundamental premise that the major portion of such interactions are initiated by reactions occurring in the gastrointestinal tract.

While it is true that certain rather spectacular events can be brought about by modifying the biochemical complexity of the tract, it is not with these reactions that we are concerned, but rather with those which separately make nothing happen but which, combined and accumulated, lead directly to the manifestations designated as aging, and finally to that ultimate irreversible reaction, death. This is not to imply that even ideal control of the internal environment of man, should this be finally possible, will lead to eternal life, but it is meant to state that proper control of this environment will significantly extend the life span.

The element of time is the key to the structure we attempt to erect. Man is, we repeat, exposed to his own gastrointestinal tract during every second of his life upon this earth. Strangely, billions of dollars and a large part of man's ingenuity are devoted to gaining greater and greater control over his external environment; very little attention is paid to his internal environment. No question is raised on the point of logic in control of the external world, but man must learn the significance and importance of the internal and far more immediate environment. It is not possible today to state the degree to which the life of man might be modified by a conditioned gastrointestinal tract, but it is certain to dwarf in significance any medical discovery to date.

The very subtle manner through which the repeated insults from the tract modify health and create pathology has probably been the major reason for the failure of this sphere of potential reward to be investigated. There is no single day, hour, period during which the attack on health is at a peak; it may be accentuated in some measure during certain situations, but in general it is an imperceptible degenerative process not characterized in any manner by immediate reactions. In the interests of clarity, it is not meant to suggest that immediate and violent bodily response cannot or does not occur to biochemical events, usually of bacterial origin, within the gut. Every physician knows that these do occur, but spectacular as such events may seem, they are of little significance relative to the major results of the slow, immediately imperceptible irreversible reactions set off in every tissue in the body by biochemical pathology in the internal milieu. It is difficult for the mind to adjust itself to thinking in terms of millions of years and to the immensity of space; it is equally difficult for the mind trained in medical research to think in terms of 50 years of constant bombardment by minor reactions. It is for this reason that the importance of the field has escaped attention. Further, the problems raised are great. Experimentally, it is most difficult to investigate processes occurring in the human body over periods of many years; even the creation of an experimental laboratory model is not easy. Study of the general process of aging has in recent years been engaging an ever increasing number of scientists. The research in geriatrics has been devoted to a comparison of the young and the old from the standpoint of some specific chemical constituent. Many differences have been found and much fine work has been done, but comparatively little study has been devoted to mechanisms for the prevention of the development of such differences. It is not desired to focus attention on aging to the exclusion of any other degenerative disease, atherosclerosis, arthritis or countless others, as these will form a portion of the pattern of bodily response to repeated insult from the gastrointestinal tract. Any one or all may logically form the basis of the experimental pattern. To repeat, it is a difficult type of research, as it ties up men, money and equipment for periods of years and carries with it no guarantee of success; but such work is being done and will be done with ever expanding concentration from the medical world.

Having stated the fundamental premise, it seems in order to review in brief the known examples of synthesis by intestinal bacteria of beneficial and harmful chemicals, and also to indicate in some measure those conditions resulting in altered permeability of the gut wall.

For orientation, let us first consider the flora of the gastrointestinal tract. In the breast-fed infant it is relatively simple, consisting largely of *L. bifidus*. This bacillus in the early weeks of life may constitute 99 per cent of the total organisms in the feces. There are in addition a few enterococci and coliform bacilli. The intestinal flora of the bottle-fed infant is not so simple. *L. bifidus* is uncommon; on the other hand, another member of the aciduric group of bacteria, *L. acidophilus,* is usually present in large numbers. Different types of coliform bacilli, enterococci, Gram-positive aerobic spore-bearing bacilli and anaerobic bacilli occur more or less abundantly. In the normal healthy adult, there are few organisms in the stomach, duodenum or upper jejunum. Organisms present in the upper part of the small intestine appear to consist chiefly of enterococci. In the lower part numerous organisms are found and in large numbers, among them coliform bacilli, staphylococci, various gelatin-liquefying organisms, sarcinae, yeasts and sometimes aciduric bacilli. In the large intestine the flora is even more complex and numerous. The following are commonly found: coliform bacilli, enterococci, staphylococci of both *aureus* and *albus* varieties, anaerobic spore-bearing organisms such as *Cl. welchii* and *Cl. putrifaciens,* aciduric bacteria including *L. acidophilus* and *L. acidophil aerogenes,* thermophilic bacteria, spirochetes and yeasts. Less frequently are found *Proteus* bacilli, *Pseudomones pyocyanea,* organisms of the Friedländer group and aerobic spore bearers such as *B. subtilis* and *B. mesentericus.* Predominant organisms are found to be obligate nonsporing anaerobes. Feces are from one-third to one-quarter bacteria, mostly dead. The intestine is sterile at birth but becomes infected both from above and below. Meconium contains organisms 4 hours after birth.

It is to be noted that in general the aciduric bacteria which metabolize carbohydrates are the ones which produce no toxic substances but do synthesize various members of the B complex. On the other hand, it is the so-called proteolytic bacteria, those metabolizing protein, which produce toxic products such as histamine and indole and which tend to destroy the various members of the B complex. The changes in the bacterial flora of the intestine with advancing years parallel the general concept. In infants the flora is mainly or almost entirely aciduric bacteria; in the adult, the flora has far more proteolytic bacteria in its composition.

VITAMIN AND AMINO ACID SYNTHESIS IN THE GASTROINTESTINAL TRACT

The synthesis of nutritional factors by intestinal bacteria is but one phase of the general problem; however, it has been studied in more recent times and the data available are clear-cut and beyond question. The simplest aspect of the subject relates to studies of synthesis, but in addition there are the interacting forces. The system must be considered ecologically; it is a bionomic sphere. No bacterium present in the intestinal tract can be considered in an isolated sense; each is in constant warfare with other bacterial forms; each derives its nutrient materials at the expense of other types. It is all very well to isolate bacteria and determine the vitamins synthesized, but this phase of study has little significance until the summation has been made, until each fragment has been placed properly and the entire picture viewed as a whole. Lazy thinking, the principle of least effort, leads immediately into the pitfall of examining the tree and never the forest. It is difficult to grasp the magnitude of the vital forces at play in our own intestines. However, the effort must be made, since with control of external environment by mankind the evolutionary force remaining presently uncontrolled is the internal milieu. One cannot lightly dismiss the potential impact of internal environment on evolution.

With this attempt to bring into the foreground the importance of summation in this field, we must now consider some of the analytical phases relative to vitamin synthesis. It is not intended to review this sphere in detail, but rather to outline it briefly. For details, the reader is referred to the articles of Najjar and Barrett (1945), Woods (1946), Johansson and Sarles (1949) and to the material contained in *Nutrition Reviews* (1946).

Thiamin

The synthesis of thiamin by the intestinal bacteria of animals was first hypothecated in 1914 by Cooper, based upon his observation that fowl and rabbit excreta contained the antineuritic factor. Subsequently, intestinal and rumen synthesis of this vitamin have been firmly established (Guerrant and Dutcher, 1932, 1934a; McElroy and Goss, 1939, 1941; Hathaway and Strom, 1946; Slater, 1946; De *et al.*, 1949). The site of maximum synthesis is the large colon, more specifically the cecum (Guerrant *et al.*, 1937). Najjar and Barrett (1945) have listed the organisms known to produce thiamin: Pfeiffer's bacillus, *B. vulgatus, B. proteus, B. subtilis, B. adhaerens, B. lactis aerogenes, B. alcaligenes,* some strains of dysentery bacilli, strains of diphtherial organisms, *B. aerogenes, B. vulgaris, B. mesentericus, Esch. coli, Ps. fluorescens, Proteus vulgaris, Cl. butyricum* and *B. bifidus.*

In the human being, the synthesis of thiamin by intestinal bacteria has been clearly established and the degree of such synthesis found to vary markedly with the individual (Najjar and Holt, 1943). Proof of such conclusion was obtained by the use of succinylsulfathiazole, which by virtue of destruction of intestinal bacteria reduced thiamin synthesis to zero. It is most interesting to note that in 1 of the 9 subjects in the Najjar and Holt experiments, reduction of thiamin intake to zero did not precipitate any clinical manifestation of beriberi. This is astonishing in that here we see clearly the power of bionomics. If an evolutionary situation existed dependent upon supply of thiamin, 1 of the 9 would survive to perpetuate his type. We have stated that the ecological aspects of intestinal flora could determine evolutionary trends, and here we see a clear-cut example proving the merit of this assertion. One must consider the bionomics of intestinal flora in terms of all animal species and not solely in terms of man and rat. Following this line of reasoning, it seems most probable that phylogenetic sequences might well have been determined in some instances by the ecological impact of intestinal flora.

It is interesting to note that disease states modify the degree of intestinal synthesis of thiamin (Alexander *et al.*, 1946). In the series of Alexander and his associates, there were 3 patients with diabetes mellitus and 1 with hyperthyroidism who deviated significantly from the normal pattern of thiamin excretion. This permits speculation relative to disease and vitamin requirements and leads directly to the conclusion that any diseased state will modify not only thiamin requirement but also the intestinal synthesis of this factor. Thus, states of health can probably be correlated with intestinal vitamin synthesis and an entire host of abnormal situations modifying the intestinal bacterial synthesis of vitamins, which in turn alter the reaction of the organismic whole to increased requirements for such nutritional factors.

The site of absorption of thiamin formed by bacterial action in the gut is apparently not the large bowel (Alexander and Landwehr, 1946). This statement is in large measure based upon experiments involving the use of enemas containing this vitamin and subsequently checking urinary excretion. While this is a valid experiment in its design, it is most probable that individuals will vary in the permeability of any mucosal surface, and further that variations will occur in the same individual from time to time during the course of any specified period of time. The answer cannot therefore be considered as established.

Riboflavin

As in the case of thiamin, riboflavin has been found to be synthesized by intestinal bacteria in animals (Guerrant and Dutcher, 1934*a*, *b*) and man (Najjar *et al.*, 1944). Once again, the colon is the major site for such activity and the bacteria capable of riboflavin synthesis include lactic acid bacilli, strains of dysentery bacilli, diphtherial organisms, *Esch. coli, B. aerogenes, Alcaligenes faecalis, B. vulgatus, B. mesentericus, B. vulgaris, Ps. fluorescens, Pr. vulgaris* and *Cl. butyricum.*

Nicotinic Acid

The pattern extends to nicotinic acid, as it has been shown that the intestinal bacteria of animals (Birch *et al.*, 1935; Pearson and Luecke, 1945; Teply *et al.*, 1947) and man (Ellinger *et al.*, 1944; Ellinger and Emmanuelowa, 1946; Najjar *et al.*, 1946) synthesize this factor. The degree of such synthesis, occurring mainly in the cecum (Mitchell and Isbell, 1942), is very high, amounting to three times the intake in animals (Shourie and Swaminathan, 1940) and to some 80 per cent of intake in man (Ellinger *et al.*, 1944). A partial list of bacteria capable of forming this factor includes: *Esch. coli, B. aerogenes, A. faecalis, B. vulgatus, B. mesentericus, Aerobacter aerogenes, Ps. fluorescens, Pr. vulgaris* and *Cl. butyricum* (Najjar and Barrett, 1945).

From the standpoint of therapeutics, it is of importance that nicotinic acid deficiencies can be precipitated either by sulfonamides (Hardwick, 1946) or by antibiotics (Ellinger and Shattock, 1946). Disturbance of the nutritional balance of the body as a result of destruction of intestinal bacteria is to be expected following the use of antibacterial agents and possibly other drugs. The result can be fatal. It would seem that reseeding the intestine with the proper flora following periods of use of antibacterials should become a routine practice. Elimination of an acute infection only to create a deficiency disease is hardly good medical practice, and such situations can be avoided by reseeding.

The diverse sequences which may follow the administration of any given drug are well illustrated by the findings of Ellinger and Emmanuelowa (1946), which clearly show that the administration of p-aminomethylbenzenesulfonamide (Ambamide) increases the intestinal synthesis of nicotinic acid. This observation was correlated with increased coliform intestinal flora and with the stimulant action of the chemical on the growth of coliform bacteria (Ellinger *et al.,* 1947). In addition, the over-all picture is modified by the *in vivo* destruction of such bacteria as *Proteus* and *Streptococcus faecalis,* which destroy or consume nicotinamide. Antibacterials of the standard variety are by no means the only chemicals which when taken orally modify the nutritional economy of the body through modification of intestinal bacterial synthesis. For example, the methyl tryptophanes both *in vitro* and *in vivo* materially reduced nicotinamide formation of *Esch. coli* (Ellinger and Kader, 1949). The probabilities are excellent that no chemical of any type, whether a food constituent or otherwise, enters the intestinal tract without in some manner modifying the ecological economy.

Benesch (1945) was among the first to study both destruction and synthesis of vitamins by the intestinal flora. He found that intestinal aerobes synthesized nicotinamide and that anaerobes destroyed it. From this he proposed the existence of an ecological system involving the aerobic and the anaerobic organisms. Shifting of the equilibrium normally existing between these forms would determine the net amount of nicotinic acid made available to the host.

Folic Acid

With folic acid as with the other B complex factors, we find essentially the same story; synthesis by intestinal bacteria in animals (Nielsen and Elvehjem, 1942; Ransone and Elvehjem, 1943; Wright and Skeggs, 1946; Carroll, 1950) and in man (Najjar and Holt, 1943). Furthermore, the list of bacteria possessing the capacity to synthesize this factor is equally impressive (Najjar and Barrett, 1945). The picture begins to take shape and will lead to the final conclusion that each and every B complex factor is synthesized in some measure by bacteria present in the intestinal tract. To establish this conclusion beyond reasonable doubt, let us examine the case for a few other factors.

Vitamin B_{12}, Cyanocobalamin

Once again, the story repeats; cyanocobalamin is synthesized by intestinal bacteria in animals (Dyke *et al.*, 1950; Davis, 1951; Hartman *et al.*, 1951) and man (Dyke *et al.*, 1950; Ludwig, 1951). Dyke and his associates (1950) state that the full requirements of man for vitamin B_{12} can be met by bacterial synthesis in the colon. In view of this statement one wonders at the frantic administration of this factor by every conceivable route to all possible types of patients.

In the case of vitamin B_{12}, the dietary content of other vitamins plays an enormous role in the degree of intestinal synthesis (Hartman *et al.*, 1951). Specifically, the factor involved seems to be riboflavin, which supplies the moiety, $1:2$-diamino-$4:5$-dimethylbenzene, also occurring in B_{12}. In view of the observations of Davis (1951), it seems probable that p-aminobenzoic acid may also be specifically related to intestinal formation of vitamin B_{12}.

While the explanation of the effect of antibiotics on growth rate in animals is not associated with the intestinal synthesis of vitamin B_{12} alone, this aspect will under certain dietary conditions be determinant. In any event, antibiotics will enhance the formation of B_{12} in the gut (Chow *et al.*, 1953; Johansson *et al.*, 1953). From the experiments of Chow and his associates (1953), it is apparent that one antibiotic may increase the synthesis of vitamin B_{12} while depressing the formation of biotin, and vice versa. Reference is made in this paper (Chow *et al.*, 1953) to the relatively poor absorption of the vitamin B_{12} formed by bacterial action in the gut. This experimental observation, doubtless correct within its design, bears little relationship to the broader problem of intestinal absorption, which will vary for different factors from hour to hour and day to day. Intestinal absorption is probably directly related to the ecological situation existing at a given time, and this is a reflection of the countless factors determining not only the intestinal flora but also the metabolic activities of that flora. It does not seem wise at present to make any sweeping conclusions relative to absorption from the intestine, as our knowledge is decidedly limited in this sphere. There are investigators who contend that no conclusive proof has been provided supporting the statement that intestinal synthesis of B complex factors results in increased absorption (Schweigert *et al.,* 1945; McGinnis *et al.,* 1950; Stokstad and Jukes, 1950; Waisman *et al.,* 1951) and there are those who believe firmly that such proof is available (Guerrant and Dutcher, 1934*a*; Najjar and Holt, 1943; Dyke *et al.,* 1950; Ludwig, 1951; Johansson *et al.,* 1953). The present author is firmly of the opinion that absorption does occur and that under certain conditions intestinal synthesis and subsequent absorption of vitamins is determinant in the nutritional economy of the host.

Essentially parallel findings have been reported for the other B complex factors, biotin (Oppel, 1942; Gardner *et al.,* 1945; Grundy *et al.,* 1947; McGregor *et al.,* 1947), pantothenic acid (McElroy and Goss, 1939; Wegner *et al.,* 1940; Mitchell and Isbell, 1942) and inositol (Woolley, 1941, 1942). Evidence is available also for the intestinal synthesis of p-aminobenzoic acid (Bloomberg, 1946), regarded as an intermediate in the synthesis of some of the other B complex factors. Thus, the pattern for the B complex vitamins is clear, but does intestinal synthesis of important nutrients extend beyond this group? The answer is in the affirmative.

Vitamin K and Other Fat-soluble Factors

Of the fat-soluble vitamins, vitamin K has been the focal point of study, and there is ample evidence of the synthesis of this factor by bacteria in the intestine of animals (Schmidt and Büsing, 1942; Day *et al.,* 1943; Kornberg *et al.,* 1943; Wakim *et al.,* 1943; Braganca and Rao, 1946; deLuca, 1947) and of man (Glavind *et al.,* 1942). The mechanism of demonstration of intestinal synthesis of vitamin K was through the use of sulfonamides (Wakim *et al.,* 1943). Further, the major site of formation was found to be the cecum (Wakim *et al.,* 1943), as cecectomy precipitated a mild increase in prothrombin times. While the cecum is probably the prime point of synthesis of this factor, the extent of such activity in other segments of the gut must be marked. The *coli* flora has been directly correlated with vitamin K formation (Orla-Jensen *et al.*, 1941; Schmidt and Büsing, 1942). It is of interest to note that the lactic acid bacteria which function so efficiently in the synthesis of B complex factors seem incapable of forming this fat-soluble vitamin (Orla-Jensen *et al.*, 1941).

Articles dealing with the intestinal synthesis of other fat-soluble factors are few in number. In the case of vitamin E, Pindborg (1949) has reported bacterial intestinal synthesis; however, Harris (1950) contends that the evidence of Pindborg demonstrated only that the feeding of sulfonamides increased the requirements of the rat for vitamin E. The divergence of results could be interpreted only if knowledge of the respective intestinal floras of the experimental animals were available. It seems probable that both investigators are entirely accurate in their observations but that these observations relate to a variable. With respect to vitamin A, the hypothesis has been advanced with some supporting evidence that intestinal synthesis occurs (LeGallic, 1950); however, future work will be required to establish the point. Intestinal synthesis does play a role in the ecological balance of the fat-soluble factors, a conclusion firmly established by reports on vitamin K. Thus, nearly the whole spectrum of vitamin factors has been demonstrated to be formed in some measure by bacterial action in the gut, and the pattern does not stop with the vitamins but extends to the amino acids.

Amino Acids

In 1944, Martin proposed the bacterial synthesis in the intestine of certain amino acids. This hypothesis was based upon the finding that rats fed on diets containing synthetic amino acid mixtures to which a sulfonamide was added did not do as well nutritionally as did those on diets containing casein or a protein hydrolysate to which had been added the same amount of a sulfonamide. Williams and Watson (1946) concluded that arginine was not synthesized in the intestine of the rat. The experimental design involved an arginine-free diet with and without added sulfonamide, with comparison of growth rates. As no difference in growth rate was noted, the experiment would seem to have established the absence of significant intestinal synthesis of this essential amino acid. Once again, the type of intestinal flora and the nature of diet could be determinant, and while under the conditions of the Williams and Watson experiments there would be no question of the results, they do not preclude possible synthesis of arginine under other conditions.

In 1950, Rose and Smith conclusively demonstrated that limited intestinal synthesis of amino acids does occur. Their experimental design involved diets containing mixtures of the ten essential amino acids alone, with added sulfonamide and with added sulfonamide plus nitrogen in the form of diammonium citrate. The latter gave growth equivalent to that observed in the absence of the sulfonamide, but the sulfonamide did cause a reduced growth rate in the animals receiving only the amino acid mixture. If the animal received an amino acid mixture containing nineteen amino acids, the addition of a sulfonamide did not alter growth rate. Rose and Smith point out that their experiments indicate a limited involvement of intestinal bacteria in amino acid nutrition, and also that their conclusions could be rendered invalid by the presence in the intestine of microorganisms not susceptible to the action of the sulfonamide used.

There can be no question concerning rumen synthesis by bacteria of amino acids and proteins from urea (Black *et al.*, 1952; Agrawala *et al.*, 1953; Duncan *et al.*, 1953). In fact, this synthesis occurs with such speed that within 6 hours after feeding, appreciable synthesis of protein from urea can be demonstrated. Black and his associates (1952) concluded that rumen microorganisms furnished the essential amino acids and that the tissues of the cow formed the nonessential factors. This is an interesting hypothesis and suggests the isolation of the responsible microorganisms with subsequent implantation and maintenance in the intestinal tract of nonruminants for purposes of amino acid synthesis.

It is the opinion of the present author that diets will contain nitrogen sources capable of conversion to amino acids and proteins by certain bacteria. The degree and significance of this in the ecological balance in man and animal remain to be determined. In considering this general problem (intestinal synthesis of nutrients) it is well to hold in mind the adaptation potentialities of bacteria. For example, Cheldelin and Nygaard (1951) indicate that lactic acid bacteria possess adaptive enzymes for the production of thiamin, p-aminobenzoic acid, vitamin B_{12} and pyridoxine phosphate. The idea to be taken from this is that intestinal bacteria might well adapt themselves to a given synthetic function in order to re-establish ecological balance.

ANTIBIOTICS

As much of the work which revealed the synthetic power of intestinal bacteria followed the discovery of insoluble sulfonamides and their application to the study, it was to have been expected that the advent of antibiotics would bring about their use for parallel purposes. It is not the author's intent to review the literature on the effects of antibiotics on intestinal flora but only to point out the impact of disturbances caused by these drugs on bionomics.

Illustrative of the effects of antibiotics on intestinal flora are the findings of Guzman-Garcia *et al.* (1953) involving rats fed penicillin-G sodium. While emphasizing the variability in the numbers and kinds of organisms in the digestive tract, they report a decrease in the concentration of anaerobes and an increase in the number of coliform organisms in the first week. By contrast, neither enterococci nor lactobacilli were significantly altered by the penicillin. From the standpoint of the favorable effect of antibiotics on growth, Guzman-Garcia and his associates favor the view that the drug increases the destruction of bacterial cells high in the intestine, thereby permitting utilization by the host of the bacterial cell content, specifically the vitamins. In other words, they do not feel that the antibiotic increases intestinal bacterial synthesis of nutrients but rather renders the amounts normally formed available. Using chicks as experimental subjects, Elam *et al.* (1953) established the growth-promoting effect of penicillin, aureomycin, bacitracin, and terramycin with an associated decrease in the total number of clostridia per gram of feces. They offer observed inhibition of toxin production by bacteria as one explanation of the growth effect.

If the growth-promoting action of antibiotics is associated with modification in intestinal flora, and if said flora varies with the diet, it should follow that the activity of these drugs with respect to growth will vary with the species of animal and with the nature of basal diet employed, and this is in accordance with observation (Cunha *et al.*, 1951).

Another explanation of the growth effect of orally administered antibiotics has been offered by Biely and March (1951), who propose that competition between microorganisms and host for marginal supplies of essential nutrients is balanced in favor of the host when the bacteria are reduced in numbers by the drug. These authors reach this conclusion as a result of experiments which showed no growth effect in chicks caused by aureomycin if the diet was optimal, and which showed a growth effect if the diet was deficient in any one of several vitamin factors, including nicotinic acid, folic acid, vitamin B_{12} and riboflavin.

Here, then, we have a situation illustrating beautifully the complexity of the ecological system with which we are dealing. The antibiotic will or will not have a growth effect, depending upon the species of the animal and upon the diet of that animal. Further, when a growth effect is demonstrated, it may be due to decreased production of toxic substances by bacteria, to increased synthesis of vitamins by intestinal microorganisms, to decreased competition by intestinal bacteria for marginal nutrient supplies, or to a host of other possible mechanisms. In any event, the complexity of this dynamic bionomic structure is astounding.

DIETARY FACTORS INFLUENCING INTESTINAL FLORA

Once again it is necessary to state that our purpose is not that of reviewing in detail the vast literature indicating the influence of dietary factors on intestinal flora but rather to cover just enough of this material to indicate the scope of the entire ecological pattern. For details the review articles of Najjar and Barrett (1945) and of Johansson and Sarles (1949) are recommended.

The dietary can be roughly subdivided into carbohydrate, protein, fat, vitamin and mineral. Each of these doubtless plays a marked role in determining the intestinal flora not only from day to day but even from hour to hour. The dynamics of the bionomic pattern dictate an ever shifting flora.

The studies of Fridericia *et al.* (1928) with reference to "refection" first directed attention to the impact of a carbohydrate, rice starch, on intestinal flora. In some animals, rice starch was the determinant factor in establishing a flora which would synthesize B complex factors. The resistance to the development of deficiency states caused by the dietary component could be transmitted from rat to rat by feeding feces. Rettger and Cheplin (1921) had reported prior to the studies of Fridericia *et al.* (1928) that diets high in lactose resulted in a flora high in lactobacilli and low in putrefying types of bacteria. Similarly, a diet high in protein and low in carbohydrate created a flora high in the coliform bacteria and low in lactobacilli.

A dietary high in carbohydrates does not automatically cause a modification in intestinal flora which will result in increased synthesis of all vitamin B factors. On the contrary, Schweigert *et al.* (1945) have observed increased formation of riboflavin but not of thiamin by intestinal bacteria in rats fed diets high in lactose, sucrose and dextrin. In general, the more complex carbohydrates tend to be most stimulatory to vitamin synthesis, and the simplest less so (Johansson and Sarles, 1949). In support of this contention is the report of Bacigalupo *et al.* (1950), which clearly shows that lactose promoted the intestinal synthesis of at least three B complex factors to a greater extent than did galactose. Guerrant *et al.* (1937) propose in explanation the greater rate of assimilation of the simpler carbohydrates, with the result that they do not remain in the intestine long enough to exert an effect on intestinal bacteria; this in direct contrast to the fate of the complex carbohydrate. In this same vein, different carbohydrates of essentially parallel molecular magnitude stimulate selectively the bacterial synthesis of B complex factors (Morgan *et al.*, 1938). Of all carbohydrate sources studied, dextrin would seem to be the most effective in creating conditions optimal for the synthesis of B complex factors (Johansson and Sarles, 1949).

Clinically, the impact of carbohydrate source on intestinal flora has been investigated and found of prime importance. In the studies of Primnig and Turkus (1943), β-lactose was found to suppress the growth of *coli* and stimulate that of *B. bifidus* in infants fed artifically. These clinicians indicate that the disappearance of *bifidus* can lead to serious gastrointestinal affections and state that artificial feeding of infants must be with β-lactose, as α-lactose will not create an intestinal flora parallelling that seen in the breast-fed infant.

The fat component of the diet markedly affects intestinal flora and vitamin synthesis. Whipple and Church (1935) observed that lard stimulated the growth of thiamin-synthesizing bacteria in the intestine of the rat. Their report was substantiated by Bacigalupo *et al.* (1950), who concluded that a high level of fat in the diet tends to increase the intestinal synthesis of at least three B complex factors. An element of selectivity seems to be operative with the fats as with the carbohydrates, as demonstrated by Teply and his associates (1947) in their report that butter fat caused more vitamin synthesis than did corn oil.

Other dietary components, proteins (Wegner *et al.*, 1941; Gall *et al.* 1951) and vitamins (Hartman *et al.*, 1951), are known to modify intestinal flora, and as a result synthesis by this flora of B complex factors. The probability is high that every dietary component will tend to modify the intestinal flora, will tend to shift the delicate ecological balance existing in the gut. Studies in the human being designed to determine the optimal intestinal flora and the dietary essential to its maintenance will be most rewarding and will probably reveal at least one essential key to defense against the chronic degenerative diseases.

DESTRUCTION OF NUTRIENTS BY INTESTINAL BACTERIA

As the pattern of the amazing bionomic complexity of the gastrointestinal tract unfolds, the aspect of nutrient destruction by intestinal bacteria assumes its important position. Unequivocally, the destruction of vitamins *in vitro* and *in vivo* by intestinal bacteria has been demonstrated. *In vitro,* the results of Young and James (1942) conclusively established the destruction of ascorbic acid by common intestinal bacteria. Parallel findings have been reported for nicotinic acid, riboflavin, pantothenic acid and thiamin. Doubtless future work will reveal the potential ability of intestinal bacteria to destroy each and every vitamin factor.

In vivo studies have been extensive, and as once again a review of such work is not intended, the discussion here will be restricted to nicotinic acid. In 1945, Benesch reported that the intestinal flora of human beings would synthesize or destroy this vitamin in accordance with the existence of aerobic or anaerobic conditions, the latter resulting in destruction. From these results, Benesch concluded that in the normal cecum an equilibrium exists between organisms which produce and those which destroy nicotinic acid. An imbalance between these bacteria could well play a part in the development of a deficiency state.

The role of drugs in modifying the ecological status is well illustrated by the results of Ellinger *et al.* (1947) showing that Ambamide (p-aminomethylbenzene sulfonamide) fed to rats increased the number of coliform bacteria known to synthesize nicotinic acid and simultaneously reduced the number of noncoliform bacteria such as *Proteus* or *Strep. faecalis* which destroy this vitamin factor. As in the case of vitamin synthesis by intestinal bacteria, vitamin destruction by this flora is altered by an equal multiplicity of factors. Commenting on the role of intestinal bacteria in nutrition, Elvehjem (1946) stated that: "We should not ignore the original ideas of Metchnikoff that certain types of bacteria in the tract may be deleterious, because they destroy certain vitamins or amino acids or because they produce toxins detrimental to health. As we learn more about intestinal flora we should be able to control both the beneficial and the detrimental types of organisms and to compensate for changes which we cannot control."

FORMATION OF TOXIC CHEMICALS BY INTESTINAL BACTERIA

The *British Medical Journal* has commented editorially (1945) that: "It was not long ago that we all believed in the evils of intestinal stasis, with its 'auto-intoxication' due to the supposed absorption of hypothetical bacterial toxins. The wheel of medical thought has turned full circle. The bacterial inhabitants of the intestine are no longer looked upon as toxin-producing parasites but as useful symbiotic organisms . . . " It will be our purpose in the next few pages to demonstrate that the turning of the wheel, while of merit in its revelation of new and useful concepts, was unfortunate in that it tended to obscure an aspect of the ecological pattern of the intestinal tract which may well be of paramount importance, namely the intestinal synthesis of toxic agents by bacteria. The intent is not to dwell on the spectacular and immediate results of the bacterial production of toxins but rather to indicate the possible significance of time and the effect of small concentrations of toxic chemicals on the body.

Many phases of this subject are controversial, and we cannot possibly review them in sufficient detail to permit conclusions; however, we can consider them in outline. For example, the significance of histamine is controversial. No investigators have questioned the formation of this toxic amine by intestinal bacteria, but it is concluded that detoxication of the amine occurs in the intestinal wall and in the liver. No question is raised concerning the validity of these conclusions within their proper limitations. However, to conclude that all of the histamine formed in the gut is detoxified would be to assume that enzymatic destruction of this factor proceeds to completion, and this cannot possibly be accurate since no enzyme reaction proceeds to completion. We can assume therefore that small amounts of histamine will pass the barriers of the intestinal wall and the liver and can exert an effect. To be sure, the result is not spectacular; no hypotension or similar pharmacological effect of the agent will follow, as the drug is not present in adequate concentrations for such effects; but it is adequate to produce minor physiological changes and it may well be present in concentration adequate to induce pathology over the course of years.

Even the adjuvant action of histamine for pathology induction cannot be overlooked. Localized intestinal production of this amine may so modify permeability of the gut wall as to permit the absorption of other toxic agents. We need not propose direct action for the pattern to form.

Histamine is formed by the action of histidine decarboxylase on the amino acid. It is destroyed by another enzyme, histaminase. Proof that conditions exist in which histaminase concentrations are lowered has been provided by Kapeller-Adler (1949). In severe toxemia of pregnancy, the histaminase activity is distinctly decreased. The ramifications of any phase of intestinal bionomics are noted with the observation of Sinclair (1952) that pyridoxal phosphate is the coenzyme for histaminase. The natural corollary is that pyridoxine deficiencies may occur in the toxemias of pregnancy, and this conclusion is in measure substantiated by the observation that pyridoxine therapy is of benefit in pregnancy toxemia (Wilson *et al.*, 1952). While the point of formation of histamine in the toxemia of pregnancy has not been established, it could well be the intestinal bacteria, and in this situation such synthesis would produce an obvious toxic effect.

One other example of acute histamine toxicity resulting from intestinal synthesis of this amine seems in order. Akerblom (1934), from his studies of the disease known as "founders," determined its cause to be histamine absorption from the gastrointestinal tract of the horse, the amine being produced from dietary histidine via decarboxylation by a specific strain of colon bacillus.

These are aspects of acute toxicity of intestinal bacterial histamine synthesis. We are not proposing for the more general pattern more than the accumulated, chronic effects of the absorption of minute amounts of such toxic agents.

The aspects of disagreement in this field are quantitative rather than qualitative. They arise from considerations based upon major degrees of toxic chemical absorption from the intestine, but even in this sphere support of the general concept seems apparent. Best and Taylor (1950), having dismissed the potentialities for the absorption of toxic products of bacterial action from the large intestine on quantitative grounds, state that: "The immunity of the body to autointoxication applies only to the large intestine. The small intestine is not equipped in the same degree to resist the passage of toxic products into the blood stream."

Normally the flora of the small intestine, due to the acid pH, is primarily aciduric, but under certain conditions proteolytic bacteria do occur; when this happens in children a toxemia results. The toxemia is corrected by eliminating the proteolytic flora and replacing it with one of the aciduric type. This can be done by feeding lactose or cultures of *B. acidophilus*.

There are investigators who ascribe alimentary intoxication in infants to guanidine or guanidinelike substances (Dodd *et al.,* 1932), and this carries with it the implication that guanidine or related substances are formed in the intestine. This subject seems to have been overlooked, as there is no direct evidence, but should the case be established there is support for the involvement of guanidine in toxemias of pregnancy (Andes *et al.,* 1937), hypertension (Major and Weber, 1927), muscular dystrophy (MacFate, 1942), epilepsy (Ellis *et al.,* 1931) and idiopathic tetany (Sharpe, 1920).

Indole and skatole are normally derived from tryptophane by the action of intestinal bacteria and are subsequently detoxified by the intestinal wall and liver to form indican. No divergence of opinion exists regarding these points, but on the issue of the toxic impact of skatole and indole few will agree. Again, it is the belief of the present author that quantitation confuses the picture. Investigators have sought evidence for the immediate induction of pathology by these chemicals in comparatively large quantities and have not studied the impact of small amounts over prolonged periods. It is with the latter aspect that we are concerned.

Alvarez (1924) in his excellent review "Intestinal Autointoxication" covers in detail the story of indole. In summary, the toxicity of indole and skatole is marked. Indican, the detoxified form, is essentially nontoxic. Clearly, there will be a correlation between the degree of formation of these toxic agents in the gut and the degree of detoxication occurring in the intestinal wall and in the liver. Injury to either the gut wall or the liver, with consequent reduction in indican formation, will result in a marked increase in the toxic manifestations caused by these chemicals. Another factor of importance is the degree of absorption from the gut, which varies with states of health and disease. Still another factor in the final picture centers around susceptibility of tissues to the nondetoxified agents. There is evidence of great variation in the impact of skatole and indole on the individual organism.

Detailed consideration of the formation by intestinal bacteria of toxic agents and the subsequent fate of these agents would require a volume in itself. Despite this, the subject has not been given adequate

study. Generally, reference is made to tyramine, histamine, indole, skatole and a few other standard examples of toxic agents produced in the
gut, but what of the countless noxious chemicals undoubtedly produced in the tract to which no study has yet been given? The approach
is experimentally a difficult one, as minute concentrations of toxic substances must be determined and the studies continued over periods of
years. In concluding, one can only state that a cloud of confusion exists
but that the pattern of participation by intestinal bacteria in degenerative disease is beginning to emerge. The significance of "conditioning"
of the internal environment is receiving study, and rich reward can
be anticipated.

Geriatrics is doubtless the field of medicine which will initially profit
the most from such studies. The aged person has greater intestinal
stasis and seeding with bacteria is facilitated by lowered secretion of
gastric acid. Orla-Jensen and his associates (1949) have reported some
remarkable correlations between intestinal bacteria and senility. In
the senile group, 48 per cent showed clostridia counts per gram of feces
above 100,000,000. By contrast, the nonsenile group gave a corresponding figure of only 9 per cent. Thus, intestinal flora of the senile group
was dominated to a greater degree by the putrefactive forms. Counts
made for *B. bifidus* showed that 9 per cent of the senile and 44 per
cent of the nonsenile patients had a count of more than 100,000,000
per gram of feces. This is a remarkable observation and illustrates the
type of research which must be carried out before we can with reasonable assurance state the nature of that bacterial flora of the gut which
is most suited to the host.

Devotion of this closing chapter to a consideration of intestinal ecological relationships has been for the goal of directing attention to
intestinal "conditioning." Ion exchange and adsorption materials will
play a major role in the ultimate resolution of this intriguing problem.
In this volume, an attempt has been made to indicate the present scope
of application of these agents and to suggest future trends.

Metchnikoff attributed the aging of mankind to putrefaction in the
colon. His thesis remains neither proved nor disproved. It is the belief
of the present author that Metchnikoff was in large measure correct,
not as to detail but in relation to the major premise. The ecological
structure existing in the intestine of man may well be the key to control
of chronic degenerative disease. Establishment and maintainence of the
proper intestinal flora is one approach to the resolution of the problem.
Unfortunately, while in broad outline we can state the nature of that

"optimal" flora, we do not yet possess adequate detailed knowledge. It is a neglected field of medical research that we consider here, but it must not remain so. It is a difficult field in which to work, due to the extreme complexity of the bionomic structure under consideration. It will be a costly and time-consuming enterprise, but out of the confusion which now clouds the entire ecological pattern will come the clarity essential to extending the life of man, physically and intellectually. Evolutionary progress for mankind in the future must be intellectual, and no greater stimulus to such progress could be forthcoming than the extension of the productive life of intelligent men.

REFERENCES

AGRAWALA, I. P., C. W. DUNCAN and C. F. HUFFMAN. *J. Nutrition,* **49:** 29, 1953.

AKERBLOM, E. *Skandinav. Arch. Physiol.,* **68** (Suppl. 3) : 1, 1934.

ALEXANDER, B., and G. LANDWEHR. *J. Clin. Investigation,* **25:** 287, 1946.

ALEXANDER, B., G. LANDWEHR, and F. MITCHELL. *J. Clin. Investigation,* **25:** 294, 1946.

ALVAREZ, W. C. *Physiol. Rev.,* **4:** 352, 1924.

ANDES, J. E., E. J. ANDES, and V. C. MYERS. *J. Lab. Clin. Med.,* **23:** 9, 1937.

BACIGALUPO, F. A., J. R. COUCH, and P. B. PEARSON. *Am. J. Physiol.,* **162:** 131, 1950.

BENESCH, R. *Lancet,* **1:** 718, 1945.

BEST, C. H., and N. B. TAYLOR. *The Physiological Basis of Medical Practice.* (5th ed.). Baltimore: Williams and Wilkins, 1950, p. 593.

BIELY, J., and B. MARCH. *Science,* **114:** 330, 1951.

BIRCH, T. W., P, GYÖRGY, and L. J. HARRIS. *Biochem. J.,* **29:** 2830, 1935.

BLACK, A. L., M. KLEIBER, and A. H. SMITH. *J. Biol. Chem.,* **197:** 365, 1952.

BLOOMBERG, B. M. *South African J. M. Sc.,* **11:** 163, 1946.

BLUM, H. F. *Time's Arrow and Evolution.* Princeton, N.J.: Princeton University Press, 1951.

BRAGANCA, B. M., and M. V. R. RAO. *Current Sc.,* **15:** 126, 1946.

Brit. M. J., Editorial, **1:** 879, 1945.

CARROLL, F. D. *J. Animal Sc.,* **9:** 139, 1950.

CHELDELIN, V. H., and A. P. NYGAARD. *J. Bact.,* **61:** 489, 1951.

CHOW, B. F., J. M. BURNETT, C. T. LING, and L. BARROWS. *J. Nutrition,* **49:** 563, 1953.

COOPER, E. A. *J. Hyg.,* **14:** 12, 1914.

CUNHA, T. J., G. B. MEADOWS, H. M. EDWARDS, R. F. SEWELL, A. M. PEARSON, and R. S. GLASSCOCK. *Arch. Biochem.,* **30:** 269, 1951.

DAVIS, B. D., *J. Bact.,* **62:** 221, 1951.

DAY, H. G., K. G. WAKIM, M. M. KRIDER, and E. E. O'BANION. *J. Nutrition*, **26**: 585, 1943.

DE, H. N., M. C. MALAKER, and A. K. PAUL. *Indian M. Gaz.*, **84**: 542, 1949.

DODD, K., A. S. MINOT, and H. CASPARIS. *Am. J. Dis. Child.*, **43**: 1, 1932.

DUNCAN, C. W., I. P. AGRAWALA, C. F. HUFFMAN, and R. W. LUECKE. *J. Nutrition*, **49**: 41, 1953.

DYKE, W. J. C., H. G. HIND, D. RIDING, and G. E. SHAW. *Lancet*, **1**: 486, 1950.

ELAM, J. F., R. L. JACOBS, W. L. TIDWELL, L. L. GEE, and J. R. COUCH. *J. Nutrition*, **49**: 307, 1953.

ELLINGER, P., and M. M. ABDEL KADER. *Biochem. J.*, **44**: 506, 1949.

ELLINGER, P., M. M. ABDEL KADER, and A. EMMANUELOWA. *Brit. J. Exper. Path.*, **28**: 261, 1947.

ELLINGER, P., R. A. COULSON, and R. BENESCH. *Nature*, **154**: 270, 1944.

ELLINGER, P., and A. EMMANUELOWA. *Lancet*, **2**: 716, 1946.

ELLINGER, P., and F. M. SHATTOCK. *Brit. M. J.*, **2**: 611, 1946.

ELLIS, M. M., M. P. NEAL, and T. R. FRAZER. *Proc. Soc. Exper. Biol. Med.*, **28**: 553, 1931.

ELVEHJEM, C. A. *J. Am. Dietet. A.*, **22**: 959, 1946.

FRIDERICIA, L. S., P. FREUDENTHAL, S. GUDJONNSSON, G. JOHANSEN, and N. SCHOUBYE. *J. Hyg.*, **27**: 70, 1928.

GALL, L. S., W. E. THOMAS, J. K. LOOSLI, and C. N. HUHTANEN. *J. Nutrition*, **44**: 113, 1951.

GARDNER, J., H. T. PARSONS, and W. H. PETERSON. *Arch. Biochem.*, **8**: 339, 1945.

GLAVIND, J., H. LARSEN, and P. PLUM. *Acta med. Scandinav.*, **112**: 198, 1942.

GRUNDY, W. E., M. FREED, H. C. JOHNSON, C. R. HENDERSON, and G. H. BERRYMAN. *Arch. Biochem.*, **15**: 187, 1947.

GUERRANT, N. B., and R. A. DUTCHER. *J. Biol. Chem.*, **98**: 225, 1932.

GUERRANT, N. B., and R. A. DUTCHER. *Proc. Soc. Exper. Biol. Med.*, **31**: 796, 1934a.

GUERRANT, N. B., and R. A. DUTCHER. *J. Nutrition*, **8**: 397, 1934b.

GUERRANT, N. B., R. A. DUTCHER, and R. A. BROWN. *J. Nutrition*, **13**: 305, 1937.

GUZMAN-GARCIA, J., W. B. SARLES, and C. A. BAUMANN. *J. Nutrition*, **49**: 647, 1953.

HARDWICK, S. W. *Lancet*, **1**: 267, 1946.

HARRIS, P. L. *Nature*, **165**: 572, 1950.

HARTMAN, A. M., L. P. DRYDEN, and C. A. CARY. *Arch. Biochem.*, **34**: 324, 1951.

HATHAWAY, M. L., and J. E. STROM. *J. Nutrition*, **32**: 1, 1946.

JOHANSSON, K. R., G. E. PETERSON, and E. C. DICK. *J. Nutrition*, **49**: 135, 1953.

JOHANSSON, K. R., and W. B. SARLES. *Bact. Rev.,* **13:** 25, 1949.

KAPELLER-ADLER, R. *Lancet,* **2:** 745, 1949.

KORNBERG, A., F. S. DAFT, and W. H. SEBRELL. *Science,* **98:** 20, 1943.

KORNBERG, A., F. S. DAFT, and W. H. SEBRELL. *J. Biol. Chem.,* **155:** 193, 1944.

LAMOREUX, W. F., and A. E. SCHUMACHER. *Poultry Sc.,* **19:** 418, 1940.

LEGALLIC, P. *Compt. rend. Soc. biol.,* **144:** 199, 1950.

DELUCA, G. *Rassegna internaz. clin. terap.,* **27:** 291, 1947.

LUDWIG, L. *Klin. Wchnschr.,* **29:** 770, 1951.

McELROY, L. W., and H. GOSS. *J. Biol. Chem.,* **130:** 437, 1939.

McELROY, L. W., and H. GOSS. *J. Nutrition,* **21:** 163, 1941.

MACFATE, R. P. *J. Lab. Clin. Med.,* **28:** 50, 1942.

McGINNIS, J., L. R. BERG, J. R. STERN, R. A. WILCOX, and G. E. BEARSE. *Poultry Sc.,* **29:** 771, 1950.

McGREGOR, M. A., H. T. PARSONS, and W. H. PETERSON. *J. Nutrition,* **33:** 517, 1947.

MAJOR, R. H., and C. J. WEBER. *Bull. Johns Hopkins Hosp.,* **40:** 85, 1927.

MARTIN, G. J. *Proc. Soc. Exper. Biol. Med.,* **55:** 182, 1944.

MITCHELL, H. K., and E. R. ISBELL. Univ. Texas Publ. No. 4237, 125, 1942.

MORGAN, A. F., B. B. COOK, and H. G. DAVISON. *J. Nutrition,* **15:** 27, 1938.

NAJJAR, V. A., and R. BARRETT. *Vitamins and Hormones,* **3:** 23, 1945.

NAJJAR, V. A., and L. E. HOLT, JR. *J. A. M. A.,* **123:** 683, 1943.

NAJJAR, V. A., L. E. HOLT, JR., G. A. JOHNS, G. C. MEDAIRY, and G. FLEISCHMANN. *Proc. Soc. Exper. Biol. Med.,* **61:** 371, 1946.

NAJJAR, V. A., G. A. JOHNS, G. C. MEDAIRY, G. FLEISCHMAN, and L. E. HOLT, JR. *J. A. M. A.,* **126:** 357, 1944.

NIELSEN, E., and C. A. ELVEHJEM. *J. Biol. Chem.,* **145:** 713, 1942.

Nutrition Rev., **4:** 310, 1946.

OPPEL, T. *Am. J. M. Sc.,* **204:** 863, 1942.

ORLA-JENSEN, S., E. OLSEN, and T. GEILL. *J. Gerontol.,* **4:** 5, 1949.

ORLA-JENSEN, S., A. D. ORLA-JENSEN, H. DAM, and J. GLAVIND. *Zentralbl. Bakt.* (Part 2), **104:** 202, 1941.

PEARSON, P. B., and R. W. LUECKE. *Arch. Biochem.,* **6:** 63, 1945.

PINDBORG, J. *Nature,* **164:** 493, 1949.

PRIMNIG, A., and M. TURKUS. *Ztschr. Kinderh.,* **63:** 595, 1943.

RANSONE, B., and C. A. ELVEHJEM. *J. Biol. Chem.,* **151:** 109, 1943.

RETTGER, L. F., and H. A. CHEPLIN. *A Treatise on the Transformation of the Intestinal Flora with Special Reference to the Implantation of Bacillus acidophilus,* New Haven: Yale University Press, 1921.

ROSE, W. C., and L. C. SMITH. *J. Biol. Chem.,* **187:** 687, 1950.

SCHMIDT, T., and K. H. BÜSING. *Klin. Wchnschr.,* **21:** 411, 1942.

SCHWEIGERT, B. S., J. M. McINTIRE, L. M. HENDERSON, and C. A. ELVEHJEM. *Arch. Biochem.,* **6:** 403, 1945.

SHARPE, J. S. *Biochem. J.*, 14: 46, 1920.

SHOURIE, K. L., and M. SWAMINATHAN. *Indian J. M. Research*, 27: 679, 1940.

SINCLAIR, H. M. *Biochem. J.*, 51: x, 1952.

SLATER, E. C. *Nature*, 157: 803, 1946.

STOKSTAD, E. L. R., and T. H. JUKES. *Poultry Sc.*, 29: 611, 1950.

TEPLY, L., W. A. KREHL, and C. A. ELVEHJEM. *Am. J. Physiol.*, 148: 98, 1947.

WAISMAN, H. A., M. GREEN, J. C. MUNOZ, A. RAMENCHIK, and J. B. RICHMOND. *Proc. Soc. Exper. Biol. Med.*, 76: 384, 1951.

WAKIM, K., M. M. KRIDER, and H. G. DAY. *Proc. Soc. Exper. Biol. Med.*, 54: 164, 1943.

WEGNER, M. I., A. N. BOOTH, C. A. ELVEHJEM, and E. B. HART. *Proc. Soc. Exper. Biol. Med.*, 45: 769, 1940.

WEGNER, M. I., A. N. BOOTH, C. A. ELVEHJEM, and E. B. HART. *Proc. Soc. Exper. Biol. Med.*, 47: 90, 1941.

WHIPPLE, D. V., and C. C. CHURCH. *J. Biol. Chem.*, 109: xcviii, 1935.

WILLIAMS, H. L., and E. M. WATSON. *Science*, 103: 654, 1946.

WILSON, D. C., and H. M. SINCLAIR, and I. SUTHERLAND. In Sinclair, H. M., Pyridoxal phosphate as coenzyme of histaminase. *Biochem. J.*, 51: x, 1952.

WOODS, R. *Borden's Rev. Nutrition Research*, 7 (May), 1946.

WOOLLEY, D. W. *J. Biol. Chem.*, 139: 29, 1941.

WOOLLEY, D. W. *J. Exper. Med.*, 75: 277, 1942.

WRIGHT, L. D., and H. R. SKEGGS. *Am. J. M. Sc.*, 212: 312, 1946.

YOUNG, R. M., and L. H. JAMES. *J. Bact.*, 44: 75, 1942.

YOUNG, R. M., and L. F. RETTGER. *J. Bact.*, 46: 351, 1943.

Index